WORKBOOK

to Accompany

Understanding Health Insurance

A Guide to Professional Billing

WORKBOOK

to Accompany

Understanding Health Insurance

A Guide to Professional Billing

6th Edition

JoAnn C. Rowell
Founder and Former Chairperson, Medical Assisting Department
Anne Arundel Community College, Arnold, MD
Currently, Adjunct Faculty
Community College of Baltimore County—Catonsville Campus Catonsville, MD

Michelle A. Green, MPS, CMA, RHIA/CTR
Professor, Department of Physical & Life Sciences
State University of New York
College of Technology at Alfred, Alfred, NY

Contributing Author

Alice Covell, CMA-A, RMA, CPC
Covell & Harwood Consultants
Kalamazoo, MI

WORKBOOK WRITTEN BY
Ruth M. Burke
Medical Billing and Coding Program Specialist at
The Community College of Baltimore County, MD
Adjunct Faculty, The Community College of Baltimore County, MD
Adjunct Faculty, Harford Community College, MD
Consultant on Administrative Procedures to Health Care Practices in Maryland and Virginia
President of the Independent Medical Billers Alliance (IMBA)
Member of the Maryland Medical Group Management Association (MGMA)

DELMAR
THOMSON LEARNING™

Australia Canada Mexico Singapore Spain United Kingdom United States

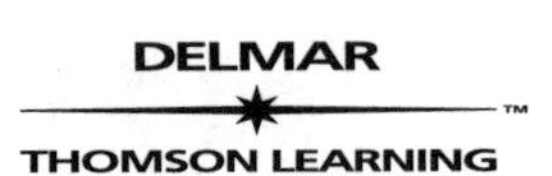

Workbook to Accompany Understanding Health Insurance

A Guide to Professional Billing 6th Edition

by Ruth Burke

Business Unit Director:
William Brottmiller

Executive Editor:
Cathy L. Esperti

Acquisitions Editor:
Maureen Muncaster

Developmental Editor:
Marjorie A. Bruce

Editorial Assistant:
Jill Korznat

Executive Marketing Manager:
Dawn F. Gerrain

Channel Manager:
Tara Carter

Project Editor
Maureen M. E. Grealish

Production Coordinator:
Anne Sherman

Art/Design Coordinator:
Connie Lundberg-Watkins

Technology Project Manager:
Laurie Davis

Printed in the United States of America
2 3 4 5 GP 06 05 04 03 02 01

For more information contact Delmar,
3 Columbia Circle, PO Box 15015,
Albany, NY 12212-5015

Or you can visit our Internet site at http://www.delmar.com or
http://www.EarlyChildEd.delmar.com

Library of Congress Cataloging-in-Publication Data
Rowell, JoAnn C., 1934–
Understanding health insurance : a guide to professional billing/
Jo Ann C. Rowell : contributing author. Michelle A. Green—6th ed.
p. cm.
Includes bibliographical references and index.
ISBN 0-7668-3206-6 (alk. paper)
1. Health insurance claims—United States. 2. Insurance, Health—United States. I. Green, Michelle A. II. Title.
HG9396 .R68 2001
368.38'2'00973—dc21
2001032396

NOTICE TO THE READER

Contents

Health Insurance Specialist—Roles and Responsibilities

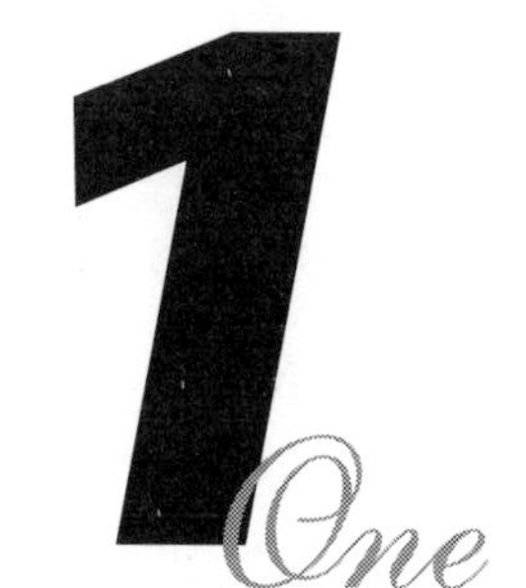

EMPLOYMENT OPPORTUNITIES

1. List three factors contributing to the increase in insurance specialist positions available in health care provider offices.

   a. ______________________

   b. ______________________

   c. ______________________

2. List six career opportunities open to health insurance specialists.

   a. ______________________

   b. ______________________

   c. ______________________

   d. ______________________

   e. ______________________

   f. ______________________

3. A consumer claim assistance professional helps private individuals ______________________

   ____

BASIC SKILL REQUIREMENTS

4. List six basic skills anyone who aspires to become a health insurance specialist must possess.

   a. ______________________

   b. ______________________

   c. ______________________

   d. ______________________

   e. ______________________

   f. ______________________

5. Health insurance specialists must draw on their knowledge of medical ____ to assign codes to the written narratives documented by the health care provider. (Circle the correct answer.)
   a. descriptions
   b. requirements
   c. terminology
   d. all of the above
6. Working with coded information requires an understanding of the ____ of these coding systems to ensure proper selection of individual codes. (Circle the correct answer.)
   a. application
   b. conventions
   c. rules
   d. all of the above
7. Misreading of any word or diagnosis may result in assignment of incorrect code numbers and the possibility of a ______________________________ or ______________________________ of a claim.
8. Insurance specialists must be comfortable discussing insurance concepts and regulations with ____. (Circle the correct answer.)
   a. health care providers
   b. insurance company personnel
   c. patients
   d. all of the above
9. Many insurance companies use Web sites to release ____________________________ and ____________________________ ____________________________ prior to adoption.

HEALTH INSURANCE SPECIALIST RESPONSIBILITIES

Critical Thinking

10. Write a paragraph describing the responsibilities of an insurance specialist.

____

____

____

____

PROFESSIONAL CERTIFICATION

11. List three professional organizations dedicated to serving health insurance specialists employed in health care provider offices.
    a. ____
    b. ____
    c. ____

CHAPTER

Introduction to Health Insurance

2 Two

WHAT IS HEALTH INSURANCE?

1. Define the following terms:

   a. insurance ______________________________

   ____

   b. health insurance ______________________________

   ____

   c. medical care ______________________________

   ____

   d. health care ______________________________

   ____

   e. preventive services ______________________________

   ____

   f. disability insurance ______________________________

   ____

   g. liability insurance ______________________________

   ____

MAJOR DEVELOPMENTS IN HEALTH INSURANCE

2. For the first 40 years of the 20th century, medical practices consisted largely of______________ ______________ in ______________ ______________.

3. A group practice is defined by the American Medical Association as:

____

____

4. What happened in the early 1950s that increased paperwork resulting in practices having to increase the size of their billing staff? ____

____

____

5. The Physician's Current Procedural Terminology (CPT) system is published by the

______________ ______________ ______________

and is currently reported on all outpatient claims in this country.

6. The standardization of diagnostic data on claims submitted by health care providers was achieved by adopting a diagnosis coding system known as the ______________________

______________________ of ______________________ .

7. List three government-sponsored health care programs established between 1965-66.

   a. ____

   b. ____

   c. ____

8. In the late 1990s CHAMPUS was reorganized and the name was changed to ________________ .

9. List the four categories of patients that medical practices were dealing with in the early 1970s.

   a. ____

   b. ____

   c. ____

   d. ____

10. Define *deductible*. ____

____

11. What attracted the attention of the general public to HMOs? ______________________

____

12. What legislation allowed the government to assist HMOs if they met specific federal requirements?

____

13. What did the Veterans Health Care Expansion Act of 1973 authorize? ________________

____

14. In 1977 the Carter administration combined the administration of the ______________________ and ______________________ programs under a single administrative agency.

15. The administrator of the Health Care Financing Administration (HCFA) is appointed by the ______________________ and reports directly to the Secretary of Health and Human Services.

16. In what year did HCFA begin to require standardization of information submitted on Medicare claims? (Circle the correct answer.)

    a. 1984
    b. 1977
    c. 1973

17. HCFA requires the use of one standard claim form known as the ____. (Circle the correct answer.)

    a. UB92
    b. HCFA-1450
    c. HCFA-1500

18. HCFA adopted the American Medical Association's existing procedure code system officially titled ______________ ______________ ______________ ______________, better known as ______________________ .

19. What forced commercial insurance companies to abandon their own customized billing forms in favor of the HCFA-1500 claim form? ______________________________________

    ____

20. In 1988, HCFA officially required the reporting of all diagnoses on claim forms using the United States version of the ______________________________________ .

21. The United States version of the World Health Organization's International Classification of Diseases is known as the ______________________________________, better known as the ______________________________________.

22. The National Correct Coding Initiative was developed to correct ______________________ coding problems.

THIRD-PARTY REIMBURSEMENT METHODS

23. List four reimbursement methods.

    a. ______________________________________
    b. ______________________________________
    c. ______________________________________
    d. ______________________________________

24. For each item, enter **T** for a true statement or **F** for a false statement on the line provided.

_______ a. Capitation is the method used by HMOs and some managed care plans to pay the health care provider a fixed amount on a per person basis.

_______ b. The capitation fee is dependent on the number of services rendered to the enrolled patients.

_______ c. Capitation is usually described in the HMO/managed care literature as the PMPM payment

_______ d. The PMPM method was initially provided to selected surgeons.

_______ e. Fee-for-service reimbursement is a relatively new form of reimbursement.

_______ f. Payment for fee-for-service claims may be made by the patient or from a third-party payer.

25. Use each of the following words or terms in a statement.

a. PMPM ____

____

b. Third-party payer ____

____

c. Utilization review ____

____

d. Episode of care ____

____

e. Global surgical fee ____

____

Know Your Acronyms

26. Define the following acronyms:

a. HMO ____

b. CPT ____

c. ICD-9-CM ____

d. HCFA ____

e. PCP ____

f. HCPCS ____

g. CCI ____

h. NPI ____

Managed Health Care

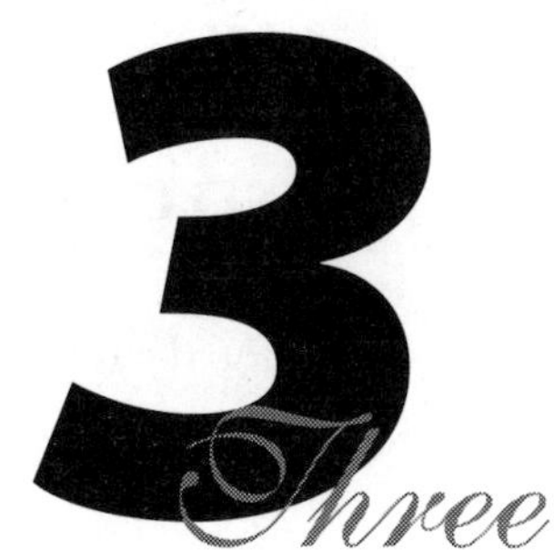

HISTORY OF MANAGED HEALTH CARE

1. Managed health care was developed as a way to provide ____ health care services to enrollees. (Circle the correct answer.)
   a. affordable
   b. comprehensive
   c. prepaid
   d. all of the above

2. The HMO Act of 1973 required most employers with more than ____ employees to offer HMO coverage if local plans were available. (Circle the correct answer.)
   a. 15
   b. 20
   c. 25
   d. 30

3. For each item, enter **T** for a true statement or **F** for a false statement on the line provided.

   _______ a. ERISA permitted small employers to self-insure employee health care benefits.

   _______ b. TEFRA defined risk contract as an arrangement among providers to provide fee-for-service health care to Medicare beneficiaries.

   _______ c. OBRA provided states with the flexibility to establish HMOs for Medicare and Medicaid programs.

   _______ d. The Preferred Provider Health Care Act of 1985 allowed subscribers to seek health care from providers inside the PPO.

   _______ e. COBRA established an employee's right to continue health care coverage beyond the scheduled benefit termination date.

   _______ f. HEDIS created standards to assess managed care systems.

   _______ g. HCFA's Office of Managed Care was established to facilitate innovation and competition among Medicare HMOs.

_______ h. HIPAA limited exclusions for pre-existing conditions.

_______ i. The Balanced Budget Act of 1997 mandated major revision of Medicare and Medicaid programs, which increased reimbursement to providers.

MANAGED CARE ORGANIZATIONS

4. A managed care organization is responsible for the health care of a group of ____. (Circle the correct answer.)
   a. employers
   b. enrollees
   c. physicians
   d. all of the above

5. Define *capitation.* ____

   ____

6. Describe the role of the primary care provider. ____

   ____

7. HEDIS consists of performance measures used to evaluate ____. (Circle the correct answer.)
   a. grievance procedures
   b. health care providers
   c. managed care plans
   d. none of the above

8. Match the terms in the first column with the description in the second column. Write the correct letter in each blank.

_______	utilization management	a.	performed to review medical necessity of inpatient care prior to the patient's admission
_______	preadmission certification	b.	used to ensure the medical necessity of tests and procedures ordered during an inpatient hospitalization
_______	preauthorization	c.	involves reviewing the appropriateness and necessity of health care provided to patients
_______	concurrent review	d.	conducted to arrange health care services required after discharge from the hospital
_______	discharge planning	e.	performed by a managed care plan, granting prior approval for reimbursement of a health care service

9. What does a utilization review organization establish? ____

   ____

   ____

10. What does case management involve? ____

____

____

11. Why do managed care plans often require a second surgical opinion? ____________________

____

____

12. What do gag clauses prevent? ____

____

____

13. Physician incentives include payments made directly, or indirectly, to health care providers to serve as encouragement to __________ or __________ services.

SIX MANAGED CARE MODELS

14. List six major MCO models available in the country today.
    a. ____
    b. ____
    c. ____
    d. ____
    e. ____
    f. ____

15. An exclusive provider organization is a managed care plan that provides benefits to subscribers if they receive services from ________________________________ providers.

16. Describe a *network provider.* ____

____

____

17. An integrated delivery system is an organization of affiliated provider sites that offer joint health care services to subscribers. List some examples of these affiliated provider sites.
    a. ____
    b. ____
    c. ____

18. What type of service does an MSO provide? ____

19. Traditional health insurance coverage is usually provided on a ____ basis. (Circle the correct answer.)

    a. capitation
    b. fee-for-service
    c. prepaid
    d. all of the above

20. HMOs provide preventive care services to promote ____. (Circle the correct answer.)

    a. easy access to medical care
    b. emergency services
    c. wellness
    d. all of the above

21. HMOs assign each subscriber to a ____ responsible for coordination of health care services and referrals to other health care providers. (Circle the correct answer.)

    a. primary care provider
    b. specialist
    c. surgeon
    d. all of the above

22. HMOs often require ____ to pay a copayment. (Circle the correct answer.)

    a. patients
    b. physicians
    c. providers
    d. all of the above

23. Define *deductible.* ______________________________

24. Match the HMO model in the first column with the description in the second column. Write the correct letter in each blank.

_______ direct contract model	a. services provided to subscribers by physicians employed by the HMO
_______ group model	b. intermediary that negotiates the HMO contract
_______ IPA	c. the HMO reimburses the physician group
_______ network model	d. services delivered to subscribers by individual physicians in the community
_______ staff model	e. services provided to subscribers by two or more physician multi-specialty group practices

25. What have some HMOs and PPOs implemented to create flexibility in managed care plans?

    ____

26. In a POS plan, patients have the freedom to use what type of providers?

    a. ______________________________
    b. ______________________________

27. A PPO is a network of physicians and hospitals that have joined together to contract with insurance companies, employers, or other organizations to provide health care to subscribers for a __________. (Circle the correct answer.)

a. premium fee

b. discounted fee

c. standard fee

d. all of the above

28. PPO premiums, deductibles, and copayments are usually ____ than those paid for HMOs. (Circle the correct answer.)

a. higher

b. lower

c. same

d. all of the above

29. A ______________ ______________ ______________ provides subscribers with a choice of HMO, PPO, or traditional health insurance plans.

ACCREDITATION OF MANAGED CARE ORGANIZATIONS

30. List two organizations that evaluate (and accredit) managed care organizations.

a. ______________________________

b. ______________________________

31. Why would a health care facility undergo NCQA accreditation? ______________________________

____

32. NCQA's current accreditation process involves almost half of the nation's HMOs in the evaluation of managed care plans based on what five areas?

a. ______________________________

b. ______________________________

c. ______________________________

d. ______________________________

e. ______________________________

EFFECTS OF MANAGED CARE ON ADMINISTRATIVE PROCEDURES IN A PHYSICIAN'S PRACTICE

33. Managed care programs have tremendous impact on a practice's administrative procedures. List a sampling of procedures that must be in place in a medical office.

a. ______________________________

b. ______________________________

c. ______________________________

d. ______________________________

e. ______________________________

f. ______________________________

Know Your Acronyms

34. Define the following acronyms:

    a. COBRA ______________________________

    b. HEDIS ______________________________

    c. HIPPA ______________________________

    d. MCO ______________________________

    e. URO ______________________________

    f. TPA ______________________________

    g. EPO ______________________________

    h. IDS ______________________________

    i. MSO ______________________________

    j. IPO ______________________________

    k. HMO ______________________________

    l. IPA ______________________________

    m. POS ______________________________

    n. PPO ______________________________

    o. NCQA ______________________________

    p. JCAHO ______________________________

CHAPTER

Life Cycle of an Insurance Claim

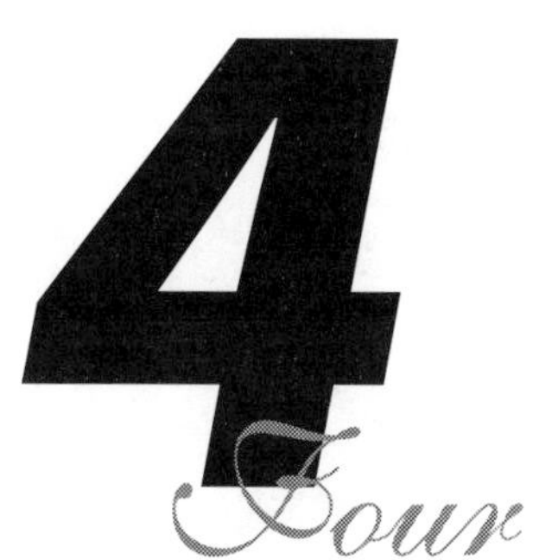

DEVELOPMENT OF THE CLAIM

1. The development of an insurance claim begins when ______________________________

____

2. List three parts of insurance claim development.

   a. ____

   b. ____

   c. ____

NEW PATIENT INTERVIEW AND CHECK-IN PROCEDURES

3. Match the terms in the first column with the definitions in the second column. Write the correct letter in each blank.

	Term	Definition
_______	primary care physician	a. a person who has not received any professional service from the health care provider within the last 36 months
_______	established patient	b. the primary policy is the one taken out by policyholder with the earliest birthday occurring in the calendar year
_______	encounter form	c. allows the office staff to gather preliminary data that ensures the patient's insurance eligibility and benefit status
_______	birthday rule	d. a medically trained person employed by a health insurance company to coordinate the health care of patients with long-term chronic conditions
_______	new patient	e. a form issued by the PCP that is either hand carried by the patient or faxed to the specialist/ancillary services provider
_______	participating provider	f. a health care provider who is not a primary care physician
_______	new patient intake interview	g. a provider who has no contractual relationship with the patient's insurance company, and has a legal right to expect the patient to pay the difference between the insurance allowed fee and the amount charged
_______	primary care referral form	
_______	nonparticipating provider	
_______	case manager	
_______	health care specialist	

(terms continue on next page)

h. a person who has been seen within the last 36 months by the health care provider or another provider of the same specialty in the same group practice

i. the financial record source document used by the health care provider to record the patient's diagnosis and services rendered during the encounter

j. a family practitioner, internist, pediatrician, and in some insurance plans, a gynecologist, responsible for providing all routine primary health care for the patient

k. a provider who has a contract with the insurance company to provide medical services to subscribers and to accept the insurance company's allowed fee for the procedure and/or service performed

4. Are retroactive treatment plans valid? ______________________________

POST CLINICAL CHECK-OUT PROCEDURES

5. Place in chronological order the following postclinical check-out procedures.

   a. Collect payment from the patient

   b. Code, if necessary, all procedures and diagnoses

   c. Post charges to the patient's ledger/account record

   d. Complete the insurance claim form

   e. Post any payment to the patient's account

   f. Enter the charges for procedures and/or services performed and total the charges

   Step 1: ____________

   Step 2: ____________

   Step 3: ____________

   Step 4: ____________

   Step 5: ____________

   Step 6: ____________

6. The ____________________ ____________________ is the permanent record of all financial transactions between the patient and practice.

7. The manual of daily accounts receivable journal, also known as the ____________________ ____________________ is a chronological summary of all transactions posted to individual patient ledgers/accounts on a specific day.

8. What is a *copay*? ______________________________

   ____

9. What is a *coinsurance payment*? ______________________________

   ____

10. State the name of the insurance claim form used to report professional and technical services. _______

___

INSURANCE COMPANY PROCESSING OF A CLAIM

11. Use each of the following terms in a statement.

Noncovered procedure ___

___

Unauthorized service ___

___

Common data file ___

___

Allowed charge ___

___

Deductible ___

___

Explanation of Benefits (EOB) ___

___

12. For each item, enter **T** for a true statement or **F** for a false statement on the line provided.

_______ a. Patients may not be billed for uncovered or noncovered procedures.

_______ b. Patients may be billed for unauthorized services.

_______ c. Any service that is considered not "medically necessary" for the submitted diagnosis code may be disallowed.

_______ d. The "allowed charge" is the maximum amount the insurance company will pay for each procedure or service, according to the patient's policy.

_______ e. Payment may sometimes be greater than the fee submitted by the provider if the allowed amount is greater than the charge.

13. List five items the Explanation of Benefits (EOB) may contain.

a. ___

b. ___

c. ___

d. ___

e. ___

14. If the claim form stated that direct payment should be made to the physician, the reimbursement check and a copy of the EOB will be mailed to the physician. List three ways to accomplish this.

    a. ______________________________

    b. ______________________________

    c. ______________________________

MAINTAINING INSURANCE CLAIM FILES

15. The federal Omnibus Budget Reconciliation Act of 1987 requires physicians to retain copies of any government insurance claim forms and all attachments filed by the provider for a period of ____. (Circle the correct answer.)

    a. 1 year

    b. 3 years

    c. 6 years

    d. forever

16. The federal Privacy Act of 1974 prohibits ____. (Circle the correct answer.)

    a. a patient from notifying the provider regarding payment or rejections of unassigned claims

    b. an insurer from notifying the provider regarding payment or rejections of unassigned claims

    c. the provider from appealing processing errors on unassigned claims

    d. an insurer from notifying the patient regarding payment or rejections of unassigned claims

Critical Thinking

17. Write a paragraph explaining the six steps that should be taken when an error in claims processing is found.

    ____

    ____

    ____

    ____

    ____

    ____

Know Your Acronyms

18. Define the following acronyms:

    a. PAR ______________________________

    b. PCP ______________________________

    c. EOB ______________________________

C H A P T E R

Legal and Regulatory Considerations

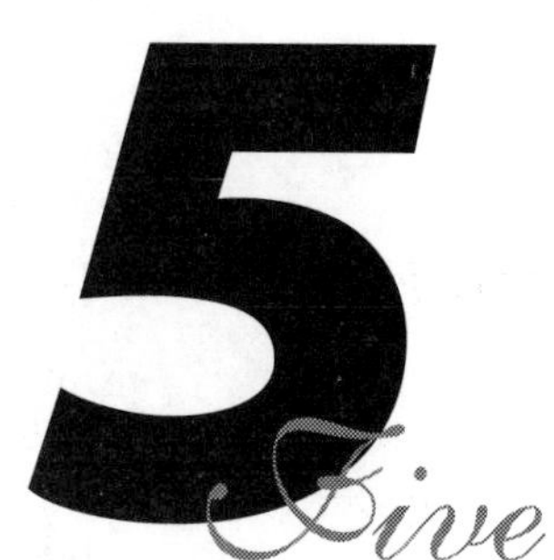

CONFIDENTIALITY OF PATIENT INFORMATION

1. Match the terms in the first column with the description in the second column. Write the correct letter in each blank.

_______	privacy	a. restricting patient information access to those with proper authorization
_______	confidentiality	b. the right of individuals to keep their information from being disclosed to others
_______	security	c. the safekeeping of patient information

2. Breach of confidentiality is often unintentional and involves the ____ release of patient information to a third party. (Circle the correct answer.)
   a. authorized
   b. intentional
   c. unauthorized
   d. none of the above

3. Match the insurance terms in the first column with the definitions in the second column. Write the correct letter in each blank.

_______	first party	a. the person or organization who is providing the service
_______	second party	b. an agreement between two or more parties to perform specific services or duties
_______	third party	c. the person designated in a contract to receive a contracted service
_______	contract	d. the person who is legally designated to be in charge of a patient's affairs
_______	guardian	e. the one who has no binding interest in a specific contract

4. For each item, enter **T** for a true statement or **F** for a false statement on the line provided.

_______ a. Breach of confidentiality cannot be charged against a health care provider if written permission to release necessary medical information to an insurance company or other third party has been obtained from the patient or guardian.

_______ b. Patients need to sign an authorization for the release of medical information statement before completing the claim form.

_______ c. A dated, signed release statement is generally considered to be in force for one year from the date stated on the form.

_______ d. The authorization for release of medical information form authorizes the processing of claim forms but the phrase "signature on file" or the patient's signature still needs to appear on each form.

_______ e. The Health Care Financing Administration (HCFA) regulations permit government programs to accept only dated authorizations.

_______ f. The federal government allows two exceptions to the required authorization for release of medical information to insurance companies: patients covered by Medicaid or Blue Cross and Blue Shield.

_______ g. When health care providers agree to treat either a Medicaid or a workers' compensation case, they agree to accept the program's payment as payment in full for covered procedures rendered to these patients.

_______ h. Patients who undergo screening for the human immunodeficiency virus (HIV) or acquired immune deficiency syndrome (AIDS) infection should not be asked to sign an additional authorization statement releasing information regarding the patient's HIV/AIDS status.

CLAIMS INFORMATION TELEPHONE INQUIRIES

Critical Thinking

5. It is very simple for a curious individual to place a call to a physician's office and claim to be an insurance company benefits clerk. Write a paragraph explaining how a physician's office can verify insurance company telephone inquiries.

____

____

____

____

____

____

____

____

6. Great care should be taken when attorneys request information over the telephone. Write a paragraph explaining how a physician's office can verify attorneys' inquiries.

____

____

____

____

____

____

____

____

FACSIMILE TRANSMISSION

7. Each facsimile transmission (FAX) of sensitive material should have a cover sheet that includes the following information:

   a. ____

   b. ____

   c. ____

   d. ____

   e. ____

   f. ____

RETENTION OF PATIENT INFORMATION AND HEALTH INSURANCE RECORDS

8. According to HCFA, patient information and health insurance records are to be maintained for a period of ____ years. (Circle the correct answer.)

   a. two

   b. five

   c. seven

   d. none of the above

9. Patient information and health insurance records must be available as references for use by ____. (Circle the correct answer.)

   a. DHHS

   b. fiscal intermediaries

   c. HCFA

   d. all of the above

10. It is acceptable to retain patient information and insurance records in a format other than original paper if the format accurately reproduces all original documents. State one retention format.

____

FEDERAL FALSE CLAIMS ACT

11. Describe *upcoding.* ____

____

12. Describe *self-referral.* ____

____

HEALTH INSURANCE PORTABILITY AND ACCOUNTABILITY ACT OF 1996

13. List four ways HIPAA provisions improve the portability and continuity of health care coverage.

    a. ____

    b. ____

    c. ____

    d. ____

14. Define *fraud.* ____

____

15. Define *abuse.* ____

____

16. Indicate whether each of the following applies to **fraud (f)** or **abuse (a)** on the line provided.

_______ a. violations of participating provider agreements

_______ b. billing for services not furnished

_______ c. falsifying medical records to justify payment

_______ d. excessive charges for services

_______ e. unbundling codes

_______ f. submitting claims that include services not medically necessary to treat the patient's stated condition

_______ g. improper billing practices that result in a payment by a government program when the claim is the legal responsibility of another third-party payer

_______ h. receiving a kickback

_______ i. misrepresenting the diagnosis to justify payment

17. A person found guilty of committing Medicare fraud faces __________, __________, and/or ________________________________ penalties.

18. Civil penalties for committing Medicare fraud are ____ per false claim. (Circle the correct answer.)

   a. $1,000 to $2,000

   b. $4,000 to $8,000

   c. $5,000 to $10,000

   d. $10,000 to $20,000

19. The Correct Coding Initiative was implemented to reduce Medicare program expenditures by detecting ________________________ coding.

20. The reporting of multiple codes to increase reimbursement from the payer, when a single combination code should be reported, is known as ________________.

21. Define *modifier.* ____

____

22. A tax-exempt trust for the purpose of paying medical expenses is known as a

______________________ ________________________ ________________________.

23. No policy can be sold as a long-term care insurance policy if it limits or excludes coverage by type of __________, __________ __________, or __________.

24. Describe the *National Provider Identifier.* ______________________________________

____

25. The process of sending data from one party to another via computer linkages is known as ________ ________ __________.

Know Your Acronyms

26. Define the following acronyms:

   a. HIPAA ____

   b. CCI ____

   c. MSA ____

   d. NPI ____

   e. EDI ____

CHAPTER

ICD-9-CM Coding

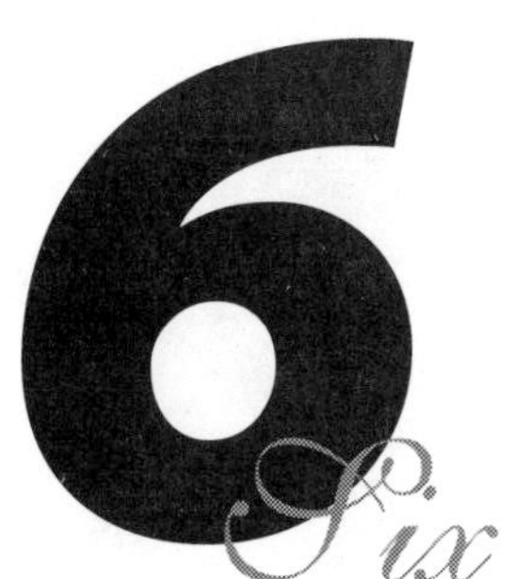

INTRODUCTION

1. Match the acronyms in the first column with their function in the second column. Write the correct letter in each blank.

_______	ICD	a. creates annual procedure classification updates for ICD-9-CM
_______	ICD-CM	b. used to code and classify mortality data
_______	HCFA	c. official system for assigning codes to diagnoses
_______	NCHS	d. used to code and classify morbidity data
_______	ICD-9-CM	e. coordinates official disease classification activities for ICD-9-CM

2. List three parts into which ICD-9-CM is organized.
   a. ____________________
   b. ____________________
   c. ____________________

3. Define *medical necessity.* ____________________

   ____

4. If a service or procedure is found "medically unnecessary" by Medicare the patient must sign a(n) __________ __________ __________.

5. New diagnosis codes officially go into effect on ____ of each year. (Circle the correct answer.)
   a. January 1
   b. March 1
   c. July 1
   d. October 1

HCFA ICD-9-CM CODING GUIDELINES

6. Explain when codes that describe symptoms and signs, as opposed to definitive diagnoses, are acceptable for reporting. ____

   ____

7. For each item, enter **T** for a true statement or **F** for a false statement on the line provided.

   _______ a. There are ICD-9-CM codes to describe conditions, symptoms, and problems.

   _______ b. ICD-9-CM does not provide codes to report encounters for circumstances other than a disease or injury.

   _______ c. The ICD-9-CM is composed of codes with either 3 or 4 digits.

   _______ d. A three-digit code is used only if it is not further subdivided.

   _______ e. Do not code diagnoses documented as "probable."

   _______ f. Code conditions that were previously treated and no longer exist.

8. Describe when historical codes (V10–V19) may be used. ______________________________________

   ____

   ____

PRIMARY VERSUS PRINCIPAL DIAGNOSIS

9. List three general classifications of facilities in which an outpatient is treated.

   a. ____

   b. ____

   c. ____

10. Define *inpatient.* ____

    ____

11. Who stipulates the inpatient admission status? ____

12. Which diagnosis is reported on physician office claims? (Circle the correct answer.)

    a. primary

    b. principal

13. Which diagnosis is reported on inpatient hospital claims? (Circle the correct answer.)

    a. primary

    b. principal

14. Which claim form is used to report physician office services and procedures? (Circle the correct answer.)

    a. HCFA-1500

    b. UB-92

15. Which claim form is used to report inpatient admissions and outpatient and emergency department services and/or procedures? (Circle the correct answer.)

    a. HCFA-1500

    b. UB-92

16. Which diagnosis is the most significant condition for which services and/or procedures were provided? (Circle the correct answer.)

    a. primary

    b. principal

17. Which diagnosis is the condition determined after study that resulted in the patient's admission to the hospital? (Circle the correct answer.)

    a. primary

    b. principal

18. Why is the HCFA-1500 paper claim form printed in red ink? ______________________________

PRIMARY VERSUS PRINCIPAL PROCEDURES

19. Hospitals are required to code all inpatient procedures using the ______________________________

    ____

20. Outpatient procedures performed in the hospital are coded using the ____. (Circle the correct answer.)

    a. Current Procedural Terminology coding system

    b. ICD-9-CM Volume III

    c. ICD-9-CM Volumes I & II

    d. any of the above

21. The definition of a *principal procedure* is ____. (Circle the correct answer.)

    a. a procedure performed to treat a complication

    b. a procedure performed for definitive treatment

    c. a procedure performed which is most closely related to the principal diagnosis

    d. any of the above

CODING QUALIFIED DIAGNOSES

22. Define *qualified diagnosis.* ______________________________

    ____

23. List five examples of qualified diagnoses. (Do not use examples found in the textbook.)

    a. ______________________________

    b. ______________________________

    c. ______________________________

    d. ______________________________

    e. ______________________________

24. Are qualified diagnoses routinely coded on claim forms submitted from health care practitioners' offices? ______________________________

25. What do HCFA regulations permit on the HCFA-1500 claim form in place of qualified diagnoses?

____

ICD-9-CM CODING SYSTEM

26. Match the coding terms in the first column with the definitions in the second column. Write the correct letter in each blank.

_______	ICD-9 Volume 1	a. Index to Procedures and Tabular List
_______	ICD-9 Volume 2	b. a numerical listing of diseases and injuries
_______	ICD-9 Volume 3	c. an alphabetic index to Volume 1

27. Match the insurance terms in the first column with the definitions in the second column. Write the correct letter in each blank.

_______	V codes	a. external causes of injury and poisoning
_______	E codes	b. tissue type of neoplasms
_______	M codes	c. factors influencing health status

28. List three sections of the Index to Diseases (Volume 2).

a. ______________________________

b. ______________________________

c. ______________________________

29. Describe *Tabular List and the Index (Volume 3).*

____

____

DISEASE INDEX ORGANIZATION

30. Main terms are printed in ______________ type and followed by the ______________ ______________.

31. A list of ______________ is indented 2 spaces under the main term.

32. Secondary qualifying conditions are indented 2 spaces under a ______________.

33. Always consult the code description in the ______________ ______________ before assigning a code.

BASIC STEPS FOR USING THE INDEX

34. What is the first step for using the index? ______________________________

____

35. Underline the main term in each of the following:
    a. Newborn anoxia
    b. Insect bite
    c. Radiation sickness
    d. Allergic bronchitis
    e. Infarction of brain stem
    f. Cranial nerve compression
    g. Erosion of the cornea
    h. Abdominal cramp

36. Assign codes to the following:
    a. Tension headache ______________
    b. Bronchial croup ______________
    c. Chronic conjunctivitis ______________
    d. Acute confusion ______________
    e. Car sickness ______________
    f. Rosacea ______________

ORGANIZATION OF THE TABULAR LIST

37. ICD-9 codes for Chapters 1 through 17 are organized according to ______________ - ______________ category codes.

38. How is specificity achieved? ______________________________
    ____

39. Match the coding conventions in the first column with the definitions in the second column. Write the correct letter in each blank.

    _______ nonessential modifiers
    _______ NEC
    _______ essential modifiers
    _______ eponyms
    _______ codes in slanted brackets

    a. not elsewhere classifiable
    b. diseases (or procedures) named for an individual
    c. listed as secondary codes because they are manifestations of other conditions
    d. subterms that are enclosed in parentheses following the main term
    e. clarifies the main term and must be contained in the diagnostic statement

40. Assign codes to the following:
    a. Pneumonia with influenza ______________
    b. Maxillary sinusitis ______________
    c. Hiatal hernia ______________

41. Assign codes to the following:
   a. Blindness due to injury NEC ____________
   b. Erythema, infectional NEC ____________
   c. Spontaneous hemorrhage NEC ____________
   d. Herpes zoster without mention of complication ____________
   e. Eruption due to other chemical products ____________

42. Assign codes to the following:
   a. Parkinson's disease ____________
   b. Skene's gland abscess ____________
   c. Stokes-Adams Syndrome ____________
   d. Sprengel's Deformity ____________
   e. Haglund's disease ____________

43. Match the coding conventions in the first column with the definitions in the second column. Write the correct letter in each blank.

_______	*See Category*	a. directs the coder to a more specific term
_______	*See also*	b. contained in boxes to further define terms, clarify index entries, and list choices for additional digits
_______	Notes	c. refers the coder to an index entry that may provide additional information
_______	*See*	d. refers the coder directly to the Tabular List category

44. When should you code directly from the index?

____

45. Assign codes to the following (remember fifth-digits):
   a. Polydactyly of fingers ____________
   b. Sickle-cell crisis, NOS ____________
   c. Closed lateral dislocation of elbow ____________
   d. Grand mal epilepsy without mention of intractable epilepsy ____________
   e. Classical migraine, intractable ____________

BASIC STEPS FOR USING THE TABULAR LIST

46. List the six basic steps for using the Tabular List.

   Step 1. ____

   Step 2. ____

   Step 3. ____

Step 4. ______________________________

Step 5. ______________________________

Step 6. ______________________________

47. Define the coding convention term *brackets.* ______________________________

48. Assign codes to the following:
    a. Abnormal electroencephalogram (EEG) ____________
    b. Pyogenic arthritis, upper arm ____________
    c. Pediculus corporis ____________
    d. Dermatitis due to poison ivy ____________

49. Assign codes to the following:
    a. Osteoarthrosis, generalized, hand ____________
    b. Allergic arthritis, multiple sites ____________
    c. Loose body in joint, shoulder region ____________
    d. Loose body in knee ____________ ________

50. Define the coding convention term *includes.* ______________________________

51. Assign codes to the following:
    a. Coccidioidomysosis, unspecified ____________
    b. Splinter, cheek, without major open wound, infected ____________
    c. Sliding inguinal hernia, with gangrene, bilateral ____________

52. Define the coding convention term *excludes.* ______________________________

53. Assign codes to the following:
    a. Smokers' cough ____________
    b. Acute gingivitis ____________
    c. Anal and rectal polyp ____________
    d. Obstruction of gallbladder ____________
    e. Situs inversus ____________

54. Define the coding convention term *braces.* ______________________________

55. Assign codes to the following:
    a. Hypertrophy of tonsils with adenoids ____________
    b. Cirrhosis of lung ____________
    c. Rupture of appendix with generalized peritonitis ____________
    d. Hiatal hernia with gangrene ____________
    e. Diverticulum of appendix ____________

56. Define the coding convention term *colon.* ______________________

57. Assign codes to the following:

a. Chronic tracheobronchitis ______________

b. Bronchopneumonia with influenza ______________

c. Dermatitis due to acids ______________

58. What does the abbreviation NOS indicate? ______________________

59. Assign codes to the following:

a. Acute sore throat NOS ______________

b. Femoral hernia, unilateral NOS ______________

c. Transfusion reaction NOS ______________

d. Acute cerebrovascular insufficiency NOS ______________

e. Unspecified peritonitis NOS ______________

60. When does a *code first underlying disease* appear? ______________________

61. Assign codes to the following case studies, giving special attention to the words "code first underlying disease " and assign codes in the correct order.

	First Code	**Second Code**
a. Patient presents with myotonic cataract resulting from Thomsen's disease	______	______
b. Patient presents with postinfectious encephalitis resulting from post-measles	______	______
c. Patient presents with cerebral degeneration in generalized lipidoses resulting from Fabry's disease	______	______
d. Patient presents with parasitic infestation of eyelid caused by pediculosis	______	______
e. Patient presents with xanthelasma of the eyelid resulting from lipoprotein deficiencies	______	______

62. Assign codes to the following case studies, giving special attention to the word "and." (Some cases may require two codes; other cases require only one code.)

	First Code	**Second Code**
a. Patient presents with degenerative disorders of eyelid and periocular area, unspecified	______	______
b. Patient presents with acute and chronic conjunctivitis	______	______
c. Patient presents with cholesteatoma of middle ear and mastoid	______	______
d. Patient presents with psoriatic arthropathy and parapsoriasis	______	______
e. Patient presents with nausea and vomiting	______	______
f. Patient presents with headache and throat pain	______	______

63. Assign codes to the following, giving special attention to the word "with."
  a. Rheumatic fever with heart involvement ________________
  b. Diverticulosis with diverticulitis ________________
  c. Acute lung edema with heart disease ________________
  d. Emphysema with acute and chronic bronchitis ________________
  e. Fracture fibula (closed) with tibia ________________
  f. Varicose vein with inflammation and ulcer ________________

WORKING WITH INDEX TABLES

64. For each item, enter **T** for a true statement or **F** for a false statement on the line provided.
  _______ a. The Hypertension/Hypertensive table contains a complete listing of hypertension codes and other conditions associated with hypertension.
  _______ b. It is not always necessary to check the Tabular List before assigning a final code for hypertension/hypertensive conditions.
  _______ c. When "with" separates two conditions in the diagnostic statement only one code is needed.
  _______ d. Secondary hypertension is a unique and separate condition listed on the table.
  _______ e. The fourth digit 9 should be used sparingly.

65. Assign codes to the following:
  a. Hypertension, benign ________________
  b. Chronic hypertension, malignant ________________
  c. Hypertension due to brain tumor, unspecified ________________
  d. Malignant hypertension with congestive heart failure ________________
  e. Newborn affected by maternal hypertension ________________

66. Define the following terms:
  a. neoplasms ____
  b. benign ____
  c. malignant ____
  d. lesion ____

67. List five examples of benign lesions.
  a. ____
  b. ____
  c. ____
  d. ____
  e. ____

68. Match the neoplasm classifications in the first column with the definitions in the second column. Write the correct letter in each blank.

_______	primary malignancy	a.	a malignant tumor that is localized
_______	secondary malignancy	b.	there is no indication of the histology or nature of the tumor
_______	carcinoma *in situ*	c.	it is not possible to predict subsequent behavior from the submitted specimen
_______	uncertain behavior	d.	the tumor has spread
_______	unspecified nature	e.	the original tumor site

69. Assign codes to the following:

a. Hodgkin's sarcoma _______________

b. Ovarian fibroma _______________

c. Bronchial adenoma _______________

d. Carcinoma of oral cavity and pharynx _______________

e. Chronic lymphecytic leukemia _______________

f. Reticulosarcoma, intrathoracic _______________

g. Adenocarcinoma of rectum and anus _______________

h. Benign lymphoma of breast _______________

i. Carcinoid small intestine _______________

j. Multiple myeloma _______________

k. Lipoma, right kidney _______________

70. What is the Table of Drugs and Chemicals used for? _______________

____

71. Define *adverse effect* or *reaction.*

____

____

72. What are E codes used for in regard to poisoning? _______________

____

73. Describe when an E code might be used as the primary code for poisoning? _______________

____

74. Assign codes to the following, using E codes where applicable.

	First Code	Second Code
a. Poisoning due to isopropyl alcohol	___________	___________
b. Poisoning due to amino acid	___________	___________
c. Suicide attempt, overdose of tranquilizers	___________	___________
d. Accidental methadone poisoning	___________	___________
e. Poisoning due to therapeutic use of codeine	___________	___________
f. Brain damage due to allergic reaction to penicillin	___________	___________

75. V codes are contained in a supplementary classification of factors influencing the person's ________________ ________________.

76. List the three V code categories.

a. ____

b. ____

c. ____

77. Assign codes to the following:

a. Exercise counseling ______________

b. History of alcoholism ______________

c. Counseling for parent/child conflict, unspecified ______________

d. Screening, cancer, unspecified ______________

e. Follow-up exam, post-surgery ______________

f. Health check, not pediatric ______________

g. Routine child health check ______________

h. Fitting of artificial eye ______________

i. Flu Shot ______________

j. Family history of breast cancer ______________

k. Observation for suspected tuberculosis ______________

CODING SPECIAL DISORDERS

78. What precautions should a coder take before entering the HIV/AIDS code on a claim form?

____

79. If the diagnostic statement does not specify whether a fracture is opened or closed, which one should the coder select? ______________________________

80. Assign codes to the following:

a. Fracture of base of skull with cerebral contusion ______________

b. Open fracture of nasal bones ______________

c. Fifth cervical vertebra fracture, closed ____________

d. Open fracture coccyx with other spinal cord injury ____________

e. Closed fracture of three ribs ____________

f. Closed fracture of clavicle ____________

g. Open finger fracture ____________

h. Bennett's fracture, closed ____________

i. Fracture of head of tibia ____________

j. Heel bone fracture, closed ____________

81. Define *late effect.* ____________

82. When coding a late effect, the primary code is the ____________ condition and the secondary code represents the ____________ condition or etiology of the late effect.

83. Assign codes to the following in the correct order:

	First Code	**Second Code**
a. Scarring due to third-degree burn of left arm	________	________
b. Nonunion fracture of neck of femur	________	________
c. Esophageal stricture due to old lye burn of esophagus	________	________
d. Hemiplegia due to old CVA	________	________

84. The percentage of total body area or surface affected by burns follows the "____________ ____________ ____________."

85. Assign codes to the following:

	First Code	**Second Code**	**Third Code**
a. Second-degree burn, right upper arm and shoulder	________	________	________
b. Third-degree burn, trunk, 35% body surface	________	________	________
c. Burn of mouth, pharynx, and esophagus	________	________	________
d. Blisters on back of hand and palm	________	________	________
e. Erythema on forearm and elbow	________	________	________
f. Deep third-degree burn with loss of thumb	________	________	________

86. Describe why a coder might report E codes on physician claims. ____________

____

____

87. Assign E codes to the following, adding a second code when the place of occurrence is provided.

	First Code	Second Code
a. Assault by hanging and strangulation	___	___
b. Unarmed fight	___	___
c. Self-inflicted injury by crashing of motor vehicle, highway	___	___
d. Exposure to noise at nightclub	___	___
e. Struck accidentally by falling rock at quarry	___	___
f. Struck by thrown ball at baseball field	___	___
g. Caught accidentally in escalator at amusement park	___	___
h. Dog bite	___	___
i. Accidental poisoning from shellfish at restaurant	___	___
j. Foreign object left in body during surgical operation	___	___
k. Fall from ladder at home	___	___
l. Accident caused by hunting rifle at rifle range	___	___

88. Codes are to be selected according to the highest level of ______________________________ .

89. Indicate which of the following codes need to be carried out to the highest level of specificity by writing the correct code in the space provided.

______________ a. 464.2 Acute laryngotracheitis without mention of obstruction

______________ b. 393 Chronic rheumatic pericarditis

______________ c. 690 Cradle cap

______________ d. 574.2 Calculus of gallbladder without mention of cholecystitis, without obstruction

______________ e. 570 Acute and subacute necrosis of liver

______________ f. 571.4 Chronic persistent hepatitis

______________ g. 914 Infected blister of the hand

90. Describe how diagnoses documented as "probable," "suspected," "questionable," or "ruled out" should be coded. ____

____

91. A 45-year-old patient presents with polyuria and polydipsia. The physician documents "suspected diabetes mellitus." Circle the correct diagnoses to be coded.

a. diabetes mellitus type II (adult-onset)
b. diabetes mellitus with other specified manifestations
c. polyuria; polydipsia; diabetes mellitus
d. polyuria; polydipsia

92. A patient presents with a blood pressure of 150/90 and is asked to rest for 10 minutes. Upon re-evaluation the blood pressure is 130/80. The patient is asked to return to the office in two weeks to rule out hypertension. Circle the correct diagnosis to be coded.

a. hypertension

b. elevated blood pressure

c. observation for suspected cardiovascular disease

d. personal history of other specified circulatory disorder

93. A patient presents with wheezing and a productive cough. The physician recorded "probable bronchitis, pending chest Xray results." Xray results confirmed bronchitis. During this visit the patient's glucose was checked to determine the status of his diabetes. The patient reported that his previous indigestion and diarrhea were currently not a problem. Circle the correct diagnoses to be coded.

a. productive cough

b. productive cough; indigestion; diarrhea

c. bronchitis; diabetes mellitus

d. bronchitis; diabetes mellitus; indigestion; diarrhea

94. A patient presents complaining of tenderness in the left breast and a family history of breast cancer. Upon examination, the physician discovers a small lump in the left breast. The patient is referred to a breast surgeon and Xray for a mammogram. The physician records questionable breast cancer of the left breast. Circle the correct diagnosis to be coded.

a. breast cancer

b. family history of breast cancer

c. breast pain; breast cancer

d. breast lump; breast pain; family history of breast cancer

CONSIDERATIONS TO ENSURE ACCURATE ICD-9-CM CODING

95. For each item, enter **T** for a true statement or **F** for a false statement on the line provided.

_______ a. M codes should be reported on the HCFA-1500 claim form.

_______ b. Code books should be purchased every other year.

_______ c. Providers and insurance specialists should be kept informed of annual coding changes.

_______ d. Preprinted diagnosis codes on encounter forms should be reviewed to verify inclusion of fifth and sixth digits.

_______ e. The postoperative diagnosis should be coded.

_______ f. Diagnosis codes should be reviewed for accuracy when updates are installed in office management software.

_______ g. Diagnosis codes should be proofread to ensure proper entry in the permanent record.

Know Your Acronyms

96. Define the following acronyms:

a. ICD-9-CM ____

b. NCHS ____

c. NEC ____

d. NOS ____

CPT Coding

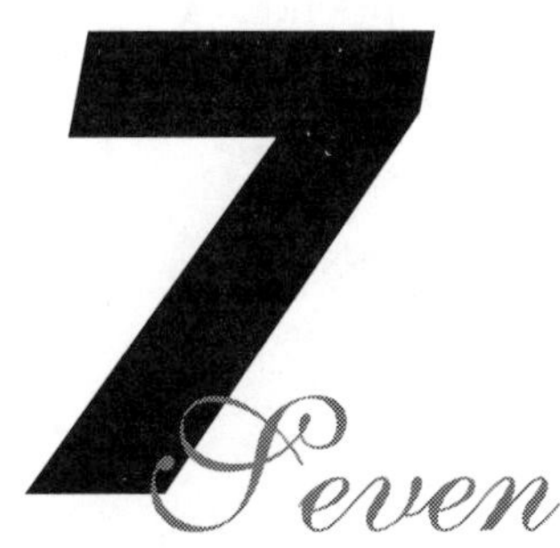

CPT CODING SYSTEM

1. CPT is a listing of descriptive terms and identifying codes for reporting ______________________ ______________________ and ______________________.

2. CPT is updated ____. (Circle the correct answer.)
   a. annually
   b. semi-annually
   c. every 2 years

3. The updated version of CPT is released in ____. (Circle the correct answer.)
   a. January
   b. late spring
   c. late fall

4. Federal programs generally implement the new codes on ____. (Circle the correct answer.)
   a. January 1
   b. June 1
   c. September 1

5. What must each procedure submitted on a claim be linked to? ______________________
____

CPT FORMAT

6. List the six sections of the CPT code book. (List in the order in which they appear.)
   a. ______________________
   b. ______________________
   c. ______________________
   d. ______________________
   e. ______________________
   f. ______________________

7. Where are the Evaluation and Management codes located? ____________________

8. Describe the contents of the following:

   Appendix A ____________________

   Appendix B ____________________

   Appendix C ____________________

   Appendix D ____________________

   Appendix E ____________________

   Appendix F ____________________

9. The CPT coding system is based on a ____ main number that describes each type of service. (Circle the correct answer.)

   a. two-digit

   b. four-digit

   c. five-digit

10. What do modifiers indicate? ____________________

CPT SYMBOLS AND CONVENTIONS

11. Match the CPT symbol in the first column with the definitions in the second column. Write the correct letter in each blank.

_______	bullet	a. the code is not to be used with modifier -51
_______	triangle	b. a new code
_______	horizontal triangles	c. an add-on code
_______	semicolon	d. surgery is billed on a fee-for-service basis
_______	asterisk	e. surround revised guidelines and notes
_______	circle with slash	f. code description revision
_______	plus symbol	g. indicates a code description revision for the current edition of CPT

TABULAR CONVENTIONS

12. Describe the function of the guidelines located at the beginning of each section in the CPT code book. ____________________

13. What is printed in boldface type? ____________________

CPT INDEX

14. The CPT index is primarily organized by ____________________.

15. Describe what *main terms* represent. ____________________

    ____

BASIC STEPS FOR CODING PROCEDURES

16. List seven basic steps for coding procedures.

Step 1: ____

____

Step 2: ____

____

Step 3: ____

Step 4: ____

____

Step 5: ____

____

Step 6: ____

____

Step 7: ____

____

17. Using only the index, write the code or range of codes to be investigated. In addition, underline the main term you referenced in the index.

a. ankle amputation ________________
b. lower arm biopsy ________________
c. artery angioplasty ________________
d. bone marrow aspiration ________________
e. bladder aspiration ________________
f. bladder neck resection ________________
g. rib resection ________________
h. salivary duct dilation ________________
i. wrist disarticulation ________________
j. drinking test for glaucoma ________________
k. Dwyer procedure ________________
l. new patient office visit ________________
m. well-baby care ________________
n. wound repair of pancreas ________________
o. inpatient hospital discharge ________________
p. house calls ________________

18. List five words/phrases used in the insurance industry that define a surgical procedure.
    a. ____________________
    b. ____________________
    c. ____________________
    d. ____________________
    e. ____________________

19. What are three questions that must be asked to code surgeries properly?
    a. ____________________
    b. ____________________
    c. ____________________

20. CPT divides surgical procedures into which two main groups? ____________________

21. List three services/procedures included in a surgical package.
    a. ____________________
    b. ____________________
    c. ____________________

22. On what basis are minor surgeries to be billed? ____________________

23. Briefly describe *unbundling*. ____________________

24. Assign codes to the following: (If an asterisk appears, include it in your answer.)
    a. removal of foreign body in tendon sheath, simple ____________
    b. puncture aspiration of cyst of breast ____________
    c. incision and drainage of thyroid gland cyst ____________
    d. abrasion, single lesion ____________
    e. destruction of four flat warts ____________
    f. incision and drainage of ankle abscess ____________
    g. incision and drainage of wrist hematoma ____________
    h. aspiration thyroid cyst ____________
    i. laparoscopy with bilateral total pelvic lymphadenenctomy and peri-aortic lymph node biopsy ____________

25. Describe when a code qualified with the phrase "separate procedure" is reported. ____________

    ____

    ____

26. Assign codes to the following, giving special attention to "separate procedure."
    a. removal of impacted vaginal foreign body ____________
    b. dilation of cervical canal, instrumental ____________
    c. pleurectomy, parietal ____________

d. thoracentesis with insertion of tube ______________

e. laryngoscopy endoscopy, indirect ______________

f. biopsy of testis, incisional ______________

27. Define *multiple surgical procedure.* ______________________________

____

28. What is added to the CPT number for each lesser surgical procedure that does not have the symbol ⊘ in front of the code? ______________________________

Critical Thinking

29. Write a paragraph describing why multiple surgical procedures are ranked into major and lesser procedures.

____

____

____

____

CODING SPECIAL SURGERY CASES

30. Define the following terms:

a. skin lesion ______________________________

b. excision of a lesion ______________________________

c. destruction of a lesion ______________________________

31. List five things you must know when reporting the excision or destruction of lesions.

a. ______________________________

b. ______________________________

c. ______________________________

d. ______________________________

e. ______________________________

32. Layered closure requires the use of two codes: one for the ____________, and one for an

____________ ____________.

33. If a physician reports the size of a lesion in inches what must the coder do? ______________

____

34. When converting the size of a lesion, one inch equals ______________________________

35. When there are multiple lacerations, which repair should be listed first? ______________

____

36. Assign codes to the following; then convert inches to centimeters.

a. excision, 1 inch benign lesion, left leg ____________ ____________

b. excision, 1/2 inch malignant lesion, finger ____________ ____________

c. simple repair of a 2 inch laceration on the right foot ____________ ____________

d. intermediate repair of a 5 inch laceration of the back ____________ ____________

e. layer closure of a 3 inch wound of the neck ____________ ____________

f. repair of laceration, 2.0 cm, anterior two-thirds of tongue ____________ ____________

37. What are six questions that must be asked to code fractures/dislocations correctly?

a. ____

b. ____

c. ____

d. ____

e. ____

f. ____

38. Match the fracture terms in the first column with the definitions in the second column. Write the correct letter in each blank.

_______ closed fracture treatment	a. the application of manually applied forces to restore normal anatomical alignment
_______ open fracture treatment	b. open reduction with internal fixation
_______ manipulation of a fracture	c. the fracture site was not surgically opened
_______ reduction of a fracture	d. the fracture site was surgically opened, bone ends visualized, aligned, and internal fixation may have been applied
_______ ORIF	e. a fixation device has been applied

39. When is arthrotomy considered the primary procedure? ____

____

40. Assign codes to the following:

a. open treatment of fracture great toe, phalanx, with external fixation ____________

b. closed treatment of nasal bone fracture with stabilization ____________

c. treatment of closed elbow dislocation; without anesthesia ____________

d. closed treatment of ulnar fracture, proximal end; with manipulation ____________

e. open treatment of maxillary fracture ____________

f. closed treatment of shoulder dislocation, with manipulation; requiring anesthesia ____________

g. Surgical elbow arthroscopy, with removal of loose body ____________

h. diagnostic hip arthroscopy, with synovial biopsy ____________

41. Endoscopy codes in CPT are classified according to: (list four)

a. ______

b. ______

c. ______

d. ______

42. Complete the following sentences:

a. Endoscopies of the digestive system are always coded to the furthest site accessed by the ______ .

b. Endoscopic guide-wire dilation involves the passage of a guide-wire through an endoscope into the ______ .

c. Indirect laryngoscopy means the larynx is visualized by using a warm laryngeal ______ .

d. Direct laryngoscopy is performed by passage of a rigid or fiberoptic endoscopy into the ______ .

43. Assign codes to the following:

a. surgical wrist endoscopy with release of transverse carpal ligament ______

b. flexible esophagoscopy with single biopsy ______

c. direct operative laryngoscopy with foreign body removal ______

d. flexible colonoscopy with biopsy ______

e. rigid proctosigmoidoscopy with dilation ______

MEDICINE SECTION OVERVIEW

44. The medicine section starts with what code? ______

45. When a physician performs only one component of a test, what modifier should be added to the global code to indicate the full procedure was not performed? ______

46. The special services and reports section is a miscellaneous section which covers services considered to be ______ as ______ to basic services provided to the patient.

47. How are psychiatric consultations reported? ______

______

48. Are psychiatric codes reserved for use only by psychiatrists? ______

49. Assign codes to the following:

a. right heart cardiac catheterization, for congenital cardiac anomalies ______

b. medical testimony ______

c. services requested between 10:00PM and 8:00AM in addition to basic service __________

d. acupuncture; one or more needles, with electrical stimulation __________

e. wheelchair management/propulsion training, 15 minutes __________

f. massage therapy, 45 min __________

g. extended medical report preparation __________

h. family psychotherapy without the patient present __________

i. hypnotherapy __________

j. nonpressurized inhalation treatment for acute airway obstruction __________

k. educational video tapes for the patient __________

l. one hour of psychological testing with interpretation and report __________

RADIOLOGY SECTION OVERVIEW

50. Define *radiologic views*. __________

51. Describe the professional component of a radiologic examination. __________

52. Describe the technical component of a radiologic examination. __________

53. Assign codes to the following:

a. complete radiologic examination of the mandible __________

b. urography, retrograde __________

c. pelvimetry __________

d. orthoroentgenogram, scanogram __________

e. chest Xray, two views, with fluoroscopy __________

f. Xray of facial bones, four views __________

g. CAT scan of the abdomen, with contrast __________

h. gastroesophageal reflux study __________

i. Xray of the cervical spine, two views __________

j. barium enema __________

k. cardiac shunt detection __________

l. splenoportography __________

m. Xray of the scapula, complete __________

n. Xray of the forearm __________

o. hip Xray, three views __________

PATHOLOGY/LABORATORY SECTION OVERVIEW

54. How would a coder locate the list of panel options? ______________________________

____

55. Describe the use of the following sections:

    a. drug testing ______________________________

    ____

    b. therapeutic drug assays ______________________________

    ____

    c. evocative/suppression testing ______________________________

    ____

56. Assign codes to the following:

    a. red blood cell count ______________
    b. blood gases pH only ______________
    c. glucose-6-phosphate dehydrogenase screen ______________
    d. glucose tolerance test, three specimens ______________
    e. KOH prep ______________
    f. HIV antibody confirmatory test ______________
    g. leptospira ______________
    h. HDL cholesterol ______________
    i. glucose reagent strip ______________
    j. occult blood, feces ______________
    k. PKU ______________
    l. rapid test for infection, screen, each antibody ______________
    m. pregnancy test, urine ______________
    n. herpes simples virus, quantification ______________
    o. urinary potassium ______________
    p. urine dip, non-automated, without microscopy ______________
    q. triglycerides ______________
    r. cholesterol, serum, total ______________
    s. TSH ______________

EVALUATION AND MANAGEMENT SECTION OVERVIEW

57. Why is the Evaluation and Management Section located at the beginning of CPT?

____

58. Define *new patient.* ______________________________

____

____

59. Define *established patient.* ______________________________

____

____

60. The E&M __________ refers to the physical location where health care is provided. (Circle the correct answer.)

    a. level of service

    b. place of service

    c. type of service

61. The E&M __________ reflects the amount of work involved in providing health care to patients. (Circle the correct answer.)

    a. level of service

    b. place of service

    c. type of service

62. The E&M __________ reflects the kind of health care services provided to patients. (Circle the correct answer.)

    a. level of service

    b. place of service

    c. type of service

63. Key components include __________. (Circle the correct answer/answers.)

    a. extent of history

    b. extent of examination

    c. complexity of medial decision making.

64. __________ key components must be considered when assigning codes for established patients. (Circle the correct answer.)

    a. One

    b. Two

    c. Three

65. __________ key components must be considered when assigning codes for new patients. (Circle the correct answer.)

    a. One

    b. Two

    c. Three

66. __________ is an assessment of the patient's organ and body systems. (Circle the correct answer.)

a. A history

b. Medical decision making

c. A physical examination

67. __________ is an interview of the patient that includes an HPI, a ROS, and a PFSH. (Circle the correct answer.)

a. A history

b. Medical decision making

c. A physical examination

68. __________ refers to the complexity of establishing a diagnosis and/or selecting a management option. (Circle the correct answer.)

a. A history

b. Medical decision making

c. A physical examination

69. List four contributory components.

a. ______________________________

b. ______________________________

c. ______________________________

d. ______________________________

70. Describe *coordination of care.* ______________________________

____

71. List five types of presenting problems.

a. ______________________________

b. ______________________________

c. ______________________________

d. ______________________________

e. ______________________________

EVALUATION AND MANAGEMENT CATEGORIES

72. For each item, enter **T** for a true statement or **F** for a false statement on the line provided.

_______ a. The hospital is required to establish a physical area of observation.

_______ b. Inpatient hospital care services cover the first hospital inpatient encounter the admitting/attending physician has with the patient for each admission.

_______ c. Subsequent hospital care includes the review of the patient's chart, the results of diagnostic studies, and/or reassessment of the patient's condition since the last assessment performed by the physician.

_______ d. Hospital discharge services do not include the final examination of the patient.

_______ e. Consultants may not initiate diagnostic and/or therapeutic services as necessary during the consultative encounter.

_______ f. A preoperative clearance is not considered a consultation when the referring physician is the patient's primary care physician.

_______ g. A confirmatory consultation is an E&M service requested by the patient.

_______ h. Nursing facility services do not include services performed at long-term care facilities.

_______ i. Domiciliary care covers E&M services provided to patients who live in custodial care or boarding home facilities that do not provide 24-hour nursing care.

73. Assign codes to the following:

a. follow-up inpatient consult, expanded _______________

b. subsequent nursing facility care, problem focused _______________

c. initial office visit, problem focused _______________

d. follow-up office visit, comprehensive _______________

e. initial observation care, detailed _______________

f. initial hospital care, low severity _______________

g. subsequent hospital care, expanded _______________

h. initial home visit, detailed _______________

i. followup home visit, comprehensive _______________

j. observation care discharge _______________

k. initial inpatient consult, detailed _______________

l. initial confirmatory consult, problem focused _______________

m. emergency dept. visit, comprehensive _______________

n. physician direction of EMS emergency care _______________

o. nursing facility assessment, comprehensive _______________

p. new patient rest home visit, expanded _______________

q. followup rest home visit, expanded _______________

r. office consult, problem focused _______________

74. Fill in the blanks using the definitions provided.

a. Medical emergency care to critically ill patients that requires the constant attendance of a physician and that is usually administered in the critical or emergency care facilities of the hospital is known as _______________________ .

b. _______________________ is used for reporting services performed by physicians for critically ill neonates/infants.

c. _______________________ is used in addition to the regular visit or consultation codes when typical treatment exceeds, by 30 minutes or more, the time described in the CPT description of the visit.

d. _______________________ allows for the reporting of cases in which the physician spends a prolonged period of time without patient contact waiting for an event to occur that will require the physician's services.

e. _______________________ is the process in which an attending physician coordinates and supervises the care provided to a patient by other health care providers.

f. ________________________________ covers the physician's time spent supervising a complex and multidisciplinary care treatment program for a specific patient who is under the care of a home health agency, hospice, or nursing facility.

g. Routine examinations or risk management counseling for children and adults exhibiting no overt signs or symptoms of a disorder while presenting to the medical office for a preventive medical physical are ________________________________ .

h. Examination of normal or high-risk neonates in the hospital or other locations, subsequent newborn care in a hospital, and resuscitation of high-risk babies is ____________________________ .

75. Assign codes to the following:

a. operative physician standby, 30 minutes ________________

b. critical care, first hour ________________

c. established well-child check-up, age 7 ________________

d. prolonged office care with direct patient contact, one hour ________________

e. complex telephone call with a distraught patient ________________

f. initial inpatient history and examination of normal newborn ________________

g. periodic preventive medicine, age 52 ________________

h. initial well-baby check-up, 6 months old ________________

i. telephone call to discuss test results in detail ________________

CPT MODIFIERS

76. Explain why modifiers are added to CPT codes. ____

____

77. Assign codes and modifiers to the following:

a. bilateral partial mastectomy ________________

b. vasovasostomy discontinued after anesthesia due to heart arrhythmia, hospital outpatient ________________

c. decision for surgery during initial office visit, comprehensive ________________

d. expanded office visit for followup to mastectomy, new onset diabetes was discovered and treated ________________

e. cholecystectomy, postoperative management only ________________

f. difficult and complicated resection of external cardiac tumor ________________

g. hemorrhoidectomy by simple ligature discontinued prior to anesthesia due to severe drop in blood pressure, hospital outpatient ________________

h. assistant surgeon, modified radical mastectomy ________________

i. total abdominal hysterectomy, preoperative management only ________________

j. total urethrectomy, including cystostomy, female, surgical care only ________________

k. simple repair of a 2 inch laceration on the right foot discontinued due to severe dizziness, physician's office ________________

78. Assign codes to the following:

	First Code	Second Code
a. tonsillectomy and adenoidectomy, age 10 and a wart removed from the patient's neck while in the OR.	___________	___________
b. excision, malignant lesion 0.6 to 1.0 cm, face and layer closure of wounds of face, 2.0 cm	___________	___________
c. incision and drainage, perianal abscess, superficial and puncture aspiration of abscess, hematoma, cyst	___________	___________

Know Your Acronyms

79. Define the following acronyms:

a. CPT ____

b. ORIF ____

c. PFSH ____

d. HPI ____

e. ROS ____

HCPCS Coding System

CHAPTER

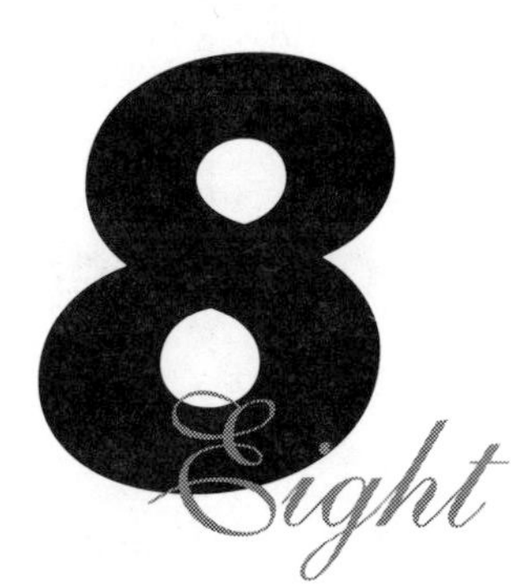

ORGANIZATION OF HCPCS CODING SYSTEM

1. How many code levels are associated with HCPCS? (Circle the correct answer.)
   a. two
   b. three
   c. four

2. Level I codes are developed and published by _____. (Circle the correct answer.)
   a. AMA
   b. HCFA
   c. LMC

3. J codes are found in which level? (Circle the correct answer.)
   a. Level I
   b. Level II
   c. Level III

4. Level II codes identify the services of _____. (Circle the correct answers.)
   a. nurse practitioners
   b. speech therapists
   c. durable medical equipment

5. J codes list _____. (Circle the correct answer.)
   a. pathology and laboratory
   b. durable medical equipment
   c. medications

6. Who is responsible for the annual updates to HCPCS Level II? (Circle the correct answer.)
   a. AMA
   b. HCFA
   c. LMC

7. Level III codes are assigned by _____. (Circle the correct answer.)
   a. AMA
   b. HCFA
   c. LMC

HCPCS NATIONAL LEVEL II CODES

8. Is HCFA responsible for errors that might occur in or from the use of private printings of HCPCS Level II Codes? ____________________

9. Which professional organization updates codes in the Level II D Series? ____________________

HCPCS NATIONAL CODES (LEVEL II) INDEX

10. Because of the wide variety of services and procedures described in HCPCS Level II, the ____________ ____________ is very helpful in finding the correct code.

11. When looking up a code in the Level II index, it is important to verify the code in the ____________ section of the codebook.

12. Assign codes to the following:

    a. injection, aminophylline, up to 250 mg ____________
    b. elbow orthosis; elastic with metal joints ____________
    c. ambulance service; BLS, non-emergency transport ____________
    d. alcohol wipes, 2 boxes ____________
    e. amputee adapter, wheelchair ____________
    f. wound cleanser ____________
    g. artificial larynx ____________
    h. ultrasonic generator filter ____________
    i. IPD supply kit ____________
    j. infusion pump, insulin ____________
    k. hypertonic saline solution ____________
    l. ambulance oxygen ____________
    m. rocking bed ____________
    n. complete upper dentures ____________
    o. breast prosthesis, adhesive skin support ____________
    p. culture sensitivity study ____________
    q. nasogastric tubing, with stylet ____________
    r. pinworm examination ____________
    s. plasma, single donor, fresh frozen ____________
    t. frames purchases ____________
    u. hearing aid, monaural, behind the ear ____________
    v. routine venipuncture for collection of specimens ____________
    w. assessment for hearing aid ____________
    x. transportation of Xray to nursing home, one patient ____________
    y. speech screening ____________
    z. noncoring needle ____________

DETERMINING CARRIER RESPONSIBILITY

13. National codes beginning with D, G, M, P, or R fall under the jurisdiction of the _____. (Circle the correct answer.)
    a. DMERC
    b. LMC
    c. DMEPOS

14. Which is responsible for Level II codes beginning with B, E, K, and L? (Circle the correct answer.)
    a. DMERC
    b. LMC
    c. DMEPOS

15. Codes beginning with A, J, Q, and V may be assigned to the____. (Circle the correct answers.)
    a. DMERC
    b. LMC
    c. DMEPOS

16. For each item, enter **T** for a true statement or **F** for a false statement on the line provided.

    _______ a. Because DME billings were out of control, HCFA decided to have all DME claims processed by only four regional carriers, the DMERCs.

    _______ b. Providers dispensing medical equipment and supplies must register with a DMERC.

    _______ c. When a Medicare patient is treated for a fractured leg and supplied with crutches, only one claim is generated and sent to the DMERC.

    _______ d. If the doctor is not registered with the DMERC, the patient is billed directly for the medical equipment.

    _______ e. Most dental procedures are included as Medicare benefits.

    _______ f. New medical and surgical services may first be assigned a Level II code because the review procedures for adding new codes to Level II is a much shorter process.

HCPCS MODIFIERS

17. Explain why Level II and Level III modifiers are added to codes. ______________________________

    ____

18. Assign codes and HCPCS modifiers to the following:
    a. family psychotherapy without the patient present, by a clinical psychologist ______________
    b. psychoanalysis, by a clinical social worker ______________
    c. initial office visit, problem focused, by a nurse practitioner in a rural area ______________
    d. new three-prong cane ______________
    e. tooth reimplantation of accidentally displaced tooth, emergency treatment ______________

f. emergency ambulance transport (BLS), all inclusive, from physician's office to hospital ______

g. dental radiographs, bitewing, single film, left side ______

h. portable whirlpool, new when rented ______

i. chemotherapy administration by infusion technique only, physician providing service in a rural HMSA ______

j. rented loop heel wheelchair ______

k. initial well-adult check-up, age 67, waiver of liability statement on file ______

l. initial home visit, detail changed to initial home visit, expanded because it was incorrect on the original claim ______

m. non-emergency ambulance transport (BLS), all inclusive from hospital to skilled nursing home ______

n. anesthesia for amputation of upper 2/3 of femur, complicated by total body hypothermia ______

o. expanded followup inpatient consult provided by a substitute physician under a reciprocal billing arrangement ______

p. custom made plastic prosthetic right eye ______

q. left ankle splint for foot drop ______

r. second opinion language screening ordered by a professional review organization ______

s. five-minute followup BP check by a physician's assistant ______

Know Your Acronyms

19. Define the following acronyms:

a. HCPCS ______

b. DME ______

c. DMERC ______

d. DMEPOS ______

e. ABN ______

f. CIM ______

g. HPSA ______

h. LMC ______

i. MCM ______

HCFA Reimbursement Issues

CHAPTER

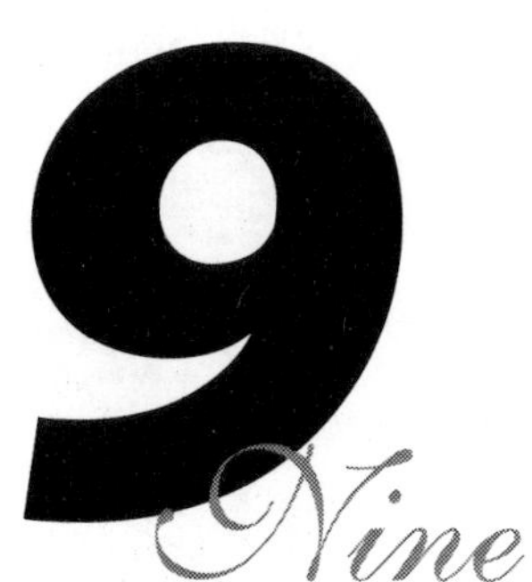

INTRODUCTION

1. Complete the following sentences:

   a. HCFA implemented the Diagnosis Related Groups Prospective Payment System to control the

   ____

   b. Medicare law requires physicians to be paid according to the ____________________

   ____

   c. The RBRVS system divides all services into relative value units or payment components of

   ____

   d. Payment for anesthesia services is based on ____________________

THE MEDICARE FEE SCHEDULE

2. Match the insurance terms in the first column with the definitions in the second column. Write the correct letter in each blank.

______ Local Medicare Carriers	a. the maximum fee a nonPAR physician may charge for services
______ limiting charge	b. publishes new payment values for procedure codes
______ "J" codes	c. establishes the payment schedule for supplies and equipment according to HCFA specified guidelines
______ federal register	d. billing adjusted amounts to beneficiaries
______ balance billing	e. assigned to medications
______ DMEPOS	f. translates the HCPCS RVUs, GPCIs, and CF into a fee schedule and distributes it to enrolled providers

HCFA REGULATIONS THAT IMPACT REIMBURSEMENT

3. Who enacts Medicare legislation? (Circle the correct answer.)
   a. local Medicare carriers
   b. Congress
   c. HCFA

4. Medicare regulations state that the ___ is responsible for knowing all rules that apply to services billed to the program. (Circle the correct answer.)
   a. patient
   b. coder
   c. provider

5. What has Medicare issued to nurse practitioners and physician assistants so that their services can be billed directly to Medicare? (Circle the correct answer.)
   a. special provider numbers
   b. a special billing address
   c. special TOS codes

6. Nurse practitioners and physician assistants are paid at ___ of the Medicare Fee Schedule. (Circle the correct answer.)
   a. 50%
   b. 75%
   c. 85%

7. Describe *constant attendance* as it relates to Medicare. ______________________________

____

MEDICARE REIMBURSEMENT

8. Define *fraud*. ______________________________

____

9. Describe the penalties for Medicare fraud. ______________________________

____

10. List the names of two manuals Medicare sends to carriers to assist in paying claims.
    a. ______________________________
    b. ______________________________

11. For each item, enter **T** for a true statement or **F** for a false statement on the line provided.

_______ a. A DRG provides a fee-for-service payment dependent on the patient's diagnosis.

_______ b. HCFA must approve a Medicare managed care plan before it is allowed to enroll Medicare beneficiaries.

_______ c. Medicare MCOs must provide coverage that is similar to a fee-for-service program.

_______ d. A CIM advises carriers on procedures for paying and denying claims.

_______ e. HCFA requested a change in CPT "visit" codes for office and hospital services as part of the 1992 RBRVS implementation.

_______ f. A properly documented patient record is an essential component of good clinical care, and supports the level of E & M service code submitted on a claim.

_______ g. Medicare regulations permit payment for preventive medicine services.

_______ h. Medicare pays for the treatment of disease.

12. List three screening services that are covered by Medicare.

    a. ______________________________

    b. ______________________________

    c. ______________________________

13. Medicare replaced the TOS indicators with ______________________________

14. The global period for each surgery includes ______________________________

15. During the global period, what modifier is used to indicate that a procedure is not related to the original service? (Circle the correct answer.)

    a. modifier -79

    b. modifier -54

    c. modifier -57

16. What modifier must be used with the consultation code to report a pre-operative evaluation? (Circle the correct answer.)

    a. modifier -79

    b. modifier -54

    c. modifier -57

17. What modifier is used with the surgical procedure code to report to Medicare that the surgeon did not provide any of the post-operative care for a surgical patient? (Circle the correct answer.)

    a. modifier -79

    b. modifier -54

    c. modifier -57

18. What modifier would a surgeon serving as an assistant surgeon use? (Circle the correct answer.)

    a. modifier -78

    b. modifier -79

    c. modifier -80

19. If a patient has to return to the OR for a related procedure during the postoperative period, what modifier would be appropriate? (Circle the correct answer.)

    a. modifier -78

    b. modifier -79

    c. modifier -80

Know Your Acronyms

20. Define the following acronyms:

    a. RBRVS ______________________________

    b. RVU ______________________________

    c. CF ______________________________

    d. GPCI ______________________________

    e. FR ______________________________

    f. MFN ______________________________

    g. NP ______________________________

    h. PA ______________________________

    i. DRG ______________________________

    j. MCO ______________________________

    k. TOS ______________________________

    l. POS ______________________________

    m. LMC ______________________________

    n. CIM ______________________________

    o. MCM ______________________________

CODING FROM SOURCE DOCUMENTS

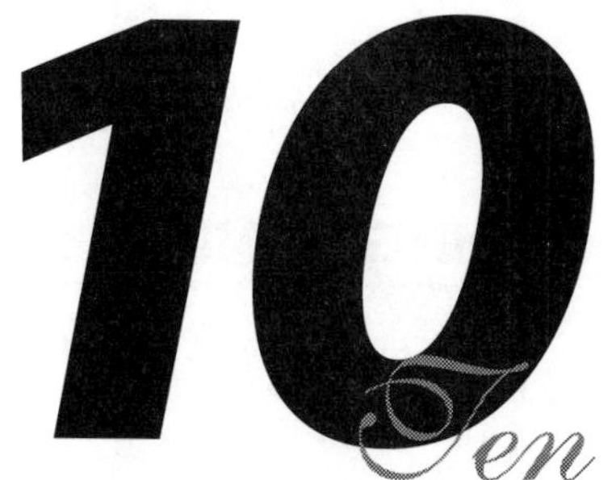

APPLYING ICD-9-CM CODING GUIDELINES

1. For each item, enter **T** for a true statement or **F** for a false statement on the line provided.

_______ a. Code and report conditions and procedures even if they are not documented in the medical report.

_______ b. Use the full range of ICD codes from 001 through 999.9 and V01 through V82.9, and E codes when warranted by circumstances.

_______ c. Code and report all conditions that are stated as questionable, suspected, or possible.

_______ d. Code to the highest level of specificity any disorder or injury that is known and documented at the time of the encounter.

_______ e. Documented symptoms should be coded and reported when they are manifestations of a reported disorder or injury.

_______ f. V codes are assigned when there is justification for the patient to seek health care but no disorder currently exists.

_______ g. Code only those problems treated during the encounter or that affect the treatment rendered.

_______ h. No more than six diagnoses can be reported on one claim form.

_______ i. Code and report all past conditions even if they are not currently active problems.

_______ j. Link each procedure or service to a condition that proves the medical necessity for performing that procedure/service.

2. Match the procedure/service in the first column with the diagnosis in the second column. Write the correct letter in each blank.

_______	EKG	a. impacted cerumin
_______	urinalysis	b. jaundice
_______	strep test	c. hay fever
_______	wrist Xray	d. bronchial asthma
_______	venipuncture	e. chest pain

_______ removal of ear wax		f. strep throat
_______ sigmoidoscopy		g. fractured wrist
_______ inhalation treatment		h. hematuria
_______ allergy test		i. rectal bleeding

CODING CLINICAL SCENARIOS

3. List eight steps for abstracting and coding clinical scenarios.
   a. ______________________________
   b. ______________________________
   c. ______________________________
   d. ______________________________
   e. ______________________________
   f. ______________________________
   g. ______________________________
   h. ______________________________

4. Assign ICD-9 and CPT codes to the following scenarios. Be sure to include all necessary CPT and/or HCPCS modifiers.

   a. A 35-year-old established patient came to the office for excessive menstruation and irregular menstrual cycle. The physician performed an expanded problem focused evaluation and cervical biopsy.

   CPT Codes **ICD-9 Codes**

   ______________________ ______________________

   b. Patient was referred to me by his primary care physician, Dr. Pearson, because of severe back pain. Dr. Pearson feels he should have surgery but the patient states the pain is relieved by regular chiropractic care and doesn't want to have back surgery. After a problem focused examination and a complete radiologic examination of the lumbosacral spine, including bending views, I consulted with Dr. Pearson and concluded the patient's degenerative disc disease is probably doing as well with a chiropractor as with orthopedic treatment. I did not recommend surgery at this time.

   CPT Codes **ICD-9 Codes**

   ______________________ ______________________

   c. Patient underwent a barium enema which included air contrast. The request form noted severe abdominal pain and diarrhea for the past two weeks. The radiology impression was diverticulitis of the colon.

   CPT Codes **ICD-9 Codes**

   ______________________ ______________________

   d. Patient presented for followup of his COPD. At this time the patient is experiencing no significant cough, no sputum, no fever, and no respiratory distress. However, there is dyspnea only with exertion, which is accompanied by angina. A detailed examination was performed and the physician spent approximately 25 minutes with the patient. Chest is clear, no wheeze or rales. Chest

Xrays, frontal and lateral, were taken to determine status of COPD. No additional treatment is required at this time.

CPT Codes **ICD-9 Codes**

_______________ _______________

e. A surgeon is called to the hospital by the emergency department physician to see a 59-year-old male who presented with an abdominal mass, left lower quadrant. The surgeon performed a comprehensive examination, admitted the patient, and scheduled an exploratory laparotomy.

CPT Codes **ICD-9 Codes**

_______________ _______________

f. On 08/12/YYYY the patient underwent an exploratory laparotomy, a left partial hepatic resection for a malignant hepatoma, and a cholecystectomy.

CPT Codes **ICD-9 Codes**

_______________ _______________

g. On 04/01/YYYY a 65-year-old patient underwent a bronchoscopy and biopsy for a left lower lobe lung mass. The biopsy revealed adenocarcinoma of the left lower lobe lung. On 04/05/YYYY the same surgeon performed a left lower lobe lobectomy and thoracic lymphadenectomy.

CPT Codes **ICD-9 Codes**

_______________ _______________

_______________ _______________

h. On 04/01/YYYY a 39-year-old female presents to her GYN office with a mass and pain in the right breast. Her mother and sister died of breast cancer. A detailed history and examination was performed. The patient was referred to a surgeon for consultation.

CPT Codes **ICD-9 Codes**

_______________ _______________

i. On 04/03/YYYY the patient presents to the surgeon's office for consultation. The patient is experiencing pain in her right breast and has noticed a lump there. She also has a family history of breast cancer. The surgeon performs a level III consultation and two breast aspirations of the right breast.

CPT Codes **ICD-9 Codes**

_______________ _______________

j. On 04/09/YYYY the patient underwent an excision of the right breast mass in the outpatient surgery center. The pathology report revealed a malignant neoplasm, central portion of the right breast. On 04/13/YYYY the patient underwent a right modified radical mastectomy by the same surgeon.

CPT Codes **ICD-9 Codes**

_______________ _______________

_______________ _______________

k. On 07/23/YYYY a four-month-old patient returned to the office for her routine well baby check-up. The following vaccines were administered by the medical assistant: Inactivated Poliovirus (IPV), Hepatitis B, Diphtheria, tetanus toxoids, and acellular pertussis. The patient is to return to the office in two months for her six-month check-up and vaccinations.

CPT Codes **ICD-9 Codes**

_______________ _______________

l. Patient returned to the office, after a five year absence, because of abdominal pain, diarrhea, and rectal bleeding which began three weeks ago. A detailed examination revealed a tense abdomen with some guarding at the right upper quadrant. Patient to be scheduled for a flexible sigmoidoscopy to R/O colon cancer.

CPT Codes ______________________ **ICD-9 Codes** ______________________

CODING MEDICAL REPORTS

5. List two major formats health care providers use for documenting clinic notes.
   a. ______________________
   b. ______________________

6. Match the SOAP terms in the first column with the definitions in the second column. Write the correct letter in each blank.

_______ subjective data	a. diagnostic statement
_______ objective data	b. how treatment will proceed
_______ assessment data	c. chief complaint and description of problem
_______ plan	d. information not relevant to treatment
	e. observations made during the physical examination and diagnostic testing

7. Assign diagnostic codes to the following SOAP Notes:

   a. S Patient complains of one week of severe epigastric pain and burning especially after eating.

   O On examination there is extreme guarding and tenderness, epigastric region, no rebound. Bowel sounds normal. BP 110/70

   A R/O gastric ulcer

   P Patient to have upper gastrointestinal series. Start on Zantac and eliminate alcohol, fried foods, and caffeine. Return to office in one week.

   ICD-9 Codes ______________________

   b. S Patient returns after undergoing an upper gastrointestinal series. She states she is still experiencing epigastric pain.

   O Upper gastrointestinal series revealed areas of ulceration.

   A Acute gastric ulcer

   P Omeprazole 10mg qd. Return for followup visit in three weeks.

   ICD-9 Codes ______________________

   c. S Patient was walking up his driveway when he slipped and fell, landing on his left arm and striking his head against his car. He was unconscious for less than ten minutes, experienced dizziness and vomiting, and felt severe pain in his left arm.

   O Examination reveals restriction of motion of his left arm and a laceration on his head.

   A Mild concussion. Laceration occipital region of scalp. Undisplaced fracture proximal left humerus (greater tuberosity)

   P Laceration repair occipital region of scalp. Patient sent to Dr. Smith for fracture care.

ICD-9 Codes ______________________________

d. S Patient complains of rectal discomfort, rectal bleeding, and severe itching.

O Examination reveals multiple soft external hemorrhoids.

A Multiple external hemorrhoids

P Suppositories after each bowel movement. Return to office in four weeks.

ICD-9 Codes ______________________________

e. S Patient presents complaining of polyuria, polydipsia, and weight loss.

O Urinalysis by dip, automated, with microscopy reveals elevated glucose.

A Possible diabetes

P Patient to have a glucose tolerance test and return in three days for blood work results

ICD-9 Codes ______________________________

CODING OPERATIVE REPORTS

8. List five items contained in an operative report.

   a. ______________________________

   b. ______________________________

   c. ______________________________

   d. ______________________________

   e. ______________________________

9. Explain why you should make a copy of the operative report before assigning codes.

   ____

10. Explain why it is important to compare the postoperative diagnosis with the biopsy report on all excised neoplasms. ______________________________

11. For each item, enter **T** for a true statement or **F** for a false statement on the line provided.

    _______ a. Because there is a monetary value for each CPT code, be sure to use multiple, separate codes to describe a procedure even if CPT has a single code that classifies all the individual components of the procedure described by the physician.

    _______ b. Never use a code number described in CPT as a "separate procedure" when it is performed within the same incision site as the primary procedure and is an integral part of a greater procedure.

    _______ c. The postoperative diagnosis should explain the medical necessity for performing the procedure(s).

    _______ d. When working in a medical practice you should code an excision even if the pathology report has not been received.

12. Assign ICD-9 and CPT codes to the following operative reports:

    a. PREOPERATIVE DIAGNOSIS: Pterygium of the right eye

    POSTOPERATIVE DIAGNOSIS: Pterygium of the right eye

    PROCEDURE PERFORMED: Pterygium excision with conjunctival autograft of the right eye

    ANESTHESIA: General endotracheal anesthesia

PROCEDURE: After the patient was prepped and draped in the usual sterile fashion, attention was directed to his right eye under the operating microscope. The area of the pterygium was viewed and an injection of lidocaine with Marcaine was placed subconjunctivally to infiltrate area of the pterygium and surrounding conjunctiva. Then, using a combination of sharp and blunt dissection with 57 Beaver blade Westcott scissors, the pterygium was lifted away from the cornea, making a plane to the cornea to achieve clarity to the cornea. Next, an area was marked with a hand-held cautery nasally through the conjunctiva. A muscle hook was inserted to identify the medial rectus muscle. Then, using Westcott scissors and .12, the head and body of the pterygium were removed noting where the medial rectus muscle was at all times. Cautery was used to achieve hemostasis. An area of conjunctiva superior to the area of the prior pterygium under the lid was isolated and an incision was made through the conjunctiva. This section of conjunctiva was then transposed and placed into position over the area of the prior pterygium, thus forming an autograft. This was sutured into place with multiple single 8-0 Vicryl sutures. The autograft was noted to be in good position. Hemostasis was noted to be well achieved. The cornea was noted to be smooth and clear in the area of the prior pterygium with the epithelial defect secondary to removal of the pterygium. Maxitrol drops were placed. The patient's eye was patched. The patient tolerated the procedure well without complications and is to follow up in our office tomorrow.

CPT Codes **ICD-9 Codes**

____________________ ____________________

b. PREOPERATIVE DIAGNOSIS: Subcutaneous mass, posterior scalp

POSTOPERATIVE DIAGNOSIS: Subcutaneous mass, posterior scalp

PROCEDURE PERFORMED: Excision, subcutaneous mass, posterior scalp

ANESTHESIA: General

PROCEDURE: After instillation of 1% Xylocaine, a transverse incision was made directly over this elongated posterior scalp lesion. Hemostasis was obtained with electrocautery and suture ligature. A fatty tumor was encountered and sharp dissection used in completely excising this lesion. Hemostasis was obtained with ties, suture ligatures, and electrocautery. The lesion was removed in its entirety. The wound was irrigated and the incision closed in layers. The skin was closed with a running nylon suture for hemostasis.

CPT Codes **ICD-9 Codes**

____________________ ____________________

c. PREOPERATIVE DIAGNOSIS: Ventral hernia

POSTOPERATIVE DIAGNOSIS: Ventral hernia

PROCEDURE PERFORMED: Repair of ventral hernia with mesh

ANESTHESIA: General

PROCEDURE: The vertical midline incision was opened. Sharp and blunt dissection was used in defining the hernia sac. The hernia sac was opened and the fascia examined. The hernia defect was sizable. Careful inspection was utilized to uncover any additional adjacent fascial defects. Small defects were observed on both sides of the major hernia and were incorporated into the main hernia. The hernia sac was dissected free of the surrounding subcutaneous tissues and retained. Prolene mesh was then fashioned to size and sutured to one side with running #0 Prolene suture. Interrupted Prolene sutures were placed on the other side and tagged untied.

The hernia sac was then sutured to the opposite side of the fascia with Vicryl suture. The Prolene sutures were passed through the interstices of the Prolene mesh and tied into place, insuring that the Prolene mesh was not placed under tension. Excess mesh was excised. Jackson-Pratt drains were placed, one on each side. Running subcutaneous suture utilizing Vicryl was placed, after which the skin was stapled.

CPT Codes **ICD-9 Codes**

____________________ ____________________

d. PREOPERATIVE DIAGNOSIS: Intermittent exotropia, alternating
Fusion with decreased stereopsis

POSTOPERATIVE DIAGNOSIS: Intermittent exotropia, alternating

Fusion with decreased stereopsis

PROCEDURE PERFORMED: Bilateral lateral rectus recession of 7.0 mm

ANESTHESIA: General endotracheal anesthesia

PROCEDURE: The patient was brought to the operating room and placed in supine position where she was prepped and draped in the usual sterile fashion for strabismus surgery. Both eyes were exposed to the surgical field. After adequate anesthesia, one drop of 2.5% Neosynephrine was placed in each eye for vasoconstriction. Forced ductions were performed on both eyes and the lateral rectus was found to be normal. An eye speculum was placed in the right eye and surgery was begun on the right eye. An inferotemporal fornix incision was performed. The right lateral rectus muscle was isolated on a muscle hook. The muscle insertion was isolated and checked ligaments were dissected back. After a series of muscle hook passes using the Steven's hook and finishing with two passes of a Green's hook, the right lateral rectus was isolated. The epimesium, as well as tenon's capsule, was dissected from the muscle insertion and the checked ligaments were lysed. The muscle was imbricated on a 6-0 Vicryl suture with an S29 needle with locking bites at either end. The muscle was detached from the globe and a distance of 7.0 mm posterior to the insertion of the muscle was marked. The muscle was then reattached 7.0 mm posterior to the original insertion using a cross-swords technique. The conjunctiva was closed using two buried sutures. Attention was then turned to the left eye where an identical procedure was performed. At the end of the case the eyes seemed slightly exotropic in position in the anesthetized state. Bounce back tests were normal. Both eyes were dressed with Tetracaine drops and Maxitrol ointment. There were no complications. The patient tolerated the procedure well, was awakened from anesthesia without difficulty, and sent to the recovery room. The patient was instructed in the use of topical antibiotics and detailed postoperative instructions were provided. The patient will be followed up within a 48-hour period in my office.

CPT Codes **ICD-9 Codes**

____________________ ____________________

Essential HCFA-1500 Claim Form Instructions

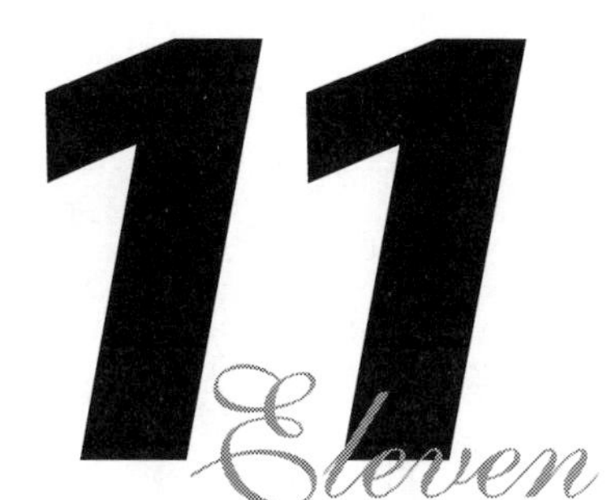

GENERAL BILLING GUIDELINES

1. Inpatient medical cases are billed on ___. (Circle the correct answer.)
   a. a fee-for-service basis
   b. a global fee basis
   c. an additional procedure basis
   d. none of the above

2. Inpatient or outpatient major surgery cases are billed on ___. (Circle the correct answer.)
   a. a fee-for-service basis
   b. a global fee basis
   c. an additional procedure basis
   d. none of the above

3. Postoperative complications requiring a return to the operating room for surgery related to the original procedure are billed on ___. (Circle the correct answer.)
   a. a fee-for-service basis
   b. a global fee basis
   c. an additional procedure basis
   d. none of the above

4. Minor surgery cases are billed on ___. (Circle the correct answer.)
   a. a fee-for-service basis
   b. a global fee basis
   c. an additional procedure basis
   d. none of the above

5. Some claims require attachments such as ___. (Circle the correct answer.)
   a. clinic notes
   b. operative reports
   c. discharge summaries
   d. all of the above

6. List four circumstances in which a "KISS" (Keep It Short and Simple) letter should be used.

   a. ______________________________

   b. ______________________________

   c. ______________________________

   d. ______________________________

7. A claim requiring attachments for clarification should ___. (Circle the correct answer.)

   a. be submitted by certified mail

   b. never be submitted by electronic mail

   c. always be submitted by electronic mail

   d. none of the above

8. Define *electronic mail.* ______________________________

   ____

9. Data on a paper-generated claim form that runs into the adjacent data blocks or appears in the wrong block will cause ____________ of ____________ .

10. Before printing a claim form, a ____________ ____________ should be run to assist with paper alignment in the printer.

OPTICAL SCANNING GUIDELINES

11. For each item, enter **T** for a true statement or **F** for a false statement on the line provided.

   _______ a. The HCFA-1500 claim form was designed to accommodate optical scanning of paper claims into the insurance company's computer system.

   _______ b. The processing time for claims prepared for optical character readers (OCR) is a little slower than for claims that must be manually entered into the insurance company's computer system.

   _______ c. The OCR guidelines were set by Medicare when the present claim form was developed.

   _______ d. The OCR guidelines are now used by all insurance carriers processing claims from the official HCFA-1500 claim form.

   _______ e. When completing a claim form, pica type (12 characters per inch) should be used.

   _______ f. When completing a claim form, all alpha characters should be typed in uppercase (capital letters).

   _______ g. When completing a claim form, a zero and the alpha character O should not be interchanged.

12. List five key strokes that can be substituted by a space when completing a claim form.

   a. ______________________________

   b. ______________________________

   c. ______________________________

   d. ______________________________

   e. ______________________________

13. Leave one ____________ ____________ between the patient/policyholder's last name, first name, and middle initial.

14. Do not use any ____________ in a patient/policyholder's provider's name, except for a hyphen in a compound name.

15. Do not use a person's title or other designations such as Sr., Jr., II, or III on a claim form unless they appear on the patient's ____________ ____________ ____________ .

16. Describe how the name on the claim form should be typed for the following patients:
    a. The name on the ID card reads: James M. Apple, II ____________
    b. The name on the ID card reads: Charles T. Treebark, Jr. ____________
    c. The name on the ID card reads: David J. Hurts, III ____________
    d. The name on the ID card reads: Jake R. Elbow, Sr. ____________

17. Describe how the birth date on the claim form should be typed for the following dates of birth:
    a. January 5, 1954: ____________
    b. March 11, 1971: ____________
    c. August 31, 1985: ____________
    d. December 2, 1994: ____________

REPORTING DIAGNOSIS: ICD-9-CM CODES

18. Diagnosis codes are placed in ___. (Circle the correct answer.)
    a. Block 24
    b. Block 33
    c. Block 21
    d. none of the above

19. The maximum number of ICD codes that may appear on a single claim form is ___. (Circle the correct answer.)
    a. four
    b. six
    c. two
    d. none of the above

20. The first ICD code listed on a claim form should be the ___. (Circle the correct answer.)
    a. qualified diagnosis
    b. possible diagnosis
    c. primary diagnosis
    d. any of the above

21. If a diagnosis not treated or addressed during an encounter is stated on the patient's record, you should ___. (Circle the correct answer.)
    a. not list the diagnosis
    b. list the diagnosis as secondary
    c. list the diagnosis as probable
    d. none of the above

22. Until a definitive diagnosis is determined, which of the following diagnoses should be used? (Circle the correct answer.)
    a. rule out
    b. suspicious for
    c. possible
    d. none of the above

REPORTING PROCEDURES AND SERVICES: HCPCS

23. Match the blocks in the first column with the definitions in the second column. Write the correct letter in each blank.

_______	Block 24A	a. Procedure Codes and Modifiers
_______	Block 24B	b. Charges
_______	Block 24C	c. COB
_______	Block 24D	d. Dates of Service
_______	Block 24E	e. Days/Units
_______	Block 24F	f. EMG
_______	Block 24G	g. Reserved for Local Use
_______	Block 24H	h. Place of Service
_______	Block 24I	i. EPSDT Family Plan
_______	Block 24J	j. Diagnosis Code
_______	Block 24K	k. Type of Service

24. The maximum number of CPT codes that may appear on a single claim form is ___. (Circle the correct answer.)
    a. four
    b. six
    c. two
    d. none of the above

25. When listing multiple procedures on the claim form, the first procedure should be the ___. (Circle the correct answer.)
    a. primary procedure
    b. procedure that took the longest
    c. procedure with the highest fee
    d. any of the above

26. Identical procedures or services may be reported on one line if the following circumstances apply. (Circle the correct answer.)
    a. Procedures were performed on consecutive days in the same month.
    b. Identical code numbers apply to all procedures.
    c. Identical charges apply.
    d. all of the above

27. The maximum number of modifiers that may be added to the right of the CPT/HCPCS code is ___. (Circle the correct answer.)
   a. four
   b. six
   c. two
   d. none of the above

Critical Thinking

28. Write a paragraph describing how to use diagnosis reference numbers.

____

____

____

____

REPORTING THE BILLING ENTITY

29. The billing entity is the ____________ ____________ ____________ of the practice.

30. If the billing entity has a group practice identification number required by the insurance carrier, this number should be typed in box number ____________ on the claim form.

PROCESSING SECONDARY CLAIMS

31. The secondary insurance claim is filed ___. (Circle the correct answer.)
   a. after the EOB from the primary claim has been received
   b. at the same time the primary claim is filed
   c. after the patient has paid his/her co-pay
   d. any of the above

32. As a general rule the secondary claim cannot be filed electronically because ___. (Circle the correct answer.)
   a. a KISS report must always accompany a secondary claim
   b. secondary insurance carriers do not accept claims electronically
   c. the primary EOB must be attached to the secondary claim
   d. all of the above

33. Supplemental plans usually cover the ___. (Circle the correct answer.)
   a. secondary procedures billed
   b. deductible and copay/coinsurance
   c. non-allowed amount
   d. none of the above

COMMON ERRORS THAT DELAY PROCESSING

34. List five common errors that delay processing of a claim.

    a. ______________________________

    b. ______________________________

    c. ______________________________

    d. ______________________________

    e. ______________________________

FINAL PROCESSING STEPS OF PAPER CLAIMS

35. List the six final processing steps of paper claims.

    a. ______________________________

    b. ______________________________

    c. ______________________________

    d. ______________________________

    e. ______________________________

    f. ______________________________

MAINTAINING INSURANCE CLAIM FILES FOR THE PRACTICE

36. The federal Omnibus Budget Reconciliation Act of 1987 requires physicians to keep copies of any ___. (Circle the correct answer.)

    a. Blue Cross/Blue Shield insurance claim forms

    b. commercial insurance claim forms

    c. government insurance claim forms

    d. all of the above

37. How do providers and billing services filing claims electronically comply with the federal regulation?

    ____

    ____

    ____

38. List four examples of the way paper claim files should be organized.

    a. ______________________________

    b. ______________________________

    c. ______________________________

    d. ______________________________

39. The ____________ ____________ ____________ of 1974 prohibits an insurance carrier from notifying the provider about payment of rejections of unassigned claims or payments sent directly to the patient/policyholder.

Critical Thinking

40. Write a paragraph describing steps that should be taken when an error in processing is found.

____

____

____

____

Know Your Acronyms

41. Define the following acronyms:
    a. EMC ____________________
    b. KISS ____________________
    c. ASC ____________________
    d. OCR ____________________
    e. EIN ____________________
    f. PIN ____________________
    g. GRP# ____________________

EXERCISES

42. Using Optical Scanning Guidelines, circle the errors found in Stanley L. Fruit's claim form on the following page.

43. Using the information provided on Stanley L. Fruit's claim form, complete the blank claim form correctly.

PLEASE
DO NOT
STAPLE
IN THIS
AREA

(SAMPLE ONLY - NOT APPROVED FOR USE)

CARRIER

PICA

HEALTH INSURANCE CLAIM FORM

PICA

1. MEDICARE (Medicare #) MEDICAID (Medicaid #) CHAMPUS (Sponsor's SSN) CHAMPVA (VA File #) GROUP HEALTH PLAN (SSN or ID) FECA BLK LUNG (SSN) OTHER [X] (ID)

1a. INSURED'S I.D. NUMBER (FOR PROGRAM IN ITEM 1): 017-09-1234

2. PATIENT'S NAME (Last Name, First Name, Middle Initial): STANLEY L. FRUIT JR.

3. PATIENT'S BIRTH DATE MM DD YY: 7 15 1954 SEX M [X] F

4. INSURED'S NAME (Last Name, First Name, Middle Initial): SAME

5. PATIENT'S ADDRESS (No. Street): 25 S. HANSON ST.

6. PATIENT RELATIONSHIP TO INSURED: Self [X] Spouse Child Other

7. INSURED'S ADDRESS (No. Street): SAME

CITY: ANYWHERE STATE: US

8. PATIENT STATUS: Single [X] Married Other; Employed [X] Full-Time Student Part-Time Student

CITY STATE

ZIP CODE: 12345 TELEPHONE (Include Area Code): (101) 112-2222

ZIP CODE TELEPHONE (INCLUDE AREA CODE) ( )

9. OTHER INSURED'S NAME (Last Name, First Name, Middle Initial): None

a. OTHER INSURED'S POLICY OR GROUP NUMBER

b. OTHER INSURED'S DATE OF BIRTH MM DD YY SEX M F

c. EMPLOYER'S NAME OR SCHOOL NAME

d. INSURANCE PLAN NAME OR PROGRAM NAME

10. IS PATIENT'S CONDITION RELATED TO:

a. EMPLOYMENT? (CURRENT OR PREVIOUS) YES [X] NO

b. AUTO ACCIDENT? PLACE (State) YES [X] NO

c. OTHER ACCIDENT? YES [X] NO

10d. RESERVED FOR LOCAL USE

11. INSURED'S POLICY GROUP OR FECA NUMBER: FED 101

a. INSURED'S DATE OF BIRTH MM DD YY SEX M F

b. EMPLOYER'S NAME OR SCHOOL NAME: U.S. POSTAL SERVICE

c. INSURANCE PLAN NAME OR PROGRAM NAME: MAILHANDLERS

d. IS THERE ANOTHER HEALTH BENEFIT PLAN? YES [X] NO If yes, return to and complete item 9 a – d.

READ BACK OF FORM BEFORE COMPLETING & SIGNING THIS FORM.

12. PATIENT'S OR AUTHORIZED PERSON'S SIGNATURE I authorize the release of any medical or other information necessary to process this claim. I also request payment of government benefits either to myself or to the party who accepts assignment below.

SIGNED SIGNATURE ON FILE DATE

13. INSURED'S OR AUTHORIZED PERSON'S SIGNATURE I authorize payment of medical benefits to the undersigned physician or supplier for services described below.

SIGNED SIGNATURE ON FILE

PATIENT AND INSURED INFORMATION

14. DATE OF CURRENT: MM DD YY ILLNESS (First symptom) OR INJURY (Accident) OR PREGNANCY (LMP)

15. IF PATIENT HAS HAD SAME OR SIMILAR ILLNESS, GIVE FIRST DATE MM DD YY

16. DATES PATIENT UNABLE TO WORK IN CURRENT OCCUPATION FROM MM DD YY TO MM DD YY

17. NAME OF REFERRING PHYSICIAN OR OTHER SOURCE

17a. I.D. NUMBER OF REFERRING PHYSICIAN

18. HOSPITALIZATION DATES RELATED TO CURRENT SERVICES FROM MM DD YY TO MM DD YY

19. RESERVED FOR LOCAL USE

20. OUTSIDE LAB? YES [X] NO $ CHARGES

21. DIAGNOSIS OR NATURE OF ILLNESS OR INJURY. (RELATE ITEMS 1, 2, 3, OR 4 TO ITEM 24E BY LINE)

1. 782.0
2. 788.41
3. ___ . __
4. ___ . __

22. MEDICAID RESUBMISSION CODE ORIGINAL REF. NO.

23. PRIOR AUTHORIZATION NUMBER

24. A DATE(S) OF SERVICE From MM DD YY	To MM DD YY	B Place of Service	C Type of Service	D PROCEDURES, SERVICES, OR SUPPLIES (Explain Unusual Circumstances) CPT/HCPCS	MODIFIER	E DIAGNOSIS CODE	F $ CHARGES	G DAYS OR UNITS	H EPSDT Family Plan	I EMG	J COB	K RESERVED FOR LOCAL USE
1 6 7 YYYY		3	1	99213		782.0	$ 60 00	1				
2												
3 6 7 YYYY		3	5	81001		788.41	$ 10 00	1				
4												
5												
6												

25. FEDERAL TAX I.D. NUMBER: 11-123456 SSN EIN [X]

26. PATIENT'S ACCOUNT NO.: 123

27. ACCEPT ASSIGNMENT? (For govt. claims, see back) [X] YES NO

28. TOTAL CHARGE: $ 70 00

29. AMOUNT PAID: $

30. BALANCE DUE: $ 70 00

31. SIGNATURE OF PHYSICIAN OR SUPPLIER INCLUDING DEGREES OR CREDENTIALS (I certify that the statements on the reverse apply to this bill and are made a part thereof.)

R.K. PAINFREE, M.D.

SIGNED DATE MMDDYYYY

32. NAME AND ADDRESS OF FACILITY WHERE SERVICES WERE RENDERED (If other than home or office)

33. PHYSICIAN'S, SUPPLIER'S BILLING NAME, ADDRESS, ZIP CODE & PHONE #

GOODMEDICINE CLINIC

PIN# 123-42 GRP# GC-12340

PHYSICIAN OR SUPPLIER INFORMATION

(SAMPLE ONLY - NOT APPROVED FOR USE)

PLEASE PRINT OR TYPE

SAMPLE FORM 1500
SAMPLE FORM 1500 SAMPLE FORM 1500

PLEASE
DO NOT
STAPLE
IN THIS
AREA

(SAMPLE ONLY - NOT APPROVED FOR USE)

CARRIER

PICA

HEALTH INSURANCE CLAIM FORM

PICA

1. MEDICARE (Medicare #) MEDICAID (Medicaid #) CHAMPUS (Sponsor's SSN) CHAMPVA (VA File #) GROUP HEALTH PLAN (SSN or ID) FECA BLK LUNG (SSN) OTHER (ID)

1a. INSURED'S I.D. NUMBER (FOR PROGRAM IN ITEM 1)

2. PATIENT'S NAME (Last Name, First Name, Middle Initial)

3. PATIENT'S BIRTH DATE MM DD YY SEX M F

4. INSURED'S NAME (Last Name, First Name, Middle Initial)

5. PATIENT'S ADDRESS (No. Street)

6. PATIENT RELATIONSHIP TO INSURED Self Spouse Child Other

7. INSURED'S ADDRESS (No. Street)

CITY STATE

8. PATIENT STATUS Single Married Other

CITY STATE

ZIP CODE TELEPHONE (Include Area Code) ( )

Employed Full-Time Student Part-Time Student

ZIP CODE TELEPHONE (INCLUDE AREA CODE) ( )

9. OTHER INSURED'S NAME (Last Name, First Name, Middle Initial)

10. IS PATIENT'S CONDITION RELATED TO:

11. INSURED'S POLICY GROUP OR FECA NUMBER

a. OTHER INSURED'S POLICY OR GROUP NUMBER

a. EMPLOYMENT? (CURRENT OR PREVIOUS) YES NO

a. INSURED'S DATE OF BIRTH MM DD YY SEX M F

b. OTHER INSURED'S DATE OF BIRTH MM DD YY SEX M F

b. AUTO ACCIDENT? PLACE (State) YES NO

b. EMPLOYER'S NAME OR SCHOOL NAME

c. EMPLOYER'S NAME OR SCHOOL NAME

c. OTHER ACCIDENT? YES NO

c. INSURANCE PLAN NAME OR PROGRAM NAME

d. INSURANCE PLAN NAME OR PROGRAM NAME

10d. RESERVED FOR LOCAL USE

d. IS THERE ANOTHER HEALTH BENEFIT PLAN? YES NO If yes, return to and complete item 9 a – d.

READ BACK OF FORM BEFORE COMPLETING & SIGNING THIS FORM.

12. PATIENT'S OR AUTHORIZED PERSON'S SIGNATURE I authorize the release of any medical or other information necessary to process this claim. I also request payment of government benefits either to myself or to the party who accepts assignment below.

SIGNED ______ DATE ______

13. INSURED'S OR AUTHORIZED PERSON'S SIGNATURE I authorize payment of medical benefits to the undersigned physician or supplier for services described below.

SIGNED ______

PATIENT AND INSURED INFORMATION

14. DATE OF CURRENT: MM DD YY ILLNESS (First symptom) OR INJURY (Accident) OR PREGNANCY (LMP)

15. IF PATIENT HAS HAD SAME OR SIMILAR ILLNESS, GIVE FIRST DATE MM DD YY

16. DATES PATIENT UNABLE TO WORK IN CURRENT OCCUPATION FROM MM DD YY TO MM DD YY

17. NAME OF REFERRING PHYSICIAN OR OTHER SOURCE

17a. I.D. NUMBER OF REFERRING PHYSICIAN

18. HOSPITALIZATION DATES RELATED TO CURRENT SERVICES FROM MM DD YY TO MM DD YY

19. RESERVED FOR LOCAL USE

20. OUTSIDE LAB? YES NO $ CHARGES

21. DIAGNOSIS OR NATURE OF ILLNESS OR INJURY. (RELATE ITEMS 1, 2, 3, OR 4 TO ITEM 24E BY LINE)

1. ___ . __ 3. ___ . __

2. ___ . __ 4. ___ . __

22. MEDICAID RESUBMISSION CODE ORIGINAL REF. NO.

23. PRIOR AUTHORIZATION NUMBER

24. A DATE(S) OF SERVICE From MM DD YY To MM DD YY	B Place of Service	C Type of Service	D PROCEDURES, SERVICES, OR SUPPLIES (Explain Unusual Circumstances) CPT/HCPCS MODIFIER	E DIAGNOSIS CODE	F $ CHARGES	G DAYS OR UNITS	H EPSDT Family Plan	I EMG	J COB	K RESERVED FOR LOCAL USE
1										
2										
3										
4										
5										
6										

25. FEDERAL TAX I.D. NUMBER SSN EIN

26. PATIENT'S ACCOUNT NO.

27. ACCEPT ASSIGNMENT? (For govt. claims, see back) YES NO

28. TOTAL CHARGE $

29. AMOUNT PAID $

30. BALANCE DUE $

31. SIGNATURE OF PHYSICIAN OR SUPPLIER INCLUDING DEGREES OR CREDENTIALS (I certify that the statements on the reverse apply to this bill and are made a part thereof.)

SIGNED DATE

32. NAME AND ADDRESS OF FACILITY WHERE SERVICES WERE RENDERED (If other than home or office)

33. PHYSICIAN'S, SUPPLIER'S BILLING NAME, ADDRESS, ZIP CODE & PHONE #

PIN# GRP#

PHYSICIAN OR SUPPLIER INFORMATION

(SAMPLE ONLY - NOT APPROVED FOR USE)

PLEASE PRINT OR TYPE

SAMPLE FORM 1500
SAMPLE FORM 1500 SAMPLE FORM 1500

CASE STUDIES

44. Using Optical Scanning Guidelines, complete the blank claim form for Jane Normal. Use the step-by-step instructions provided in the textbook to properly fill out the form.

DATE	REMARKS
02/05/YYYY	

PATIENT		CHART #	SEX	BIRTHDATE
Jane Normal	121-01-2179		F	02/07/1953

MAILING ADDRESS	CITY	STATE	ZIP	HOME PHONE	WORK PHONE
534 Robin St.	Anywhere	US	12345	(410) 123 1234	(301) 321 4321

EMPLOYER	ADDRESS	PATIENT STATUS
Dress Barn	576 Fleet St.	X MARRIED DIVORCED SINGLE STUDENT OTHER

INSURANCE: PRIMARY	ID#	GROUP	SECONDARY POLICY
Metropolitan	121-01-2179	C26	

POLICYHOLDER NAME	BIRTHDATE	RELATIONSHIP	POLICYHOLDER NAME	BIRTHDATE	RELATIONSHIP
		Self			

SUPPLEMENTAL PLAN	EMPLOYER

POLICYHOLDER NAME	BIRTHDATE	RELATIONSHIP	DIAGNOSIS	CODE
			1. Sinusitis, frontal	461.1
EMPLOYER			2.	
			3.	
REFERRING PHYSICIAN UPIN/SSN			4.	

PLACE OF SERVICE Office

PROCEDURES	CODE	CHARGE
1. Established patient OV level II	99212	$65.00
2.		
3.		
4.		
5.		
6.		

SPECIAL NOTES

TOTAL CHARGES	PAYMENTS	ADJUSTMENTS	BALANCE
$65.00	-0-	-0-	$65.00

RETURN VISIT	PHYSICIAN SIGNATURE
PRN	Donald L. Givings, M.D.

MEDICARE D1234
MEDICAID DLG1234
BCBS 12345

DONALD L. GIVINGS, M.D.
11350 MEDICAL DRIVE, ANYWHERE US 12345
PHONE NUMBER (101)111-5555

EIN 11-123456
SSN 123-12-1234
PIN DG1234
GRP DG12345

PLEASE
DO NOT
STAPLE
IN THIS
AREA

(SAMPLE ONLY - NOT APPROVED FOR USE)

CARRIER

PICA

HEALTH INSURANCE CLAIM FORM

PICA

PATIENT AND INSURED INFORMATION

1. MEDICARE ☐ (Medicare #) MEDICAID ☐ (Medicaid #) CHAMPUS ☐ (Sponsor's SSN) CHAMPVA ☐ (VA File #) GROUP HEALTH PLAN ☐ (SSN or ID) FECA BLK LUNG ☐ (SSN) OTHER ☐ (ID)

1a. INSURED'S I.D. NUMBER (FOR PROGRAM IN ITEM 1)

2. PATIENT'S NAME (Last Name, First Name, Middle Initial)

3. PATIENT'S BIRTH DATE MM DD YY SEX M ☐ F ☐

4. INSURED'S NAME (Last Name, First Name, Middle Initial)

5. PATIENT'S ADDRESS (No. Street)

6. PATIENT RELATIONSHIP TO INSURED Self ☐ Spouse ☐ Child ☐ Other ☐

7. INSURED'S ADDRESS (No. Street)

CITY STATE

8. PATIENT STATUS Single ☐ Married ☐ Other ☐

CITY STATE

ZIP CODE TELEPHONE (Include Area Code) ( )

Employed ☐ Full-Time Student ☐ Part-Time Student ☐

ZIP CODE TELEPHONE (INCLUDE AREA CODE) ( )

9. OTHER INSURED'S NAME (Last Name, First Name, Middle Initial)

10. IS PATIENT'S CONDITION RELATED TO:

11. INSURED'S POLICY GROUP OR FECA NUMBER

a. OTHER INSURED'S POLICY OR GROUP NUMBER

a. EMPLOYMENT? (CURRENT OR PREVIOUS) ☐ YES ☐ NO

a. INSURED'S DATE OF BIRTH MM DD YY SEX M ☐ F ☐

b. OTHER INSURED'S DATE OF BIRTH MM DD YY SEX M ☐ F ☐

b. AUTO ACCIDENT? ☐ YES ☐ NO PLACE (State)

b. EMPLOYER'S NAME OR SCHOOL NAME

c. EMPLOYER'S NAME OR SCHOOL NAME

c. OTHER ACCIDENT? ☐ YES ☐ NO

c. INSURANCE PLAN NAME OR PROGRAM NAME

d. INSURANCE PLAN NAME OR PROGRAM NAME

10d. RESERVED FOR LOCAL USE

d. IS THERE ANOTHER HEALTH BENEFIT PLAN? ☐ YES ☐ NO If yes, return to and complete item 9 a – d.

READ BACK OF FORM BEFORE COMPLETING & SIGNING THIS FORM.

12. PATIENT'S OR AUTHORIZED PERSON'S SIGNATURE I authorize the release of any medical or other information necessary to process this claim. I also request payment of government benefits either to myself or to the party who accepts assignment below.

SIGNED ______________________ DATE ____________

13. INSURED'S OR AUTHORIZED PERSON'S SIGNATURE I authorize payment of medical benefits to the undersigned physician or supplier for services described below.

SIGNED ______________________

PHYSICIAN OR SUPPLIER INFORMATION

14. DATE OF CURRENT: MM DD YY ◀ ILLNESS (First symptom) OR INJURY (Accident) OR PREGNANCY (LMP)

15. IF PATIENT HAS HAD SAME OR SIMILAR ILLNESS, GIVE FIRST DATE MM DD YY

16. DATES PATIENT UNABLE TO WORK IN CURRENT OCCUPATION MM DD YY FROM MM DD YY TO

17. NAME OF REFERRING PHYSICIAN OR OTHER SOURCE

17a. I.D. NUMBER OF REFERRING PHYSICIAN

18. HOSPITALIZATION DATES RELATED TO CURRENT SERVICES MM DD YY FROM MM DD YY TO

19. RESERVED FOR LOCAL USE

20. OUTSIDE LAB? ☐ YES ☐ NO $ CHARGES

21. DIAGNOSIS OR NATURE OF ILLNESS OR INJURY. (RELATE ITEMS 1, 2, 3, OR 4 TO ITEM 24E BY LINE)

1. ___ . __ 3. ___ . __

2. ___ . __ 4. ___ . __

22. MEDICAID RESUBMISSION CODE ORIGINAL REF. NO.

23. PRIOR AUTHORIZATION NUMBER

	24. A DATE(S) OF SERVICE From MM DD YY To MM DD YY	B Place of Service	C Type of Service	D PROCEDURES, SERVICES, OR SUPPLIES (Explain Unusual Circumstances) CPT/HCPCS MODIFIER	E DIAGNOSIS CODE	F $ CHARGES	G DAYS OR UNITS	H EPSDT Family Plan	I EMG	J COB	K RESERVED FOR LOCAL USE
1											
2											
3											
4											
5											
6											

25. FEDERAL TAX I.D. NUMBER SSN EIN ☐ ☐

26. PATIENT'S ACCOUNT NO.

27. ACCEPT ASSIGNMENT? (For govt. claims, see back) ☐ YES ☐ NO

28. TOTAL CHARGE $

29. AMOUNT PAID $

30. BALANCE DUE $

31. SIGNATURE OF PHYSICIAN OR SUPPLIER INCLUDING DEGREES OR CREDENTIALS (I certify that the statements on the reverse apply to this bill and are made a part thereof.)

SIGNED DATE

32. NAME AND ADDRESS OF FACILITY WHERE SERVICES WERE RENDERED (If other than home or office)

33. PHYSICIAN'S, SUPPLIER'S BILLING NAME, ADDRESS, ZIP CODE & PHONE #

PIN# GRP#

(SAMPLE ONLY - NOT APPROVED FOR USE)

PLEASE PRINT OR TYPE

SAMPLE FORM 1500
SAMPLE FORM 1500 SAMPLE FORM 1500

45. Using Optical Scanning Guidelines, complete the blank claim for Thomas J. Meekes. Use the step-by-step instructions provided in the textbook to properly fill out the form.

DATE	REMARKS
08/13/YYYY	

PATIENT		CHART #	SEX	BIRTHDATE
Thomas J. Meekes	441-44-1111		M	12/10/1949

MAILING ADDRESS	CITY	STATE	ZIP	HOME PHONE	WORK PHONE
39567 Aliceville Rd.	Anywhere	US	12345	(101) 333 4444	576 2222

EMPLOYER	ADDRESS	PATIENT STATUS
Western Auto	7928 James St.	X MARRIED DIVORCED SINGLE STUDENT OTHER

INSURANCE: PRIMARY	ID#	GROUP	SECONDARY POLICY
Atlantic Plus	411-44-1111	J276	

POLICYHOLDER NAME	BIRTHDATE	RELATIONSHIP	POLICYHOLDER NAME	BIRTHDATE	RELATIONSHIP
		Self			

SUPPLEMENTAL PLAN	EMPLOYER

POLICYHOLDER NAME	BIRTHDATE	RELATIONSHIP	DIAGNOSIS	CODE
			1. Bronchial Pneumonia	485
EMPLOYER			2.	
			3.	
REFERRING PHYSICIAN UPIN/SSN			4.	

PLACE OF SERVICE Mercy Hospital Anywhere Street Anywhere US 12345

PROCEDURES		CODE	CHARGE
1. Initial Hospital Care Level I	08/09/YYYY	99221	$75.00
2. Subsequent Hospital Care Level I	08/10/YYYY	99231	$50.00
3. Subsequent Hospital Care Level I	08/11/YYYY	99231	$50.00
4. Subsequent Hospital Care Level I	08/12/YYYY	99231	$50.00
5. Discharge, 30 min.	08/13/YYYY	99238	$75.00
6.			

SPECIAL NOTES

TOTAL CHARGES	PAYMENTS	ADJUSTMENTS	BALANCE
$300.00	-0-	-0-	$300.00

RETURN VISIT	PHYSICIAN SIGNATURE
Pt will call to set up appointment within one week	Donald L. Givings, M.D.

MEDICARE D1234
MEDICAID DLG1234
BCBS 12345

DONALD L. GIVINGS, M.D.
11350 MEDICAL DRIVE, ANYWHERE US 12345
PHONE NUMBER (101)111-5555

EIN 11-123456
SSN 123-12-1234
PIN DG1234
GRP DG12345

PLEASE
DO NOT
STAPLE
IN THIS
AREA

(SAMPLE ONLY - NOT APPROVED FOR USE)

CARRIER

PICA

HEALTH INSURANCE CLAIM FORM

PICA

1. MEDICARE (Medicare #) MEDICAID (Medicaid #) CHAMPUS (Sponsor's SSN) CHAMPVA (VA File #) GROUP HEALTH PLAN (SSN or ID) FECA BLK LUNG (SSN) OTHER (ID)

1a. INSURED'S I.D. NUMBER (FOR PROGRAM IN ITEM 1)

2. PATIENT'S NAME (Last Name, First Name, Middle Initial)

3. PATIENT'S BIRTH DATE MM DD YY SEX M F

4. INSURED'S NAME (Last Name, First Name, Middle Initial)

5. PATIENT'S ADDRESS (No. Street)

6. PATIENT RELATIONSHIP TO INSURED Self Spouse Child Other

7. INSURED'S ADDRESS (No. Street)

CITY STATE

8. PATIENT STATUS Single Married Other

CITY STATE

ZIP CODE TELEPHONE (Include Area Code) ( )

Employed Full-Time Student Part-Time Student

ZIP CODE TELEPHONE (INCLUDE AREA CODE) ( )

9. OTHER INSURED'S NAME (Last Name, First Name, Middle Initial)

10. IS PATIENT'S CONDITION RELATED TO:

11. INSURED'S POLICY GROUP OR FECA NUMBER

a. OTHER INSURED'S POLICY OR GROUP NUMBER

a. EMPLOYMENT? (CURRENT OR PREVIOUS) YES NO

a. INSURED'S DATE OF BIRTH MM DD YY SEX M F

b. OTHER INSURED'S DATE OF BIRTH MM DD YY SEX M F

b. AUTO ACCIDENT? PLACE (State) YES NO

b. EMPLOYER'S NAME OR SCHOOL NAME

c. EMPLOYER'S NAME OR SCHOOL NAME

c. OTHER ACCIDENT? YES NO

c. INSURANCE PLAN NAME OR PROGRAM NAME

d. INSURANCE PLAN NAME OR PROGRAM NAME

10d. RESERVED FOR LOCAL USE

d. IS THERE ANOTHER HEALTH BENEFIT PLAN? YES NO If yes, return to and complete item 9 a – d.

READ BACK OF FORM BEFORE COMPLETING & SIGNING THIS FORM.

12. PATIENT'S OR AUTHORIZED PERSON'S SIGNATURE I authorize the release of any medical or other information necessary to process this claim. I also request payment of government benefits either to myself or to the party who accepts assignment below.

SIGNED DATE

13. INSURED'S OR AUTHORIZED PERSON'S SIGNATURE I authorize payment of medical benefits to the undersigned physician or supplier for services described below.

SIGNED

PATIENT AND INSURED INFORMATION

14. DATE OF CURRENT: MM DD YY ILLNESS (First symptom) OR INJURY (Accident) OR PREGNANCY (LMP)

15. IF PATIENT HAS HAD SAME OR SIMILAR ILLNESS, GIVE FIRST DATE MM DD YY

16. DATES PATIENT UNABLE TO WORK IN CURRENT OCCUPATION FROM MM DD YY TO MM DD YY

17. NAME OF REFERRING PHYSICIAN OR OTHER SOURCE

17a. I.D. NUMBER OF REFERRING PHYSICIAN

18. HOSPITALIZATION DATES RELATED TO CURRENT SERVICES FROM MM DD YY TO MM DD YY

19. RESERVED FOR LOCAL USE

20. OUTSIDE LAB? YES NO $ CHARGES

21. DIAGNOSIS OR NATURE OF ILLNESS OR INJURY. (RELATE ITEMS 1, 2, 3, OR 4 TO ITEM 24E BY LINE)

1. ___ . __
2. ___ . __
3. ___ . __
4. ___ . __

22. MEDICAID RESUBMISSION CODE ORIGINAL REF. NO.

23. PRIOR AUTHORIZATION NUMBER

24. A DATE(S) OF SERVICE From MM DD YY To MM DD YY	B Place of Service	C Type of Service	D PROCEDURES, SERVICES, OR SUPPLIES (Explain Unusual Circumstances) CPT/HCPCS MODIFIER	E DIAGNOSIS CODE	F $ CHARGES	G DAYS OR UNITS	H EPSDT Family Plan	I EMG	J COB	K RESERVED FOR LOCAL USE
1										
2										
3										
4										
5										
6										

25. FEDERAL TAX I.D. NUMBER SSN EIN

26. PATIENT'S ACCOUNT NO.

27. ACCEPT ASSIGNMENT? (For govt. claims, see back) YES NO

28. TOTAL CHARGE $

29. AMOUNT PAID $

30. BALANCE DUE $

31. SIGNATURE OF PHYSICIAN OR SUPPLIER INCLUDING DEGREES OR CREDENTIALS (I certify that the statements on the reverse apply to this bill and are made a part thereof.)

SIGNED DATE

32. NAME AND ADDRESS OF FACILITY WHERE SERVICES WERE RENDERED (If other than home or office)

33. PHYSICIAN'S, SUPPLIER'S BILLING NAME, ADDRESS, ZIP CODE & PHONE #

PIN# GRP#

PHYSICIAN OR SUPPLIER INFORMATION

(SAMPLE ONLY - NOT APPROVED FOR USE)

PLEASE PRINT OR TYPE

SAMPLE FORM 1500
SAMPLE FORM 1500 SAMPLE FORM 1500

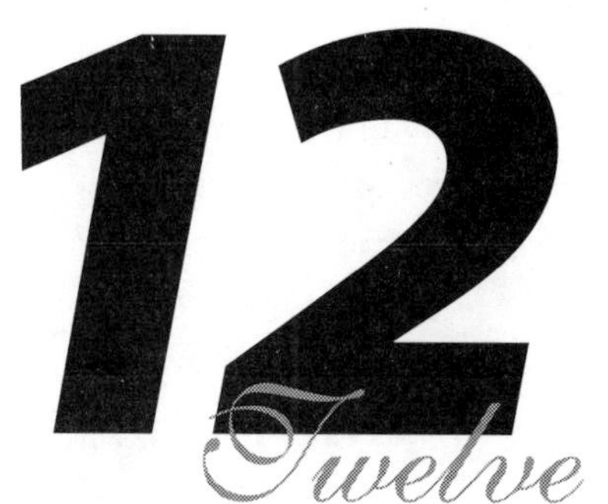

Filing Commercial Claims

PATIENT AND POLICY IDENTIFICATION

1. Describe the information to be provided in Block 4 if the patient is not the policyholder.

2. When completing Block 8, what information must be filed with the first claim when the patient is between the ages of 19 and 23, is a dependent on a family policy, and is a full-time student?

3. What does an "X" in the YES box of Block 10A indicate?

4. What does a patient's signature appearing in Block 13 authorize?

5. In Blocks 12 and 13, what phrase is acceptable if the patient has signed an Authorization for Release of Medical Information Form?

DIAGNOSTIC AND TREATMENT DATA

6. When would it be appropriate to complete Block 17?

7. When would it be appropriate to complete Block 18? ____________________

____

____

8. What does an "X" in the YES box of Block 20 indicate? ____________________

____

____

9. When would it be appropriate to complete Block 23? ____________________

____

____

10. Indicate the *place of service* code number that should appear in Block 24B if the service reported was performed in the
    a. provider's office ________
    b. hospital (inpatient) ________
    c. hospital (outpatient) ________
    d. nursing home ________

11. Indicate the *type of service* code number that should appear in Block 24C if the service reported was
    a. consultation ________
    b. medical care ________
    c. diagnostic laboratory ________
    d. surgery ________
    e. diagnostic Xray ________

12. When would it be appropriate to place an "X" in Block 24I? ____________________

____

____

PROVIDER/BILLING ENTITY IDENTIFICATION

13. Describe the significance of entering an "X" in the YES box of Block 27. ____________________

____

____

14. Describe what an "X" in the NO box of Block 27 indicates. ____________________

____

____

15. When is it appropriate for a negative charge to appear in Block 28? ____________________

16. In which block would payment toward a patient's deductible for procedures appear? __________

17. When would it be appropriate to complete Block 32? ____________________

____

____

EXERCISES

18. Complete Case Studies 12-a through 12-j using the blank claim forms provided. Follow the step-by-step instructions in the textbook to properly complete the claim form. If a patient has secondary insurance, complete an additional claim form using secondary directions from the textbook. You may choose to use a pencil so corrections can be made.

Case Study 12-a

DATE	REMARKS
05/10/YYYY	Patient prefers to be addressed as Bob

PATIENT		CHART #	SEX	BIRTHDATE
Wayne L. Carrie	444-55-6666	12-a	M	02/12/1967

MAILING ADDRESS	CITY	STATE	ZIP	HOME PHONE	WORK PHONE
663 Hilltop Drive	Anywhere	US	12345	(101) 333 4445	576 2225

EMPLOYER	ADDRESS	PATIENT STATUS
Superfresh Foods	187 East Avenue	MARRIED DIVORCED SINGLE (X) STUDENT OTHER

INSURANCE: PRIMARY	ID#	GROUP	SECONDARY POLICY
North West Health	444-55-6666	SF123	

POLICYHOLDER NAME	BIRTHDATE	RELATIONSHIP	POLICYHOLDER NAME	BIRTHDATE	RELATIONSHIP
		Self			

SUPPLEMENTAL PLAN	EMPLOYER

POLICYHOLDER NAME	BIRTHDATE	RELATIONSHIP

EMPLOYER

REFERRING PHYSICIAN UPIN/SSN

DIAGNOSIS	CODE
1. Headache, facial pain	784.0
2. Cough	786.2
3.	
4.	

PLACE OF SERVICE Office

PROCEDURES	CODE	CHARGE
1. Est. patient OV Level II	99212	$ 65.00
2.		
3.		
4.		
5.		
6.		

SPECIAL NOTES

TOTAL CHARGES	PAYMENTS	ADJUSTMENTS	BALANCE
$65.00	-0-	-0-	$65.00

RETURN VISIT	PHYSICIAN SIGNATURE
2 weeks	Donald L. Givings, M.D.

MEDICARE D1234
MEDICAID DLG1234
BCBS 12345

DONALD L. GIVINGS, M.D.
11350 MEDICAL DRIVE, ANYWHERE US 12345
PHONE NUMBER (101)111-5555

EIN 11-123456
SSN 123-12-1234
PIN DG1234
GRP DG12345

PLEASE
DO NOT
STAPLE
IN THIS
AREA

(SAMPLE ONLY - NOT APPROVED FOR USE)

CARRIER

PICA

HEALTH INSURANCE CLAIM FORM

PICA

1. MEDICARE MEDICAID CHAMPUS CHAMPVA GROUP HEALTH PLAN FECA BLK LUNG OTHER
(Medicare #) (Medicaid #) (Sponsor's SSN) (VA File #) (SSN or ID) (SSN) (ID)

1a. INSURED'S I.D. NUMBER (FOR PROGRAM IN ITEM 1)

2. PATIENT'S NAME (Last Name, First Name, Middle Initial)

3. PATIENT'S BIRTH DATE MM DD YY SEX M F

4. INSURED'S NAME (Last Name, First Name, Middle Initial)

5. PATIENT'S ADDRESS (No. Street)

6. PATIENT RELATIONSHIP TO INSURED Self Spouse Child Other

7. INSURED'S ADDRESS (No. Street)

CITY STATE

8. PATIENT STATUS Single Married Other

CITY STATE

ZIP CODE TELEPHONE (Include Area Code) ( )

Employed Full-Time Student Part-Time Student

ZIP CODE TELEPHONE (INCLUDE AREA CODE) ( )

9. OTHER INSURED'S NAME (Last Name, First Name, Middle Initial)

10. IS PATIENT'S CONDITION RELATED TO:

11. INSURED'S POLICY GROUP OR FECA NUMBER

a. OTHER INSURED'S POLICY OR GROUP NUMBER

a. EMPLOYMENT? (CURRENT OR PREVIOUS) YES NO

a. INSURED'S DATE OF BIRTH MM DD YY SEX M F

b. OTHER INSURED'S DATE OF BIRTH MM DD YY SEX M F

b. AUTO ACCIDENT? PLACE (State) YES NO

b. EMPLOYER'S NAME OR SCHOOL NAME

c. EMPLOYER'S NAME OR SCHOOL NAME

c. OTHER ACCIDENT? YES NO

c. INSURANCE PLAN NAME OR PROGRAM NAME

d. INSURANCE PLAN NAME OR PROGRAM NAME

10d. RESERVED FOR LOCAL USE

d. IS THERE ANOTHER HEALTH BENEFIT PLAN? YES NO If yes, return to and complete item 9 a – d.

READ BACK OF FORM BEFORE COMPLETING & SIGNING THIS FORM.

12. PATIENT'S OR AUTHORIZED PERSON'S SIGNATURE I authorize the release of any medical or other information necessary to process this claim. I also request payment of government benefits either to myself or to the party who accepts assignment below.

SIGNED ______ DATE ______

13. INSURED'S OR AUTHORIZED PERSON'S SIGNATURE I authorize payment of medical benefits to the undersigned physician or supplier for services described below.

SIGNED ______

PATIENT AND INSURED INFORMATION

14. DATE OF CURRENT: MM DD YY ◀ ILLNESS (First symptom) OR INJURY (Accident) OR PREGNANCY (LMP)

15. IF PATIENT HAS HAD SAME OR SIMILAR ILLNESS, GIVE FIRST DATE MM DD YY

16. DATES PATIENT UNABLE TO WORK IN CURRENT OCCUPATION FROM MM DD YY TO MM DD YY

17. NAME OF REFERRING PHYSICIAN OR OTHER SOURCE

17a. I.D. NUMBER OF REFERRING PHYSICIAN

18. HOSPITALIZATION DATES RELATED TO CURRENT SERVICES FROM MM DD YY TO MM DD YY

19. RESERVED FOR LOCAL USE

20. OUTSIDE LAB? YES NO $ CHARGES

21. DIAGNOSIS OR NATURE OF ILLNESS OR INJURY. (RELATE ITEMS 1, 2, 3, OR 4 TO ITEM 24E BY LINE)

1. ___ . __
2. ___ . __
3. ___ . __
4. ___ . __

22. MEDICAID RESUBMISSION CODE ORIGINAL REF. NO.

23. PRIOR AUTHORIZATION NUMBER

24. A DATE(S) OF SERVICE From MM DD YY To MM DD YY	B Place of Service	C Type of Service	D PROCEDURES, SERVICES, OR SUPPLIES (Explain Unusual Circumstances) CPT/HCPCS | MODIFIER	E DIAGNOSIS CODE	F $ CHARGES	G DAYS OR UNITS	H EPSDT Family Plan	I EMG	J COB	K RESERVED FOR LOCAL USE
1										
2										
3										
4										
5										
6										

25. FEDERAL TAX I.D. NUMBER SSN EIN

26. PATIENT'S ACCOUNT NO.

27. ACCEPT ASSIGNMENT? (For govt. claims, see back) YES NO

28. TOTAL CHARGE $

29. AMOUNT PAID $

30. BALANCE DUE $

31. SIGNATURE OF PHYSICIAN OR SUPPLIER INCLUDING DEGREES OR CREDENTIALS (I certify that the statements on the reverse apply to this bill and are made a part thereof.)

SIGNED DATE

32. NAME AND ADDRESS OF FACILITY WHERE SERVICES WERE RENDERED (If other than home or office)

33. PHYSICIAN'S, SUPPLIER'S BILLING NAME, ADDRESS, ZIP CODE & PHONE #

PIN# GRP#

PHYSICIAN OR SUPPLIER INFORMATION

(SAMPLE ONLY - NOT APPROVED FOR USE)

PLEASE PRINT OR TYPE

SAMPLE FORM 1500
SAMPLE FORM 1500 SAMPLE FORM 1500

Case Study 12-b

DATE	REMARKS
12/04/YYYY	

PATIENT		CHART #	SEX	BIRTHDATE
Bethany L. Branch	333-99-3434	12-b	F	05/03/1986

MAILING ADDRESS	CITY	STATE	ZIP	HOME PHONE	WORK PHONE
401 Cartvalley Court	Anywhere	US	12345	(101) 333 4466	333 5656

EMPLOYER	ADDRESS	PATIENT STATUS
		MARRIED DIVORCED SINGLE (X) STUDENT OTHER

INSURANCE: PRIMARY	ID#	GROUP	SECONDARY POLICY
Metropolitan	212-22-4545	GW292	

POLICYHOLDER NAME	BIRTHDATE	RELATIONSHIP	POLICYHOLDER NAME	BIRTHDATE	RELATIONSHIP
John L. Branch	10/10/54	Father			

SUPPLEMENTAL PLAN	EMPLOYER

POLICYHOLDER NAME	BIRTHDATE	RELATIONSHIP

EMPLOYER: Gateway Computers Inc.

REFERRING PHYSICIAN UPIN/SSN: James R. Feltbetter, M.D. 777887878

DIAGNOSIS	CODE
1. Bronchitis	466.0
2. Strep Throat	034.0
3.	
4.	

PLACE OF SERVICE: Office

PROCEDURES	CODE	CHARGE
1. Office Consult Level II	99242	$ 75.00
2. Quick Strep Test	86403	12.00
3.		
4.		
5.		
6.		

SPECIAL NOTES

TOTAL CHARGES	PAYMENTS	ADJUSTMENTS	BALANCE
$87.00	-0-	-0-	$87.00

RETURN VISIT	PHYSICIAN SIGNATURE
PRN	Donald L. Givings, M.D.

MEDICARE D1234 MEDICAID DLG1234 BCBS 12345	**DONALD L. GIVINGS, M.D.** **11350 MEDICAL DRIVE, ANYWHERE US 12345** **PHONE NUMBER (101)111-5555**	EIN 11-123456 SSN 123-12-1234 PIN DG1234 GRP DG12345

PLEASE
DO NOT
STAPLE
IN THIS
AREA

(SAMPLE ONLY - NOT APPROVED FOR USE)

CARRIER

PICA

HEALTH INSURANCE CLAIM FORM

PICA

1. MEDICARE (Medicare #) MEDICAID (Medicaid #) CHAMPUS (Sponsor's SSN) CHAMPVA (VA File #) GROUP HEALTH PLAN (SSN or ID) FECA BLK LUNG (SSN) OTHER (ID)

1a. INSURED'S I.D. NUMBER (FOR PROGRAM IN ITEM 1)

2. PATIENT'S NAME (Last Name, First Name, Middle Initial)

3. PATIENT'S BIRTH DATE MM DD YY SEX M F

4. INSURED'S NAME (Last Name, First Name, Middle Initial)

5. PATIENT'S ADDRESS (No. Street)

6. PATIENT RELATIONSHIP TO INSURED Self Spouse Child Other

7. INSURED'S ADDRESS (No. Street)

CITY STATE

8. PATIENT STATUS Single Married Other Employed Full-Time Student Part-Time Student

CITY STATE

ZIP CODE TELEPHONE (Include Area Code) ( )

ZIP CODE TELEPHONE (INCLUDE AREA CODE) ( )

9. OTHER INSURED'S NAME (Last Name, First Name, Middle Initial)

10. IS PATIENT'S CONDITION RELATED TO:

11. INSURED'S POLICY GROUP OR FECA NUMBER

a. OTHER INSURED'S POLICY OR GROUP NUMBER

a. EMPLOYMENT? (CURRENT OR PREVIOUS) YES NO

a. INSURED'S DATE OF BIRTH MM DD YY SEX M F

b. OTHER INSURED'S DATE OF BIRTH MM DD YY SEX M F

b. AUTO ACCIDENT? PLACE (State) YES NO

b. EMPLOYER'S NAME OR SCHOOL NAME

c. EMPLOYER'S NAME OR SCHOOL NAME

c. OTHER ACCIDENT? YES NO

c. INSURANCE PLAN NAME OR PROGRAM NAME

d. INSURANCE PLAN NAME OR PROGRAM NAME

10d. RESERVED FOR LOCAL USE

d. IS THERE ANOTHER HEALTH BENEFIT PLAN? YES NO If yes, return to and complete item 9 a – d.

READ BACK OF FORM BEFORE COMPLETING & SIGNING THIS FORM.

12. PATIENT'S OR AUTHORIZED PERSON'S SIGNATURE I authorize the release of any medical or other information necessary to process this claim. I also request payment of government benefits either to myself or to the party who accepts assignment below.

SIGNED ______ DATE ______

13. INSURED'S OR AUTHORIZED PERSON'S SIGNATURE I authorize payment of medical benefits to the undersigned physician or supplier for services described below.

SIGNED ______

PATIENT AND INSURED INFORMATION

14. DATE OF CURRENT: MM DD YY ILLNESS (First symptom) OR INJURY (Accident) OR PREGNANCY (LMP)

15. IF PATIENT HAS HAD SAME OR SIMILAR ILLNESS, GIVE FIRST DATE MM DD YY

16. DATES PATIENT UNABLE TO WORK IN CURRENT OCCUPATION FROM MM DD YY TO MM DD YY

17. NAME OF REFERRING PHYSICIAN OR OTHER SOURCE

17a. I.D. NUMBER OF REFERRING PHYSICIAN

18. HOSPITALIZATION DATES RELATED TO CURRENT SERVICES FROM MM DD YY TO MM DD YY

19. RESERVED FOR LOCAL USE

20. OUTSIDE LAB? YES NO $ CHARGES

21. DIAGNOSIS OR NATURE OF ILLNESS OR INJURY. (RELATE ITEMS 1, 2, 3, OR 4 TO ITEM 24E BY LINE)

1. ___ . __ 3. ___ . __

2. ___ . __ 4. ___ . __

22. MEDICAID RESUBMISSION CODE ORIGINAL REF. NO.

23. PRIOR AUTHORIZATION NUMBER

24.	A DATE(S) OF SERVICE From MM DD YY To MM DD YY	B Place of Service	C Type of Service	D PROCEDURES, SERVICES, OR SUPPLIES (Explain Unusual Circumstances) CPT/HCPCS MODIFIER	E DIAGNOSIS CODE	F $ CHARGES	G DAYS OR UNITS	H EPSDT Family Plan	I EMG	J COB	K RESERVED FOR LOCAL USE
1											
2											
3											
4											
5											
6											

25. FEDERAL TAX I.D. NUMBER SSN EIN

26. PATIENT'S ACCOUNT NO.

27. ACCEPT ASSIGNMENT? (For govt. claims, see back) YES NO

28. TOTAL CHARGE $

29. AMOUNT PAID $

30. BALANCE DUE $

31. SIGNATURE OF PHYSICIAN OR SUPPLIER INCLUDING DEGREES OR CREDENTIALS (I certify that the statements on the reverse apply to this bill and are made a part thereof.)

SIGNED DATE

32. NAME AND ADDRESS OF FACILITY WHERE SERVICES WERE RENDERED (If other than home or office)

33. PHYSICIAN'S, SUPPLIER'S BILLING NAME, ADDRESS, ZIP CODE & PHONE #

PIN# GRP#

PHYSICIAN OR SUPPLIER INFORMATION

(SAMPLE ONLY - NOT APPROVED FOR USE)

PLEASE PRINT OR TYPE

SAMPLE FORM 1500
SAMPLE FORM 1500 SAMPLE FORM 1500

Case Study 12-c

DATE	REMARKS
10/28/YYYY	

PATIENT		CHART #	SEX	BIRTHDATE
Laurie P. Reed	456-78-6969	12-c	F	06/05/1964

MAILING ADDRESS	CITY	STATE	ZIP	HOME PHONE	WORK PHONE
579 Vacation Drive	Anywhere	US	12345	(101) 333 5555	444 5555

EMPLOYER	ADDRESS	PATIENT STATUS
The Learning Center	Anywhere, US	MARRIED DIVORCED SINGLE (X) STUDENT OTHER

INSURANCE: PRIMARY	ID#	GROUP	SECONDARY POLICY
US Health	C748593	TLC45	

POLICYHOLDER NAME	BIRTHDATE	RELATIONSHIP	POLICYHOLDER NAME	BIRTHDATE	RELATIONSHIP
		Self			

SUPPLEMENTAL PLAN	EMPLOYER

POLICYHOLDER NAME	BIRTHDATE	RELATIONSHIP

EMPLOYER

REFERRING PHYSICIAN UPIN/SSN

DIAGNOSIS	CODE
1. Allergic Rhinitis	477.9
2.	
3.	
4.	

PLACE OF SERVICE Office

PROCEDURES	CODE	CHARGE
1. Est. patient OV Level I	99211	$ 55.00
2.		
3.		
4.		
5.		
6.		

SPECIAL NOTES

TOTAL CHARGES	PAYMENTS	ADJUSTMENTS	BALANCE
$55.00	$55.00	-0-	-0-

RETURN VISIT	PHYSICIAN SIGNATURE
PRN	Donald L. Givings, M.D.

MEDICARE D1234
MEDICAID DLG1234
BCBS 12345

DONALD L. GIVINGS, M.D.
11350 MEDICAL DRIVE, ANYWHERE US 12345
PHONE NUMBER (101)111-5555

EIN 11-123456
SSN 123-12-1234
PIN DG1234
GRP DG12345

PLEASE DO NOT STAPLE IN THIS AREA

(SAMPLE ONLY - NOT APPROVED FOR USE)

CARRIER

PICA

HEALTH INSURANCE CLAIM FORM

PICA

1. MEDICARE (Medicare #) MEDICAID (Medicaid #) CHAMPUS (Sponsor's SSN) CHAMPVA (VA File #) GROUP HEALTH PLAN (SSN or ID) FECA BLK LUNG (SSN) OTHER (ID)

1a. INSURED'S I.D. NUMBER (FOR PROGRAM IN ITEM 1)

2. PATIENT'S NAME (Last Name, First Name, Middle Initial)

3. PATIENT'S BIRTH DATE MM DD YY SEX M F

4. INSURED'S NAME (Last Name, First Name, Middle Initial)

5. PATIENT'S ADDRESS (No. Street)

6. PATIENT RELATIONSHIP TO INSURED Self Spouse Child Other

7. INSURED'S ADDRESS (No. Street)

CITY STATE

8. PATIENT STATUS Single Married Other

CITY STATE

ZIP CODE TELEPHONE (Include Area Code) ( )

Employed Full-Time Student Part-Time Student

ZIP CODE TELEPHONE (INCLUDE AREA CODE) ( )

9. OTHER INSURED'S NAME (Last Name, First Name, Middle Initial)

10. IS PATIENT'S CONDITION RELATED TO:

11. INSURED'S POLICY GROUP OR FECA NUMBER

a. OTHER INSURED'S POLICY OR GROUP NUMBER

a. EMPLOYMENT? (CURRENT OR PREVIOUS) YES NO

a. INSURED'S DATE OF BIRTH MM DD YY SEX M F

b. OTHER INSURED'S DATE OF BIRTH MM DD YY SEX M F

b. AUTO ACCIDENT? PLACE (State) YES NO

b. EMPLOYER'S NAME OR SCHOOL NAME

c. EMPLOYER'S NAME OR SCHOOL NAME

c. OTHER ACCIDENT? YES NO

c. INSURANCE PLAN NAME OR PROGRAM NAME

d. INSURANCE PLAN NAME OR PROGRAM NAME

10d. RESERVED FOR LOCAL USE

d. IS THERE ANOTHER HEALTH BENEFIT PLAN? YES NO If yes, return to and complete item 9 a – d.

READ BACK OF FORM BEFORE COMPLETING & SIGNING THIS FORM.

12. PATIENT'S OR AUTHORIZED PERSON'S SIGNATURE I authorize the release of any medical or other information necessary to process this claim. I also request payment of government benefits either to myself or to the party who accepts assignment below.

SIGNED DATE

13. INSURED'S OR AUTHORIZED PERSON'S SIGNATURE I authorize payment of medical benefits to the undersigned physician or supplier for services described below.

SIGNED

PATIENT AND INSURED INFORMATION

14. DATE OF CURRENT: MM DD YY ILLNESS (First symptom) OR INJURY (Accident) OR PREGNANCY (LMP)

15. IF PATIENT HAS HAD SAME OR SIMILAR ILLNESS, GIVE FIRST DATE MM DD YY

16. DATES PATIENT UNABLE TO WORK IN CURRENT OCCUPATION FROM MM DD YY TO MM DD YY

17. NAME OF REFERRING PHYSICIAN OR OTHER SOURCE

17a. I.D. NUMBER OF REFERRING PHYSICIAN

18. HOSPITALIZATION DATES RELATED TO CURRENT SERVICES FROM MM DD YY TO MM DD YY

19. RESERVED FOR LOCAL USE

20. OUTSIDE LAB? YES NO $ CHARGES

21. DIAGNOSIS OR NATURE OF ILLNESS OR INJURY. (RELATE ITEMS 1, 2, 3, OR 4 TO ITEM 24E BY LINE)

1. ___ . __

3. ___ . __

2. ___ . __

4. ___ . __

22. MEDICAID RESUBMISSION CODE ORIGINAL REF. NO.

23. PRIOR AUTHORIZATION NUMBER

24. A DATE(S) OF SERVICE From MM DD YY To MM DD YY	B Place of Service	C Type of Service	D PROCEDURES, SERVICES, OR SUPPLIES (Explain Unusual Circumstances) CPT/HCPCS MODIFIER	E DIAGNOSIS CODE	F $ CHARGES	G DAYS OR UNITS	H EPSDT Family Plan	I EMG	J COB	K RESERVED FOR LOCAL USE
1										
2										
3										
4										
5										
6										

25. FEDERAL TAX I.D. NUMBER SSN EIN

26. PATIENT'S ACCOUNT NO.

27. ACCEPT ASSIGNMENT? (For govt. claims, see back) YES NO

28. TOTAL CHARGE $

29. AMOUNT PAID $

30. BALANCE DUE $

31. SIGNATURE OF PHYSICIAN OR SUPPLIER INCLUDING DEGREES OR CREDENTIALS (I certify that the statements on the reverse apply to this bill and are made a part thereof.)

SIGNED DATE

32. NAME AND ADDRESS OF FACILITY WHERE SERVICES WERE RENDERED (If other than home or office)

33. PHYSICIAN'S, SUPPLIER'S BILLING NAME, ADDRESS, ZIP CODE & PHONE #

PIN# GRP#

PHYSICIAN OR SUPPLIER INFORMATION

(SAMPLE ONLY - NOT APPROVED FOR USE)

PLEASE PRINT OR TYPE

SAMPLE FORM 1500
SAMPLE FORM 1500 SAMPLE FORM 1500

Case Study 12-d

DATE	REMARKS				
07/04/YYYY	Prior Authorization #27901				

PATIENT		CHART #	SEX	BIRTHDATE
Pamela Sharp	212-77-8989	12-d	F	05/09/1970

MAILING ADDRESS	CITY	STATE	ZIP	HOME PHONE	WORK PHONE
678 Heather Avenue	Anywhere	US	12345	(101) 333 5559	444 5556

EMPLOYER	ADDRESS	PATIENT STATUS
Design Consultants	Anywhere US	MARRIED DIVORCED SINGLE (X) STUDENT OTHER

INSURANCE: PRIMARY	ID#	GROUP	SECONDARY POLICY
Cigna	123-66-6666	DC22	

POLICYHOLDER NAME	BIRTHDATE	RELATIONSHIP	POLICYHOLDER NAME	BIRTHDATE	RELATIONSHIP
		Self			

SUPPLEMENTAL PLAN	EMPLOYER

POLICYHOLDER NAME	BIRTHDATE	RELATIONSHIP

EMPLOYER

REFERRING PHYSICIAN UPIN/SSN: Ledger Masters, M.D. 595-33-4959

DIAGNOSIS	CODE
1. Chronic Obstructive Asthma	493.21
2. Bronchial Pneumonia	485
3.	
4.	

PLACE OF SERVICE Office

PROCEDURES		CODE	CHARGE
1. Initial Hospital Level I	06/28/YYYY	99221	$ 75.00
2. Subsequent Hospital Level I	06/29/YYYY	99231	50.00
3. Subsequent Hospital Level I	06/30/YYYY	99231	50.00
4. Subsequent Hospital Level I	07/01/YYYY	99231	50.00
5. Subsequent Hospital Level I	07/02/YYYY	99231	50.00
6. Discharge 30 Min.	07/03/YYYY	99238	75.00

SPECIAL NOTES

TOTAL CHARGES	PAYMENTS	ADJUSTMENTS	BALANCE
$350.00	-0-	-0-	$350.00

RETURN VISIT

PHYSICIAN SIGNATURE: Donald L. Givings, M.D.

DONALD L. GIVINGS, M.D.
11350 MEDICAL DRIVE, ANYWHERE US 12345
PHONE NUMBER (101)111-5555

MEDICARE D1234
MEDICAID DLG1234
BCBS 12345

EIN 11-123456
SSN 123-12-1234
PIN DG1234
GRP DG12345

PLEASE DO NOT STAPLE IN THIS AREA

(SAMPLE ONLY - NOT APPROVED FOR USE)

CARRIER

PICA

HEALTH INSURANCE CLAIM FORM

PICA

1. MEDICARE (Medicare #) MEDICAID (Medicaid #) CHAMPUS (Sponsor's SSN) CHAMPVA (VA File #) GROUP HEALTH PLAN (SSN or ID) FECA BLK LUNG (SSN) OTHER (ID)

1a. INSURED'S I.D. NUMBER (FOR PROGRAM IN ITEM 1)

2. PATIENT'S NAME (Last Name, First Name, Middle Initial)

3. PATIENT'S BIRTH DATE MM DD YY SEX M F

4. INSURED'S NAME (Last Name, First Name, Middle Initial)

5. PATIENT'S ADDRESS (No. Street)

6. PATIENT RELATIONSHIP TO INSURED Self Spouse Child Other

7. INSURED'S ADDRESS (No. Street)

CITY STATE

8. PATIENT STATUS Single Married Other

CITY STATE

ZIP CODE TELEPHONE (Include Area Code) ( )

Employed Full-Time Student Part-Time Student

ZIP CODE TELEPHONE (INCLUDE AREA CODE) ( )

9. OTHER INSURED'S NAME (Last Name, First Name, Middle Initial)

10. IS PATIENT'S CONDITION RELATED TO:

11. INSURED'S POLICY GROUP OR FECA NUMBER

a. OTHER INSURED'S POLICY OR GROUP NUMBER

a. EMPLOYMENT? (CURRENT OR PREVIOUS) YES NO

a. INSURED'S DATE OF BIRTH MM DD YY SEX M F

b. OTHER INSURED'S DATE OF BIRTH MM DD YY SEX M F

b. AUTO ACCIDENT? PLACE (State) YES NO

b. EMPLOYER'S NAME OR SCHOOL NAME

c. EMPLOYER'S NAME OR SCHOOL NAME

c. OTHER ACCIDENT? YES NO

c. INSURANCE PLAN NAME OR PROGRAM NAME

d. INSURANCE PLAN NAME OR PROGRAM NAME

10d. RESERVED FOR LOCAL USE

d. IS THERE ANOTHER HEALTH BENEFIT PLAN? YES NO If yes, return to and complete item 9 a – d.

READ BACK OF FORM BEFORE COMPLETING & SIGNING THIS FORM.

12. PATIENT'S OR AUTHORIZED PERSON'S SIGNATURE I authorize the release of any medical or other information necessary to process this claim. I also request payment of government benefits either to myself or to the party who accepts assignment below.

SIGNED DATE

13. INSURED'S OR AUTHORIZED PERSON'S SIGNATURE I authorize payment of medical benefits to the undersigned physician or supplier for services described below.

SIGNED

PATIENT AND INSURED INFORMATION

14. DATE OF CURRENT: MM DD YY ILLNESS (First symptom) OR INJURY (Accident) OR PREGNANCY (LMP)

15. IF PATIENT HAS HAD SAME OR SIMILAR ILLNESS, GIVE FIRST DATE MM DD YY

16. DATES PATIENT UNABLE TO WORK IN CURRENT OCCUPATION FROM MM DD YY TO MM DD YY

17. NAME OF REFERRING PHYSICIAN OR OTHER SOURCE

17a. I.D. NUMBER OF REFERRING PHYSICIAN

18. HOSPITALIZATION DATES RELATED TO CURRENT SERVICES FROM MM DD YY TO MM DD YY

19. RESERVED FOR LOCAL USE

20. OUTSIDE LAB? YES NO $ CHARGES

21. DIAGNOSIS OR NATURE OF ILLNESS OR INJURY. (RELATE ITEMS 1, 2, 3, OR 4 TO ITEM 24E BY LINE)

1. ___ . __

3. ___ . __

2. ___ . __

4. ___ . __

22. MEDICAID RESUBMISSION CODE ORIGINAL REF. NO.

23. PRIOR AUTHORIZATION NUMBER

24. A DATE(S) OF SERVICE From MM DD YY To MM DD YY	B Place of Service	C Type of Service	D PROCEDURES, SERVICES, OR SUPPLIES (Explain Unusual Circumstances) CPT/HCPCS MODIFIER	E DIAGNOSIS CODE	F $ CHARGES	G DAYS OR UNITS	H EPSDT Family Plan	I EMG	J COB	K RESERVED FOR LOCAL USE
1										
2										
3										
4										
5										
6										

25. FEDERAL TAX I.D. NUMBER SSN EIN

26. PATIENT'S ACCOUNT NO.

27. ACCEPT ASSIGNMENT? (For govt. claims, see back) YES NO

28. TOTAL CHARGE $

29. AMOUNT PAID $

30. BALANCE DUE $

31. SIGNATURE OF PHYSICIAN OR SUPPLIER INCLUDING DEGREES OR CREDENTIALS (I certify that the statements on the reverse apply to this bill and are made a part thereof.)

SIGNED DATE

32. NAME AND ADDRESS OF FACILITY WHERE SERVICES WERE RENDERED (If other than home or office)

33. PHYSICIAN'S, SUPPLIER'S BILLING NAME, ADDRESS, ZIP CODE & PHONE #

PIN# GRP#

PHYSICIAN OR SUPPLIER INFORMATION

(SAMPLE ONLY - NOT APPROVED FOR USE)

PLEASE PRINT OR TYPE

SAMPLE FORM 1500
SAMPLE FORM 1500 SAMPLE FORM 1500

Case Study 12-e

DATE	REMARKS			
02/03/YYYY				

PATIENT		CHART #	SEX	BIRTHDATE
James R. Brandt	576-66-9997	12-e	M	12/05/1948

MAILING ADDRESS	CITY	STATE	ZIP	HOME PHONE	WORK PHONE
95 Commission Circle	Anywhere	US	12345	(101) 223 5555	224 5555

EMPLOYER	ADDRESS	PATIENT STATUS
The Yard Guard	Anywhere US	X (above DIVORCED) — MARRIED DIVORCED SINGLE STUDENT OTHER

INSURANCE: PRIMARY	ID#	GROUP	SECONDARY POLICY
Prudential	555-66-7777	YG4	

POLICYHOLDER NAME	BIRTHDATE	RELATIONSHIP	POLICYHOLDER NAME	BIRTHDATE	RELATIONSHIP
		Self			

SUPPLEMENTAL PLAN	EMPLOYER

POLICYHOLDER NAME	BIRTHDATE	RELATIONSHIP

EMPLOYER

REFERRING PHYSICIAN UPIN/SSN: Rita M. Michaels, M.D. 343-54-7979

DIAGNOSIS	CODE
1. Diabetes, Type II	250.00
2. Hypertension, Benign	401.1
3. Gout	274.0
4.	

PLACE OF SERVICE Office

PROCEDURES		CODE	CHARGE
1. New patient OV Level IV	02/02/YYYY	99204	$ 100.00
2. EKG	02/02/YYYY	93000	50.00
3. Glucose	02/02/YYYY	82947	10.00
4. Est. patient OV Level III	02/03/YYYY	99213	75.00
5. Glucose	02/03/YYYY	82947	10.00
6.			

SPECIAL NOTES

Onset 02/02/YYYY

TOTAL CHARGES	PAYMENTS	ADJUSTMENTS	BALANCE
$245.00	-0-	-0-	$245.00

RETURN VISIT	PHYSICIAN SIGNATURE
2 weeks	Donald L. Givings, M.D.

MEDICARE D1234
MEDICAID DLG1234
BCBS 12345

DONALD L. GIVINGS, M.D.
11350 MEDICAL DRIVE, ANYWHERE US 12345
PHONE NUMBER (101)111-5555

EIN 11-123456
SSN 123-12-1234
PIN DG1234
GRP DG12345

PLEASE
DO NOT
STAPLE
IN THIS
AREA

(SAMPLE ONLY - NOT APPROVED FOR USE)

CARRIER

PICA

HEALTH INSURANCE CLAIM FORM

PICA

1. MEDICARE (Medicare #) MEDICAID (Medicaid #) CHAMPUS (Sponsor's SSN) CHAMPVA (VA File #) GROUP HEALTH PLAN (SSN or ID) FECA BLK LUNG (SSN) OTHER (ID)

1a. INSURED'S I.D. NUMBER (FOR PROGRAM IN ITEM 1)

2. PATIENT'S NAME (Last Name, First Name, Middle Initial)

3. PATIENT'S BIRTH DATE MM DD YY SEX M F

4. INSURED'S NAME (Last Name, First Name, Middle Initial)

5. PATIENT'S ADDRESS (No. Street)

6. PATIENT RELATIONSHIP TO INSURED Self Spouse Child Other

7. INSURED'S ADDRESS (No. Street)

CITY STATE

8. PATIENT STATUS Single Married Other

CITY STATE

ZIP CODE TELEPHONE (Include Area Code) ( )

Employed Full-Time Student Part-Time Student

ZIP CODE TELEPHONE (INCLUDE AREA CODE) ( )

9. OTHER INSURED'S NAME (Last Name, First Name, Middle Initial)

10. IS PATIENT'S CONDITION RELATED TO:

11. INSURED'S POLICY GROUP OR FECA NUMBER

a. OTHER INSURED'S POLICY OR GROUP NUMBER

a. EMPLOYMENT? (CURRENT OR PREVIOUS) YES NO

a. INSURED'S DATE OF BIRTH MM DD YY SEX M F

b. OTHER INSURED'S DATE OF BIRTH MM DD YY SEX M F

b. AUTO ACCIDENT? YES NO PLACE (State)

b. EMPLOYER'S NAME OR SCHOOL NAME

c. EMPLOYER'S NAME OR SCHOOL NAME

c. OTHER ACCIDENT? YES NO

c. INSURANCE PLAN NAME OR PROGRAM NAME

d. INSURANCE PLAN NAME OR PROGRAM NAME

10d. RESERVED FOR LOCAL USE

d. IS THERE ANOTHER HEALTH BENEFIT PLAN? YES NO If yes, return to and complete item 9 a – d.

READ BACK OF FORM BEFORE COMPLETING & SIGNING THIS FORM.

12. PATIENT'S OR AUTHORIZED PERSON'S SIGNATURE I authorize the release of any medical or other information necessary to process this claim. I also request payment of government benefits either to myself or to the party who accepts assignment below.

SIGNED ____________ DATE ____________

13. INSURED'S OR AUTHORIZED PERSON'S SIGNATURE I authorize payment of medical benefits to the undersigned physician or supplier for services described below.

SIGNED ____________

PATIENT AND INSURED INFORMATION

14. DATE OF CURRENT: MM DD YY ILLNESS (First symptom) OR INJURY (Accident) OR PREGNANCY (LMP)

15. IF PATIENT HAS HAD SAME OR SIMILAR ILLNESS, GIVE FIRST DATE MM DD YY

16. DATES PATIENT UNABLE TO WORK IN CURRENT OCCUPATION FROM MM DD YY TO MM DD YY

17. NAME OF REFERRING PHYSICIAN OR OTHER SOURCE

17a. I.D. NUMBER OF REFERRING PHYSICIAN

18. HOSPITALIZATION DATES RELATED TO CURRENT SERVICES FROM MM DD YY TO MM DD YY

19. RESERVED FOR LOCAL USE

20. OUTSIDE LAB? YES NO $ CHARGES

21. DIAGNOSIS OR NATURE OF ILLNESS OR INJURY. (RELATE ITEMS 1, 2, 3, OR 4 TO ITEM 24E BY LINE)

1. ___ . __
2. ___ . __
3. ___ . __
4. ___ . __

22. MEDICAID RESUBMISSION CODE ORIGINAL REF. NO.

23. PRIOR AUTHORIZATION NUMBER

24.	A DATE(S) OF SERVICE From MM DD YY	To MM DD YY	B Place of Service	C Type of Service	D PROCEDURES, SERVICES, OR SUPPLIES (Explain Unusual Circumstances) CPT/HCPCS MODIFIER	E DIAGNOSIS CODE	F $ CHARGES	G DAYS OR UNITS	H EPSDT Family Plan	I EMG	J COB	K RESERVED FOR LOCAL USE
1												
2												
3												
4												
5												
6												

25. FEDERAL TAX I.D. NUMBER SSN EIN

26. PATIENT'S ACCOUNT NO.

27. ACCEPT ASSIGNMENT? (For govt. claims, see back) YES NO

28. TOTAL CHARGE $

29. AMOUNT PAID $

30. BALANCE DUE $

31. SIGNATURE OF PHYSICIAN OR SUPPLIER INCLUDING DEGREES OR CREDENTIALS (I certify that the statements on the reverse apply to this bill and are made a part thereof.)

SIGNED DATE

32. NAME AND ADDRESS OF FACILITY WHERE SERVICES WERE RENDERED (If other than home or office)

33. PHYSICIAN'S, SUPPLIER'S BILLING NAME, ADDRESS, ZIP CODE & PHONE #

PIN# GRP#

PHYSICIAN OR SUPPLIER INFORMATION

(SAMPLE ONLY - NOT APPROVED FOR USE)

PLEASE PRINT OR TYPE

SAMPLE FORM 1500
SAMPLE FORM 1500 SAMPLE FORM 1500

Case Study 12-f

DATE	REMARKS			
04/23/YYYY	Patient has a $10 Copay			

PATIENT		CHART #	SEX	BIRTHDATE
Judy R. Hudnet	212-34-1414	12-f	F	03/28/1950

MAILING ADDRESS	CITY	STATE	ZIP	HOME PHONE	WORK PHONE
548 Dayton Terr.	Anywhere	US	12345	(101) 333 5555	444 5555

EMPLOYER	ADDRESS	PATIENT STATUS
Printers "R" Us	Anywhere, US	MARRIED DIVORCED SINGLE (X) STUDENT OTHER

INSURANCE: PRIMARY	ID#	GROUP	SECONDARY POLICY
Great West	21785		

POLICYHOLDER NAME	BIRTHDATE	RELATIONSHIP	POLICYHOLDER NAME	BIRTHDATE	RELATIONSHIP
		Self			

SUPPLEMENTAL PLAN	EMPLOYER

POLICYHOLDER NAME	BIRTHDATE	RELATIONSHIP

EMPLOYER

REFERRING PHYSICIAN UPIN/SSN

DIAGNOSIS	CODE
1. Incontinence of urine	788.30
2. Polyuria	788.42
3.	
4.	

PLACE OF SERVICE Office

PROCEDURES	CODE	CHARGE
1. Est. patient OV Level II	99212	$ 65.00
2. Urinalysis	81000	10.00
3.		
4.		
5.		
6.		

SPECIAL NOTES

Patient to be scheduled at St. John's Hospital for surgery

TOTAL CHARGES	PAYMENTS	ADJUSTMENTS	BALANCE
$75.00	$10.00	-0-	$65.00

RETURN VISIT	PHYSICIAN SIGNATURE
Refer to Dr. Stream	Donald L. Givings, M.D.

MEDICARE D1234
MEDICAID DLG1234
BCBS 12345

DONALD L. GIVINGS, M.D.
11350 MEDICAL DRIVE, ANYWHERE US 12345
PHONE NUMBER (101)111-5555

EIN 11-123456
SSN 123-12-1234
PIN DG1234
GRP DG12345

PLEASE
DO NOT
STAPLE
IN THIS
AREA

(SAMPLE ONLY - NOT APPROVED FOR USE)

CARRIER

PICA

HEALTH INSURANCE CLAIM FORM

PICA

1. MEDICARE (Medicare #) MEDICAID (Medicaid #) CHAMPUS (Sponsor's SSN) CHAMPVA (VA File #) GROUP HEALTH PLAN (SSN or ID) FECA BLK LUNG (SSN) OTHER (ID)

1a. INSURED'S I.D. NUMBER (FOR PROGRAM IN ITEM 1)

2. PATIENT'S NAME (Last Name, First Name, Middle Initial)

3. PATIENT'S BIRTH DATE MM DD YY SEX M F

4. INSURED'S NAME (Last Name, First Name, Middle Initial)

5. PATIENT'S ADDRESS (No. Street)

6. PATIENT RELATIONSHIP TO INSURED Self Spouse Child Other

7. INSURED'S ADDRESS (No. Street)

CITY STATE

8. PATIENT STATUS Single Married Other

CITY STATE

ZIP CODE TELEPHONE (Include Area Code) ( )

Employed Full-Time Student Part-Time Student

ZIP CODE TELEPHONE (INCLUDE AREA CODE) ( )

9. OTHER INSURED'S NAME (Last Name, First Name, Middle Initial)

10. IS PATIENT'S CONDITION RELATED TO:

11. INSURED'S POLICY GROUP OR FECA NUMBER

a. OTHER INSURED'S POLICY OR GROUP NUMBER

a. EMPLOYMENT? (CURRENT OR PREVIOUS) YES NO

a. INSURED'S DATE OF BIRTH MM DD YY SEX M F

b. OTHER INSURED'S DATE OF BIRTH MM DD YY SEX M F

b. AUTO ACCIDENT? YES NO PLACE (State)

b. EMPLOYER'S NAME OR SCHOOL NAME

c. EMPLOYER'S NAME OR SCHOOL NAME

c. OTHER ACCIDENT? YES NO

c. INSURANCE PLAN NAME OR PROGRAM NAME

d. INSURANCE PLAN NAME OR PROGRAM NAME

10d. RESERVED FOR LOCAL USE

d. IS THERE ANOTHER HEALTH BENEFIT PLAN? YES NO If yes, return to and complete item 9 a – d.

READ BACK OF FORM BEFORE COMPLETING & SIGNING THIS FORM.

12. PATIENT'S OR AUTHORIZED PERSON'S SIGNATURE I authorize the release of any medical or other information necessary to process this claim. I also request payment of government benefits either to myself or to the party who accepts assignment below.

SIGNED DATE

13. INSURED'S OR AUTHORIZED PERSON'S SIGNATURE I authorize payment of medical benefits to the undersigned physician or supplier for services described below.

SIGNED

PATIENT AND INSURED INFORMATION

14. DATE OF CURRENT: MM DD YY ILLNESS (First symptom) OR INJURY (Accident) OR PREGNANCY (LMP)

15. IF PATIENT HAS HAD SAME OR SIMILAR ILLNESS, GIVE FIRST DATE MM DD YY

16. DATES PATIENT UNABLE TO WORK IN CURRENT OCCUPATION FROM MM DD YY TO MM DD YY

17. NAME OF REFERRING PHYSICIAN OR OTHER SOURCE

17a. I.D. NUMBER OF REFERRING PHYSICIAN

18. HOSPITALIZATION DATES RELATED TO CURRENT SERVICES FROM MM DD YY TO MM DD YY

19. RESERVED FOR LOCAL USE

20. OUTSIDE LAB? YES NO $ CHARGES

21. DIAGNOSIS OR NATURE OF ILLNESS OR INJURY. (RELATE ITEMS 1, 2, 3, OR 4 TO ITEM 24E BY LINE)

1. ___ . __
2. ___ . __
3. ___ . __
4. ___ . __

22. MEDICAID RESUBMISSION CODE ORIGINAL REF. NO.

23. PRIOR AUTHORIZATION NUMBER

24.	A DATE(S) OF SERVICE From MM DD YY	To MM DD YY	B Place of Service	C Type of Service	D PROCEDURES, SERVICES, OR SUPPLIES (Explain Unusual Circumstances) CPT/HCPCS MODIFIER	E DIAGNOSIS CODE	F $ CHARGES	G DAYS OR UNITS	H EPSDT Family Plan	I EMG	J COB	K RESERVED FOR LOCAL USE
1												
2												
3												
4												
5												
6												

25. FEDERAL TAX I.D. NUMBER SSN EIN

26. PATIENT'S ACCOUNT NO.

27. ACCEPT ASSIGNMENT? (For govt. claims, see back) YES NO

28. TOTAL CHARGE $

29. AMOUNT PAID $

30. BALANCE DUE $

31. SIGNATURE OF PHYSICIAN OR SUPPLIER INCLUDING DEGREES OR CREDENTIALS (I certify that the statements on the reverse apply to this bill and are made a part thereof.)

SIGNED DATE

32. NAME AND ADDRESS OF FACILITY WHERE SERVICES WERE RENDERED (If other than home or office)

33. PHYSICIAN'S, SUPPLIER'S BILLING NAME, ADDRESS, ZIP CODE & PHONE #

PIN# GRP#

PHYSICIAN OR SUPPLIER INFORMATION

(SAMPLE ONLY - NOT APPROVED FOR USE)

PLEASE PRINT OR TYPE

SAMPLE FORM 1500
SAMPLE FORM 1500 SAMPLE FORM 1500

Case Study 12-g

DATE	REMARKS
05/12/YYYY	Prior Authorization #29704/Onset of symptoms 4/23/YYYY

PATIENT		CHART #	SEX	BIRTHDATE
Judy R. Hudnet	212-34-1414	12-g	F	03/28/1950

MAILING ADDRESS	CITY	STATE	ZIP	HOME PHONE	WORK PHONE
548 Dayton Terr.	Anywhere	US	12345	(101) 333 5555	444 5555

EMPLOYER	ADDRESS	PATIENT STATUS
Printers "R" Us	Anywhere, US	MARRIED DIVORCED SINGLE (X) STUDENT OTHER

INSURANCE: PRIMARY	ID#	GROUP	SECONDARY POLICY
Great West	21785		

POLICYHOLDER NAME	BIRTHDATE	RELATIONSHIP	POLICYHOLDER NAME	BIRTHDATE	RELATIONSHIP
		Self			

SUPPLEMENTAL PLAN	EMPLOYER

POLICYHOLDER NAME	BIRTHDATE	RELATIONSHIP

EMPLOYER

REFERRING PHYSICIAN UPIN/SSN	
Donald L. Givings, MD	123-12-1234

DIAGNOSIS	CODE
1. Incontinence of urine	788.30
2. Polyuria	788.42
3.	
4.	

PLACE OF SERVICE Office

PROCEDURES	CODE	CHARGE
1. Office Consultation Level III	99243	$ 85.00
2. Urinalysis, with Microscopy	81001	10.00
3.		
4.		
5.		
6.		

SPECIAL NOTES

Patient to be scheduled at St. John's Hospital for surgery

TOTAL CHARGES	PAYMENTS	ADJUSTMENTS	BALANCE
$95.00	-0-	-0-	$95.00

RETURN VISIT	PHYSICIAN SIGNATURE
	Paul R. Stream, M.D.

MEDICARE P1234
MEDICAID PRS1234
BCBS 12345

PAUL R. STREAM, M.D. UROLOGY
456 HOSPITAL DRIVE, ANYWHERE US 12345
PHONE NUMBER (101)111-5555

EIN 11223344
SSN 555-12-1234
PIN PS1234
GRP PS12345

PLEASE
DO NOT
STAPLE
IN THIS
AREA

(SAMPLE ONLY - NOT APPROVED FOR USE)

CARRIER

PICA

HEALTH INSURANCE CLAIM FORM

PICA

1. MEDICARE (Medicare #) MEDICAID (Medicaid #) CHAMPUS (Sponsor's SSN) CHAMPVA (VA File #) GROUP HEALTH PLAN (SSN or ID) FECA BLK LUNG (SSN) OTHER (ID)

1a. INSURED'S I.D. NUMBER (FOR PROGRAM IN ITEM 1)

2. PATIENT'S NAME (Last Name, First Name, Middle Initial)

3. PATIENT'S BIRTH DATE MM DD YY SEX M F

4. INSURED'S NAME (Last Name, First Name, Middle Initial)

5. PATIENT'S ADDRESS (No. Street)

6. PATIENT RELATIONSHIP TO INSURED Self Spouse Child Other

7. INSURED'S ADDRESS (No. Street)

CITY STATE

8. PATIENT STATUS Single Married Other

CITY STATE

ZIP CODE TELEPHONE (Include Area Code) ( )

Employed Full-Time Student Part-Time Student

ZIP CODE TELEPHONE (INCLUDE AREA CODE) ( )

9. OTHER INSURED'S NAME (Last Name, First Name, Middle Initial)

10. IS PATIENT'S CONDITION RELATED TO:

11. INSURED'S POLICY GROUP OR FECA NUMBER

a. OTHER INSURED'S POLICY OR GROUP NUMBER

a. EMPLOYMENT? (CURRENT OR PREVIOUS) YES NO

a. INSURED'S DATE OF BIRTH MM DD YY SEX M F

b. OTHER INSURED'S DATE OF BIRTH MM DD YY SEX M F

b. AUTO ACCIDENT? YES NO PLACE (State)

b. EMPLOYER'S NAME OR SCHOOL NAME

c. EMPLOYER'S NAME OR SCHOOL NAME

c. OTHER ACCIDENT? YES NO

c. INSURANCE PLAN NAME OR PROGRAM NAME

d. INSURANCE PLAN NAME OR PROGRAM NAME

10d. RESERVED FOR LOCAL USE

d. IS THERE ANOTHER HEALTH BENEFIT PLAN? YES NO If yes, return to and complete item 9 a – d.

READ BACK OF FORM BEFORE COMPLETING & SIGNING THIS FORM.

12. PATIENT'S OR AUTHORIZED PERSON'S SIGNATURE I authorize the release of any medical or other information necessary to process this claim. I also request payment of government benefits either to myself or to the party who accepts assignment below.

SIGNED ____________ DATE ____________

13. INSURED'S OR AUTHORIZED PERSON'S SIGNATURE I authorize payment of medical benefits to the undersigned physician or supplier for services described below.

SIGNED ____________

PATIENT AND INSURED INFORMATION

14. DATE OF CURRENT: MM DD YY ◀ ILLNESS (First symptom) OR INJURY (Accident) OR PREGNANCY (LMP)

15. IF PATIENT HAS HAD SAME OR SIMILAR ILLNESS, GIVE FIRST DATE MM DD YY

16. DATES PATIENT UNABLE TO WORK IN CURRENT OCCUPATION FROM MM DD YY TO MM DD YY

17. NAME OF REFERRING PHYSICIAN OR OTHER SOURCE

17a. I.D. NUMBER OF REFERRING PHYSICIAN

18. HOSPITALIZATION DATES RELATED TO CURRENT SERVICES FROM MM DD YY TO MM DD YY

19. RESERVED FOR LOCAL USE

20. OUTSIDE LAB? YES NO $ CHARGES

21. DIAGNOSIS OR NATURE OF ILLNESS OR INJURY. (RELATE ITEMS 1, 2, 3, OR 4 TO ITEM 24E BY LINE)

1. ___ . __
2. ___ . __
3. ___ . __
4. ___ . __

22. MEDICAID RESUBMISSION CODE ORIGINAL REF. NO.

23. PRIOR AUTHORIZATION NUMBER

24. A DATE(S) OF SERVICE From MM DD YY To MM DD YY	B Place of Service	C Type of Service	D PROCEDURES, SERVICES, OR SUPPLIES (Explain Unusual Circumstances) CPT/HCPCS MODIFIER	E DIAGNOSIS CODE	F $ CHARGES	G DAYS OR UNITS	H EPSDT Family Plan	I EMG	J COB	K RESERVED FOR LOCAL USE
1										
2										
3										
4										
5										
6										

25. FEDERAL TAX I.D. NUMBER SSN EIN

26. PATIENT'S ACCOUNT NO.

27. ACCEPT ASSIGNMENT? (For govt. claims, see back) YES NO

28. TOTAL CHARGE $

29. AMOUNT PAID $

30. BALANCE DUE $

31. SIGNATURE OF PHYSICIAN OR SUPPLIER INCLUDING DEGREES OR CREDENTIALS (I certify that the statements on the reverse apply to this bill and are made a part thereof.)

SIGNED DATE

32. NAME AND ADDRESS OF FACILITY WHERE SERVICES WERE RENDERED (If other than home or office)

33. PHYSICIAN'S, SUPPLIER'S BILLING NAME, ADDRESS, ZIP CODE & PHONE #

PIN# GRP#

PHYSICIAN OR SUPPLIER INFORMATION

(SAMPLE ONLY - NOT APPROVED FOR USE)

PLEASE PRINT OR TYPE

SAMPLE FORM 1500
SAMPLE FORM 1500 SAMPLE FORM 1500

Case Study 12-h

DATE	REMARKS
05/19/YYYY	Prior Authorization #29948/Onset of symptoms 4/23/YYYY

PATIENT		CHART #	SEX	BIRTHDATE
Judy R. Hudnet	212-34-1414	12-h	F	03/28/1950

MAILING ADDRESS	CITY	STATE	ZIP	HOME PHONE	WORK PHONE
548 Dayton Terr.	Anywhere	US	12345	(101) 333 5555	444 5555

EMPLOYER	ADDRESS	PATIENT STATUS
Printers "R" Us	Anywhere, US	MARRIED DIVORCED SINGLE (X) STUDENT OTHER

INSURANCE: PRIMARY	ID#	GROUP	SECONDARY POLICY
Great West	21785		

POLICYHOLDER NAME	BIRTHDATE	RELATIONSHIP	POLICYHOLDER NAME	BIRTHDATE	RELATIONSHIP
		Self			

SUPPLEMENTAL PLAN	EMPLOYER

POLICYHOLDER NAME | BIRTHDATE | RELATIONSHIP

EMPLOYER

REFERRING PHYSICIAN UPIN/SSN: Donald L. Givings, MD 123-12-1234

DIAGNOSIS	CODE
1. Bladder tumor, anterior wall	239.4
2.	
3.	
4.	

PLACE OF SERVICE St. Johns Hospital 456 Hospital Drive Anywhere US 12345

PROCEDURES	CODE	CHARGE
1. Cystourethroscopy w/ fulguration of bladder tumor 05/19/YYYY	52235	$ 1200.00
2.		
3.		
4.		
5.		
6.		

SPECIAL NOTES

TOTAL CHARGES	PAYMENTS	ADJUSTMENTS	BALANCE
$1200.00	-0-	-0-	$1200.00

RETURN VISIT	PHYSICIAN SIGNATURE
	Paul R. Stream, M.D.

MEDICARE P1234
MEDICAID PRS1234
BCBS 12345

PAUL R. STREAM, M.D. UROLOGY
456 HOSPITAL DRIVE, ANYWHERE US 12345
PHONE NUMBER (101)111-5555

EIN 11223344
SSN 555-12-1234
PIN PS1234
GRP PS12345

PLEASE
DO NOT
STAPLE
IN THIS
AREA

(SAMPLE ONLY - NOT APPROVED FOR USE)

CARRIER

PICA

HEALTH INSURANCE CLAIM FORM

PICA

1. MEDICARE (Medicare #) MEDICAID (Medicaid #) CHAMPUS (Sponsor's SSN) CHAMPVA (VA File #) GROUP HEALTH PLAN (SSN or ID) FECA BLK LUNG (SSN) OTHER (ID)

1a. INSURED'S I.D. NUMBER (FOR PROGRAM IN ITEM 1)

2. PATIENT'S NAME (Last Name, First Name, Middle Initial)

3. PATIENT'S BIRTH DATE MM DD YY SEX M F

4. INSURED'S NAME (Last Name, First Name, Middle Initial)

5. PATIENT'S ADDRESS (No. Street)

6. PATIENT RELATIONSHIP TO INSURED Self Spouse Child Other

7. INSURED'S ADDRESS (No. Street)

CITY STATE

8. PATIENT STATUS Single Married Other

CITY STATE

ZIP CODE TELEPHONE (Include Area Code) ( )

Employed Full-Time Student Part-Time Student

ZIP CODE TELEPHONE (INCLUDE AREA CODE) ( )

9. OTHER INSURED'S NAME (Last Name, First Name, Middle Initial)

10. IS PATIENT'S CONDITION RELATED TO:

11. INSURED'S POLICY GROUP OR FECA NUMBER

a. OTHER INSURED'S POLICY OR GROUP NUMBER

a. EMPLOYMENT? (CURRENT OR PREVIOUS) YES NO

a. INSURED'S DATE OF BIRTH MM DD YY SEX M F

b. OTHER INSURED'S DATE OF BIRTH MM DD YY SEX M F

b. AUTO ACCIDENT? YES NO PLACE (State)

b. EMPLOYER'S NAME OR SCHOOL NAME

c. EMPLOYER'S NAME OR SCHOOL NAME

c. OTHER ACCIDENT? YES NO

c. INSURANCE PLAN NAME OR PROGRAM NAME

d. INSURANCE PLAN NAME OR PROGRAM NAME

10d. RESERVED FOR LOCAL USE

d. IS THERE ANOTHER HEALTH BENEFIT PLAN? YES NO If yes, return to and complete item 9 a – d.

READ BACK OF FORM BEFORE COMPLETING & SIGNING THIS FORM.

12. PATIENT'S OR AUTHORIZED PERSON'S SIGNATURE I authorize the release of any medical or other information necessary to process this claim. I also request payment of government benefits either to myself or to the party who accepts assignment below.

SIGNED DATE

13. INSURED'S OR AUTHORIZED PERSON'S SIGNATURE I authorize payment of medical benefits to the undersigned physician or supplier for services described below.

SIGNED

PATIENT AND INSURED INFORMATION

14. DATE OF CURRENT: MM DD YY ILLNESS (First symptom) OR INJURY (Accident) OR PREGNANCY (LMP)

15. IF PATIENT HAS HAD SAME OR SIMILAR ILLNESS, GIVE FIRST DATE MM DD YY

16. DATES PATIENT UNABLE TO WORK IN CURRENT OCCUPATION FROM MM DD YY TO MM DD YY

17. NAME OF REFERRING PHYSICIAN OR OTHER SOURCE

17a. I.D. NUMBER OF REFERRING PHYSICIAN

18. HOSPITALIZATION DATES RELATED TO CURRENT SERVICES FROM MM DD YY TO MM DD YY

19. RESERVED FOR LOCAL USE

20. OUTSIDE LAB? YES NO $ CHARGES

21. DIAGNOSIS OR NATURE OF ILLNESS OR INJURY. (RELATE ITEMS 1, 2, 3, OR 4 TO ITEM 24E BY LINE)

1. ___ . __
2. ___ . __
3. ___ . __
4. ___ . __

22. MEDICAID RESUBMISSION CODE ORIGINAL REF. NO.

23. PRIOR AUTHORIZATION NUMBER

24. A DATE(S) OF SERVICE From MM DD YY	To MM DD YY	B Place of Service	C Type of Service	D PROCEDURES, SERVICES, OR SUPPLIES (Explain Unusual Circumstances) CPT/HCPCS MODIFIER	E DIAGNOSIS CODE	F $ CHARGES	G DAYS OR UNITS	H EPSDT Family Plan	I EMG	J COB	K RESERVED FOR LOCAL USE
1											
2											
3											
4											
5											
6											

25. FEDERAL TAX I.D. NUMBER SSN EIN

26. PATIENT'S ACCOUNT NO.

27. ACCEPT ASSIGNMENT? (For govt. claims, see back) YES NO

28. TOTAL CHARGE $

29. AMOUNT PAID $

30. BALANCE DUE $

31. SIGNATURE OF PHYSICIAN OR SUPPLIER INCLUDING DEGREES OR CREDENTIALS (I certify that the statements on the reverse apply to this bill and are made a part thereof.)

SIGNED DATE

32. NAME AND ADDRESS OF FACILITY WHERE SERVICES WERE RENDERED (If other than home or office)

33. PHYSICIAN'S, SUPPLIER'S BILLING NAME, ADDRESS, ZIP CODE & PHONE #

PIN# GRP#

PHYSICIAN OR SUPPLIER INFORMATION

(SAMPLE ONLY - NOT APPROVED FOR USE)

PLEASE PRINT OR TYPE

SAMPLE FORM 1500
SAMPLE FORM 1500 SAMPLE FORM 1500

Case Study 12-i

DATE	REMARKS
09/03/YYYY	

PATIENT		CHART #	SEX	BIRTHDATE
Ben A. Hanson	334-55-8686	12-i	M	08/09/1975

MAILING ADDRESS	CITY	STATE	ZIP	HOME PHONE	WORK PHONE
632 Greenvalley Ct.	Anywhere	US	12345	(101) 333 5555	444 5555

EMPLOYER	ADDRESS	PATIENT STATUS
Ace Plumbing Service	Anywhere, US	X MARRIED DIVORCED SINGLE STUDENT OTHER

INSURANCE: PRIMARY	ID#	GROUP	SECONDARY POLICY	ID#	GROUP
Guardian	334-55-8686	4596	Liberty Mutual	334-88-7788	DD12

POLICYHOLDER NAME	BIRTHDATE	RELATIONSHIP	POLICYHOLDER NAME	BIRTHDATE	RELATIONSHIP
		Self	Joy M. Hanson	10/10/77	Wife

SUPPLEMENTAL PLAN	EMPLOYER
	Dew Drop Inn

POLICYHOLDER NAME	BIRTHDATE	RELATIONSHIP

EMPLOYER

REFERRING PHYSICIAN UPIN/SSN

DIAGNOSIS	CODE
1. Painful respiration	786.52
2. Chest tightness	786.59
3.	
4.	

PLACE OF SERVICE Office

PROCEDURES	CODE	CHARGE
1. Est. patient OV Level III	99213	$ 75.00
2. EKG	93000	50.00
3.		
4.		
5.		
6.		

SPECIAL NOTES

Refer to Dr. Stanley M. Hart

TOTAL CHARGES	PAYMENTS	ADJUSTMENTS	BALANCE
$125.00	-0-	-0-	$125.00

RETURN VISIT	PHYSICIAN SIGNATURE
2 weeks after seeing Dr. Hart	Donald L. Givings, M.D.

MEDICARE D1234
MEDICAID DLG1234
BCBS 12345

DONALD L. GIVINGS, M.D.
11350 MEDICAL DRIVE, ANYWHERE US 12345
PHONE NUMBER (101)111-5555

EIN 11-123456
SSN 123-12-1234
PIN DG1234
GRP DG12345

Case Study 12-i Primary

PLEASE DO NOT STAPLE IN THIS AREA

(SAMPLE ONLY - NOT APPROVED FOR USE)

CARRIER

PICA

HEALTH INSURANCE CLAIM FORM

PICA

1. MEDICARE (Medicare #) MEDICAID (Medicaid #) CHAMPUS (Sponsor's SSN) CHAMPVA (VA File #) GROUP HEALTH PLAN (SSN or ID) FECA BLK LUNG (SSN) OTHER (ID)

1a. INSURED'S I.D. NUMBER (FOR PROGRAM IN ITEM 1)

2. PATIENT'S NAME (Last Name, First Name, Middle Initial)

3. PATIENT'S BIRTH DATE MM DD YY SEX M F

4. INSURED'S NAME (Last Name, First Name, Middle Initial)

5. PATIENT'S ADDRESS (No. Street)

6. PATIENT RELATIONSHIP TO INSURED Self Spouse Child Other

7. INSURED'S ADDRESS (No. Street)

CITY STATE

8. PATIENT STATUS Single Married Other

CITY STATE

ZIP CODE TELEPHONE (Include Area Code) ( )

Employed Full-Time Student Part-Time Student

ZIP CODE TELEPHONE (INCLUDE AREA CODE) ( )

9. OTHER INSURED'S NAME (Last Name, First Name, Middle Initial)

10. IS PATIENT'S CONDITION RELATED TO:

11. INSURED'S POLICY GROUP OR FECA NUMBER

a. OTHER INSURED'S POLICY OR GROUP NUMBER

a. EMPLOYMENT? (CURRENT OR PREVIOUS) YES NO

a. INSURED'S DATE OF BIRTH MM DD YY SEX M F

b. OTHER INSURED'S DATE OF BIRTH MM DD YY SEX M F

b. AUTO ACCIDENT? YES NO PLACE (State)

b. EMPLOYER'S NAME OR SCHOOL NAME

c. EMPLOYER'S NAME OR SCHOOL NAME

c. OTHER ACCIDENT? YES NO

c. INSURANCE PLAN NAME OR PROGRAM NAME

d. INSURANCE PLAN NAME OR PROGRAM NAME

10d. RESERVED FOR LOCAL USE

d. IS THERE ANOTHER HEALTH BENEFIT PLAN? YES NO If yes, return to and complete item 9 a – d.

READ BACK OF FORM BEFORE COMPLETING & SIGNING THIS FORM.

12. PATIENT'S OR AUTHORIZED PERSON'S SIGNATURE I authorize the release of any medical or other information necessary to process this claim. I also request payment of government benefits either to myself or to the party who accepts assignment below.

SIGNED ______ DATE ______

13. INSURED'S OR AUTHORIZED PERSON'S SIGNATURE I authorize payment of medical benefits to the undersigned physician or supplier for services described below.

SIGNED ______

PATIENT AND INSURED INFORMATION

14. DATE OF CURRENT: MM DD YY ILLNESS (First symptom) OR INJURY (Accident) OR PREGNANCY (LMP)

15. IF PATIENT HAS HAD SAME OR SIMILAR ILLNESS, GIVE FIRST DATE MM DD YY

16. DATES PATIENT UNABLE TO WORK IN CURRENT OCCUPATION FROM MM DD YY TO MM DD YY

17. NAME OF REFERRING PHYSICIAN OR OTHER SOURCE

17a. I.D. NUMBER OF REFERRING PHYSICIAN

18. HOSPITALIZATION DATES RELATED TO CURRENT SERVICES FROM MM DD YY TO MM DD YY

19. RESERVED FOR LOCAL USE

20. OUTSIDE LAB? YES NO $ CHARGES

21. DIAGNOSIS OR NATURE OF ILLNESS OR INJURY. (RELATE ITEMS 1, 2, 3, OR 4 TO ITEM 24E BY LINE)

1. ___ . __ 3. ___ . __

2. ___ . __ 4. ___ . __

22. MEDICAID RESUBMISSION CODE ORIGINAL REF. NO.

23. PRIOR AUTHORIZATION NUMBER

24. A DATE(S) OF SERVICE From MM DD YY	To MM DD YY	B Place of Service	C Type of Service	D PROCEDURES, SERVICES, OR SUPPLIES (Explain Unusual Circumstances) CPT/HCPCS MODIFIER	E DIAGNOSIS CODE	F $ CHARGES	G DAYS OR UNITS	H EPSDT Family Plan	I EMG	J COB	K RESERVED FOR LOCAL USE
1											
2											
3											
4											
5											
6											

25. FEDERAL TAX I.D. NUMBER SSN EIN

26. PATIENT'S ACCOUNT NO.

27. ACCEPT ASSIGNMENT? (For govt. claims, see back) YES NO

28. TOTAL CHARGE $

29. AMOUNT PAID $

30. BALANCE DUE $

31. SIGNATURE OF PHYSICIAN OR SUPPLIER INCLUDING DEGREES OR CREDENTIALS (I certify that the statements on the reverse apply to this bill and are made a part thereof.)

SIGNED DATE

32. NAME AND ADDRESS OF FACILITY WHERE SERVICES WERE RENDERED (If other than home or office)

33. PHYSICIAN'S, SUPPLIER'S BILLING NAME, ADDRESS, ZIP CODE & PHONE #

PIN# GRP#

PHYSICIAN OR SUPPLIER INFORMATION

(SAMPLE ONLY - NOT APPROVED FOR USE)

PLEASE PRINT OR TYPE

SAMPLE FORM 1500
SAMPLE FORM 1500 SAMPLE FORM 1500

Case Study 12-i Secondary

PLEASE DO NOT STAPLE IN THIS AREA

(SAMPLE ONLY - NOT APPROVED FOR USE)

CARRIER

PICA

HEALTH INSURANCE CLAIM FORM

PICA

1. MEDICARE (Medicare #) MEDICAID (Medicaid #) CHAMPUS (Sponsor's SSN) CHAMPVA (VA File #) GROUP HEALTH PLAN (SSN or ID) FECA BLK LUNG (SSN) OTHER (ID)

1a. INSURED'S I.D. NUMBER (FOR PROGRAM IN ITEM 1)

2. PATIENT'S NAME (Last Name, First Name, Middle Initial)

3. PATIENT'S BIRTH DATE MM DD YY SEX M F

4. INSURED'S NAME (Last Name, First Name, Middle Initial)

5. PATIENT'S ADDRESS (No. Street)

6. PATIENT RELATIONSHIP TO INSURED Self Spouse Child Other

7. INSURED'S ADDRESS (No. Street)

CITY STATE

8. PATIENT STATUS Single Married Other

CITY STATE

ZIP CODE TELEPHONE (Include Area Code) ( )

Employed Full-Time Student Part-Time Student

ZIP CODE TELEPHONE (INCLUDE AREA CODE) ( )

9. OTHER INSURED'S NAME (Last Name, First Name, Middle Initial)

10. IS PATIENT'S CONDITION RELATED TO:

11. INSURED'S POLICY GROUP OR FECA NUMBER

a. OTHER INSURED'S POLICY OR GROUP NUMBER

a. EMPLOYMENT? (CURRENT OR PREVIOUS) YES NO

a. INSURED'S DATE OF BIRTH MM DD YY SEX M F

b. OTHER INSURED'S DATE OF BIRTH MM DD YY SEX M F

b. AUTO ACCIDENT? PLACE (State) YES NO

b. EMPLOYER'S NAME OR SCHOOL NAME

c. EMPLOYER'S NAME OR SCHOOL NAME

c. OTHER ACCIDENT? YES NO

c. INSURANCE PLAN NAME OR PROGRAM NAME

d. INSURANCE PLAN NAME OR PROGRAM NAME

10d. RESERVED FOR LOCAL USE

d. IS THERE ANOTHER HEALTH BENEFIT PLAN? YES NO If yes, return to and complete item 9 a – d.

READ BACK OF FORM BEFORE COMPLETING & SIGNING THIS FORM.

12. PATIENT'S OR AUTHORIZED PERSON'S SIGNATURE I authorize the release of any medical or other information necessary to process this claim. I also request payment of government benefits either to myself or to the party who accepts assignment below.

SIGNED ______ DATE ______

13. INSURED'S OR AUTHORIZED PERSON'S SIGNATURE I authorize payment of medical benefits to the undersigned physician or supplier for services described below.

SIGNED ______

PATIENT AND INSURED INFORMATION

14. DATE OF CURRENT: MM DD YY ILLNESS (First symptom) OR INJURY (Accident) OR PREGNANCY (LMP)

15. IF PATIENT HAS HAD SAME OR SIMILAR ILLNESS, GIVE FIRST DATE MM DD YY

16. DATES PATIENT UNABLE TO WORK IN CURRENT OCCUPATION FROM MM DD YY TO MM DD YY

17. NAME OF REFERRING PHYSICIAN OR OTHER SOURCE

17a. I.D. NUMBER OF REFERRING PHYSICIAN

18. HOSPITALIZATION DATES RELATED TO CURRENT SERVICES FROM MM DD YY TO MM DD YY

19. RESERVED FOR LOCAL USE

20. OUTSIDE LAB? YES NO $ CHARGES

21. DIAGNOSIS OR NATURE OF ILLNESS OR INJURY. (RELATE ITEMS 1, 2, 3, OR 4 TO ITEM 24E BY LINE)

1. ___ . __ 3. ___ . __

2. ___ . __ 4. ___ . __

22. MEDICAID RESUBMISSION CODE ORIGINAL REF. NO.

23. PRIOR AUTHORIZATION NUMBER

24.	A DATE(S) OF SERVICE From MM DD YY	To MM DD YY	B Place of Service	C Type of Service	D PROCEDURES, SERVICES, OR SUPPLIES (Explain Unusual Circumstances) CPT/HCPCS MODIFIER	E DIAGNOSIS CODE	F $ CHARGES	G DAYS OR UNITS	H EPSDT Family Plan	I EMG	J COB	K RESERVED FOR LOCAL USE
1												
2												
3												
4												
5												
6												

25. FEDERAL TAX I.D. NUMBER SSN EIN

26. PATIENT'S ACCOUNT NO.

27. ACCEPT ASSIGNMENT? (For govt. claims, see back) YES NO

28. TOTAL CHARGE $

29. AMOUNT PAID $

30. BALANCE DUE $

31. SIGNATURE OF PHYSICIAN OR SUPPLIER INCLUDING DEGREES OR CREDENTIALS (I certify that the statements on the reverse apply to this bill and are made a part thereof.)

SIGNED DATE

32. NAME AND ADDRESS OF FACILITY WHERE SERVICES WERE RENDERED (If other than home or office)

33. PHYSICIAN'S, SUPPLIER'S BILLING NAME, ADDRESS, ZIP CODE & PHONE #

PIN# GRP#

PHYSICIAN OR SUPPLIER INFORMATION

(SAMPLE ONLY - NOT APPROVED FOR USE)

PLEASE PRINT OR TYPE

SAMPLE FORM 1500

SAMPLE FORM 1500 SAMPLE FORM 1500

Case Study 12-j

DATE	REMARKS
09/03/YYYY	Prior Authorization #659427

PATIENT		CHART #	SEX	BIRTHDATE
Ben A. Hanson	334-55-8686	12-j	M	08/09/1975

MAILING ADDRESS	CITY	STATE	ZIP	HOME PHONE	WORK PHONE
632 Greenvalley Ct.	Anywhere	US	12345	(101) 333 5555	444 5555

EMPLOYER	ADDRESS	PATIENT STATUS
Ace Plumbing Service	Anywhere, US	X MARRIED DIVORCED SINGLE STUDENT OTHER

INSURANCE: PRIMARY	ID#	GROUP	SECONDARY POLICY	ID#	GROUP
Guardian	334-55-8686	4596	Liberty Mutual	334-88-7788	DD12

POLICYHOLDER NAME	BIRTHDATE	RELATIONSHIP	POLICYHOLDER NAME	BIRTHDATE	RELATIONSHIP
		Self	Joy M. Hanson	10/10/77	Wife

SUPPLEMENTAL PLAN	EMPLOYER
	Dew Drop Inn

POLICYHOLDER NAME	BIRTHDATE	RELATIONSHIP

EMPLOYER

REFERRING PHYSICIAN UPIN/SSN: Donald L. Givings, M.D.

DIAGNOSIS	CODE
1. Painful respiration	786.52
2. Chest tightness	786.59
3. Abnormal chest sounds	786.7
4.	

PLACE OF SERVICE: Office

PROCEDURES	CODE	CHARGE
1. Office consult Level II	99242	$ 75.00
2. Cardiovascular stress test, with interpretation and report	93015	150.00
3.		
4.		
5.		
6.		

SPECIAL NOTES

TOTAL CHARGES	PAYMENTS	ADJUSTMENTS	BALANCE
$225.00	-0-	-0-	$225.00

RETURN VISIT	PHYSICIAN SIGNATURE
PRN	Stanley M. Hart, M.D.

MEDICARE S1234
MEDICAID SMH1234
BCBS 12388

STANLEY M. HART, M.D. CARDIOLOGY
316 GRACE WAY, SUITE 102, ANYWHERE US 12345
PHONE NUMBER (101)111-5555

EIN 11785678
SSN 133-12-1254
PIN SH1234
GRP SH12345

Case Study 12-j Primary

PLEASE DO NOT STAPLE IN THIS AREA

(SAMPLE ONLY - NOT APPROVED FOR USE)

CARRIER

PICA

HEALTH INSURANCE CLAIM FORM

PICA

1. MEDICARE (Medicare #) MEDICAID (Medicaid #) CHAMPUS (Sponsor's SSN) CHAMPVA (VA File #) GROUP HEALTH PLAN (SSN or ID) FECA BLK LUNG (SSN) OTHER (ID)

1a. INSURED'S I.D. NUMBER (FOR PROGRAM IN ITEM 1)

2. PATIENT'S NAME (Last Name, First Name, Middle Initial)

3. PATIENT'S BIRTH DATE MM DD YY SEX M F

4. INSURED'S NAME (Last Name, First Name, Middle Initial)

5. PATIENT'S ADDRESS (No. Street)

6. PATIENT RELATIONSHIP TO INSURED Self Spouse Child Other

7. INSURED'S ADDRESS (No. Street)

CITY STATE

8. PATIENT STATUS Single Married Other

CITY STATE

ZIP CODE TELEPHONE (Include Area Code) ( )

Employed Full-Time Student Part-Time Student

ZIP CODE TELEPHONE (INCLUDE AREA CODE) ( )

9. OTHER INSURED'S NAME (Last Name, First Name, Middle Initial)

10. IS PATIENT'S CONDITION RELATED TO:

11. INSURED'S POLICY GROUP OR FECA NUMBER

a. OTHER INSURED'S POLICY OR GROUP NUMBER

a. EMPLOYMENT? (CURRENT OR PREVIOUS) YES NO

a. INSURED'S DATE OF BIRTH MM DD YY SEX M F

b. OTHER INSURED'S DATE OF BIRTH MM DD YY SEX M F

b. AUTO ACCIDENT? PLACE (State) YES NO

b. EMPLOYER'S NAME OR SCHOOL NAME

c. EMPLOYER'S NAME OR SCHOOL NAME

c. OTHER ACCIDENT? YES NO

c. INSURANCE PLAN NAME OR PROGRAM NAME

d. INSURANCE PLAN NAME OR PROGRAM NAME

10d. RESERVED FOR LOCAL USE

d. IS THERE ANOTHER HEALTH BENEFIT PLAN? YES NO If yes, return to and complete item 9 a – d.

READ BACK OF FORM BEFORE COMPLETING & SIGNING THIS FORM.

12. PATIENT'S OR AUTHORIZED PERSON'S SIGNATURE I authorize the release of any medical or other information necessary to process this claim. I also request payment of government benefits either to myself or to the party who accepts assignment below.

SIGNED ______ DATE ______

13. INSURED'S OR AUTHORIZED PERSON'S SIGNATURE I authorize payment of medical benefits to the undersigned physician or supplier for services described below.

SIGNED ______

PATIENT AND INSURED INFORMATION

14. DATE OF CURRENT: MM DD YY ILLNESS (First symptom) OR INJURY (Accident) OR PREGNANCY (LMP)

15. IF PATIENT HAS HAD SAME OR SIMILAR ILLNESS, GIVE FIRST DATE MM DD YY

16. DATES PATIENT UNABLE TO WORK IN CURRENT OCCUPATION FROM MM DD YY TO MM DD YY

17. NAME OF REFERRING PHYSICIAN OR OTHER SOURCE

17a. I.D. NUMBER OF REFERRING PHYSICIAN

18. HOSPITALIZATION DATES RELATED TO CURRENT SERVICES FROM MM DD YY TO MM DD YY

19. RESERVED FOR LOCAL USE

20. OUTSIDE LAB? YES NO $ CHARGES

21. DIAGNOSIS OR NATURE OF ILLNESS OR INJURY. (RELATE ITEMS 1, 2, 3, OR 4 TO ITEM 24E BY LINE)

1. ___ . __ 3. ___ . __

2. ___ . __ 4. ___ . __

22. MEDICAID RESUBMISSION CODE ORIGINAL REF. NO.

23. PRIOR AUTHORIZATION NUMBER

24. A DATE(S) OF SERVICE From MM DD YY To MM DD YY	B Place of Service	C Type of Service	D PROCEDURES, SERVICES, OR SUPPLIES (Explain Unusual Circumstances) CPT/HCPCS MODIFIER	E DIAGNOSIS CODE	F $ CHARGES	G DAYS OR UNITS	H EPSDT Family Plan	I EMG	J COB	K RESERVED FOR LOCAL USE
1										
2										
3										
4										
5										
6										

PHYSICIAN OR SUPPLIER INFORMATION

25. FEDERAL TAX I.D. NUMBER SSN EIN

26. PATIENT'S ACCOUNT NO.

27. ACCEPT ASSIGNMENT? (For govt. claims, see back) YES NO

28. TOTAL CHARGE $

29. AMOUNT PAID $

30. BALANCE DUE $

31. SIGNATURE OF PHYSICIAN OR SUPPLIER INCLUDING DEGREES OR CREDENTIALS (I certify that the statements on the reverse apply to this bill and are made a part thereof.)

SIGNED DATE

32. NAME AND ADDRESS OF FACILITY WHERE SERVICES WERE RENDERED (If other than home or office)

33. PHYSICIAN'S, SUPPLIER'S BILLING NAME, ADDRESS, ZIP CODE & PHONE #

PIN# GRP#

(SAMPLE ONLY - NOT APPROVED FOR USE)

PLEASE PRINT OR TYPE

SAMPLE FORM 1500
SAMPLE FORM 1500 SAMPLE FORM 1500

Case Study 12-j Secondary

PLEASE DO NOT STAPLE IN THIS AREA

(SAMPLE ONLY - NOT APPROVED FOR USE)

CARRIER

PICA

HEALTH INSURANCE CLAIM FORM

PICA

1. MEDICARE (Medicare #) MEDICAID (Medicaid #) CHAMPUS (Sponsor's SSN) CHAMPVA (VA File #) GROUP HEALTH PLAN (SSN or ID) FECA BLK LUNG (SSN) OTHER (ID)

1a. INSURED'S I.D. NUMBER (FOR PROGRAM IN ITEM 1)

2. PATIENT'S NAME (Last Name, First Name, Middle Initial)

3. PATIENT'S BIRTH DATE MM DD YY SEX M F

4. INSURED'S NAME (Last Name, First Name, Middle Initial)

5. PATIENT'S ADDRESS (No. Street)

6. PATIENT RELATIONSHIP TO INSURED Self Spouse Child Other

7. INSURED'S ADDRESS (No. Street)

CITY STATE

8. PATIENT STATUS Single Married Other

CITY STATE

ZIP CODE TELEPHONE (Include Area Code) ( )

Employed Full-Time Student Part-Time Student

ZIP CODE TELEPHONE (INCLUDE AREA CODE) ( )

9. OTHER INSURED'S NAME (Last Name, First Name, Middle Initial)

10. IS PATIENT'S CONDITION RELATED TO:

11. INSURED'S POLICY GROUP OR FECA NUMBER

a. OTHER INSURED'S POLICY OR GROUP NUMBER

a. EMPLOYMENT? (CURRENT OR PREVIOUS) YES NO

a. INSURED'S DATE OF BIRTH MM DD YY SEX M F

b. OTHER INSURED'S DATE OF BIRTH MM DD YY SEX M F

b. AUTO ACCIDENT? YES NO PLACE (State)

b. EMPLOYER'S NAME OR SCHOOL NAME

c. EMPLOYER'S NAME OR SCHOOL NAME

c. OTHER ACCIDENT? YES NO

c. INSURANCE PLAN NAME OR PROGRAM NAME

d. INSURANCE PLAN NAME OR PROGRAM NAME

10d. RESERVED FOR LOCAL USE

d. IS THERE ANOTHER HEALTH BENEFIT PLAN? YES NO If yes, return to and complete item 9 a – d.

READ BACK OF FORM BEFORE COMPLETING & SIGNING THIS FORM.

12. PATIENT'S OR AUTHORIZED PERSON'S SIGNATURE I authorize the release of any medical or other information necessary to process this claim. I also request payment of government benefits either to myself or to the party who accepts assignment below.

SIGNED DATE

13. INSURED'S OR AUTHORIZED PERSON'S SIGNATURE I authorize payment of medical benefits to the undersigned physician or supplier for services described below.

SIGNED

PATIENT AND INSURED INFORMATION

14. DATE OF CURRENT: MM DD YY ILLNESS (First symptom) OR INJURY (Accident) OR PREGNANCY (LMP)

15. IF PATIENT HAS HAD SAME OR SIMILAR ILLNESS, GIVE FIRST DATE MM DD YY

16. DATES PATIENT UNABLE TO WORK IN CURRENT OCCUPATION FROM MM DD YY TO MM DD YY

17. NAME OF REFERRING PHYSICIAN OR OTHER SOURCE

17a. I.D. NUMBER OF REFERRING PHYSICIAN

18. HOSPITALIZATION DATES RELATED TO CURRENT SERVICES FROM MM DD YY TO MM DD YY

19. RESERVED FOR LOCAL USE

20. OUTSIDE LAB? YES NO $ CHARGES

21. DIAGNOSIS OR NATURE OF ILLNESS OR INJURY. (RELATE ITEMS 1, 2, 3, OR 4 TO ITEM 24E BY LINE)

1. ___ . __

2. ___ . __

3. ___ . __

4. ___ . __

22. MEDICAID RESUBMISSION CODE ORIGINAL REF. NO.

23. PRIOR AUTHORIZATION NUMBER

24. A DATE(S) OF SERVICE From MM DD YY To MM DD YY	B Place of Service	C Type of Service	D PROCEDURES, SERVICES, OR SUPPLIES (Explain Unusual Circumstances) CPT/HCPCS MODIFIER	E DIAGNOSIS CODE	F $ CHARGES	G DAYS OR UNITS	H EPSDT Family Plan	I EMG	J COB	K RESERVED FOR LOCAL USE
1										
2										
3										
4										
5										
6										

25. FEDERAL TAX I.D. NUMBER SSN EIN

26. PATIENT'S ACCOUNT NO.

27. ACCEPT ASSIGNMENT? (For govt. claims, see back) YES NO

28. TOTAL CHARGE $

29. AMOUNT PAID $

30. BALANCE DUE $

31. SIGNATURE OF PHYSICIAN OR SUPPLIER INCLUDING DEGREES OR CREDENTIALS (I certify that the statements on the reverse apply to this bill and are made a part thereof.)

SIGNED DATE

32. NAME AND ADDRESS OF FACILITY WHERE SERVICES WERE RENDERED (If other than home or office)

33. PHYSICIAN'S, SUPPLIER'S BILLING NAME, ADDRESS, ZIP CODE & PHONE #

PIN# GRP#

PHYSICIAN OR SUPPLIER INFORMATION

(SAMPLE ONLY - NOT APPROVED FOR USE)

PLEASE PRINT OR TYPE

SAMPLE FORM 1500
SAMPLE FORM 1500 SAMPLE FORM 1500

Blue Cross and Blue Shield Plans

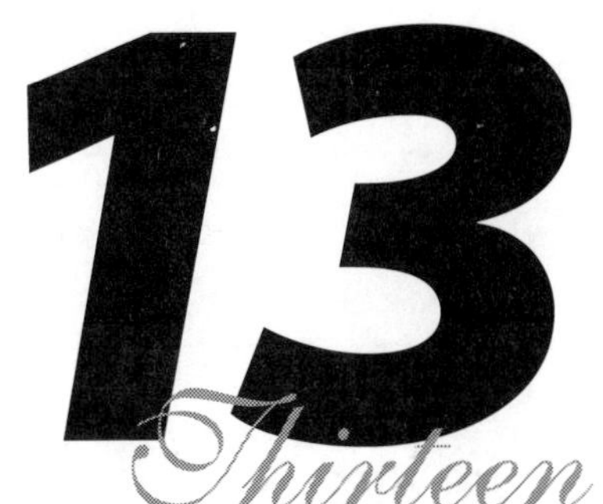

BRIEF HISTORY

1. The forerunner of what is known today as the Blue Cross plan began when Baylor University Hospital approached ___. (Circle the correct answer.)
   a. doctors
   b. teachers
   c. hospital employees
   d. none of the above

2. The Blue Cross Association grew out of what need? (Circle the correct answer.)
   a. additional national coordination among plans
   b. additional member hospitals
   c. additional participating physicians
   d. all of the above

3. The Blue Shield plans began as a resolution passed by the House of Delegates at a meeting of the ___. (Circle the correct answer.)
   a. Blue Cross Association
   b. American Hospital Association
   c. American Medical Association
   d. none of the above

4. The first Blue Shield plan was formed in 1939 and was known as ___. (Circle the correct answer.)
   a. California Physicians' Service
   b. Blue Shield of California
   c. Blue Cross Association
   d. none of the above

5. The Blue Shield design was first used as a trademark by the ___. (Circle the correct answer.)
   a. California Physicians' Service
   b. Buffalo, New York plan
   c. American Medical Association
   d. none of the above

6. Blue Cross plans originally covered only ______________________ bills.

7. Blue Shield plans were set up to cover fees for __________________ services.

8. Define *nonprofit corporation.* ____

____

9. Define *for-profit corporation.* ____

____

BCBS ASSOCIATION

10. List four functions of the Blue Cross and Blue Shield Association (BCBSA).

    a. ____

    b. ____

    c. ____

    d. ____

11. BCBSA is the registered owner of the BC and BS ________________________________ .

BCBS DISTINCTIVE FEATURES

12. The "Blues" were pioneers in _____ prepaid health care. (Circle the correct answer.)

    a. profit

    b. nonprofit

    c. premium

    d. all of the above

13. The "Blues" agreed to perform which of the following service(s)? (Circle the correct answer.)

    a. make prompt, direct payments of claims

    b. maintain regional professional representatives to assist participating providers with claim problems

    c. provide educational seminars, workshops, billing manuals, and newsletters

    d. all of the above

14. BCBS plans are forbidden by state law from __________________ ______________________ for an individual because he or she is in poor health or BCBS payments to providers have far exceeded the average.

15. Describe when a BCBS policy can be canceled or an individual disenrolled. ____________________

____

____

16. BCBS plans must obtain approval for any rate increase or benefit change from the ___. (Circle the correct answer.)
   a. State Insurance Commissioner
   b. American Hospital Association
   c. American Medical Association
   d. all of the above

PARTICIPATING PROVIDERS

17. When a health care provider elects to become a participating provider (PAR), that provider enters into a contract with a BCBS corporation and agrees to ___. (Circle the correct answer.)
   a. submit insurance claims for all BCBS subscribers
   b. write off the difference between the amount charged and the approved fee
   c. bill patients for only the deductible and copay/coinsurance amounts and the full fee for any uncovered service
   d. all of the above

18. List five services BCBS agrees to provide to PAR providers.
   a. ______________________________
   b. ______________________________
   c. ______________________________
   d. ______________________________
   e. ______________________________

NONPARTICIPATING PROVIDERS

19. Nonparticipating Providers ___. (Circle the correct answer.)
   a. have not signed participating provider contracts
   b. expect to be paid the full amount of the fee charged for services they perform
   c. understand the insurance company will send payment for claims directly to the patient
   d. all of the above

Critical Thinking

20. Write a paragraph describing the basic differences between a participating provider and a nonparticipating provider.

____

____

____

____

____

TRADITIONAL FEE-FOR-SERVICE COVERAGE

21. Name two types of coverage into which many of the large group contracts are subdivided.
    a. ______________________________
    b. ______________________________

22. List seven benefits routinely included under BCBS basic coverage.
    a. ______________________________
    b. ______________________________
    c. ______________________________
    d. ______________________________
    e. ______________________________
    f. ______________________________
    g. ______________________________

23. List seven benefits routinely included under the BCBS major medical plan.
    a. ______________________________
    b. ______________________________
    c. ______________________________
    d. ______________________________
    e. ______________________________
    f. ______________________________
    g. ______________________________

24. Major Medical services are usually subject to patient ______________ and ______________ requirements.

Critical Thinking

25. Write a paragraph describing riders; include special accidental injury riders and medical emergency care riders.

____

____

____

____

____

____

____

____

NATIONAL ACCOUNTS AND BLUECARD PROGRAM

26. Which health insurance contract covers company employees who are located in more than one geographic area? (Circle the correct answer.)
    a. BlueCard Program
    b. BlueCard WorldWide
    c. National Account
    d. none of the above

27. Describe the symbol that is found on a National Account ID card. ________________________________

    ____

28. National Accounts claims are filed with the ___. (Circle the correct answer.)
    a. local BCBS agencies
    b. national Blue Cross and Blue Shield Association in Chicago
    c. state insurance commissioner's office
    d. all of the above

29. Those who are allowed to receive their local Blue plan health care benefits while traveling or living outside of their plan's area include ___ subscribers. (Circle the correct answer.)
    a. BlueCard Program
    b. BlueCard WorldWide
    c. National Account
    d. none of the above

30. BlueCard patients have identification numbers that begin with a(n) ___. (Circle the correct answer.)
    a. numerical prefix
    b. asterisk as a prefix
    c. alpha prefix
    d. none of the above

31. Which program allows subscribers who travel or live abroad to receive covered inpatient hospital care and physician services from a network of hospitals and doctors around the world? (Circle the correct answer.)
    a. BlueCard Program
    b. BlueCard WorldWide
    c. National Account
    d. none of the above

32. Match the insurance terms in the first column with the definitions in the second column. Write the correct letter in each blank.

_______	PPO	a. assumes responsibility for coordinating all the subscriber's medical care
_______	subscriber	b. subscriber-driven program
_______	Point-of-Service Plan	c. provides benefits to over nine million federal employees and dependents
_______	primary care physician	d. policyholder
_______	Federal Employee Program	e. managed care plan that provides a full range of inpatient and outpatient services

33. The primary care physician is often referred to as the ______________________ of the patient's medical care.

34. For each item, enter **T** for a true statement or **F** for a false statement on the line provided.

_______ a. The subscriber is responsible for remaining within the network of PPO providers.

_______ b. An exclusive provider organization does not cover out-of-network care.

_______ c. In the POS plan, subscribers choose a PCP from the local telephone directory.

_______ d. Written referral notices issued by the PCP must be attached to all paper claims for services.

_______ e. In the POS plan, the patient is responsible for obtaining authorizations for all inpatient hospitalizations.

_______ f. The BCBS Federal Employee Program ID number begins with the letter "F" followed by eight digits.

_______ g. FEP cards contain the phrase "Government-Wide Service Benefit Plan."

35. The Outpatient Pretreatment Authorization Plan requires preauthorization of outpatient ___. (Circle the correct answer.)
   a. physical therapy services
   b. occupational therapy services
   c. speech therapy services
   d. all of the above

36. The mandatory second surgical opinion requirement is necessary when a patient is considering ___. (Circle the correct answer.)
   a. emergency surgical care
   b. elective, non-emergency surgical care
   c. non-emergency surgical care
   d. all of the above

37. The Coordinated Home Health and Hospice Care program allows patients with this option to elect an alternative to the ___. (Circle the correct answer.)
   a. acute care setting
   b. second surgical opinion requirement
   c. urgent care center
   d. none of the above

38. All BCBS corporations offer at least one ______________ ______________ ______________ plan.

MEDICARE SUPPLEMENTAL PLANS

39. BCBS corporations offer several of the federally-designed and regulated Medicare Supplemental plans which augment the Medicare program by paying for Medicare ______________ and ______________ .

40. These plans are better known throughout the industry as ______________ ______________ .

BILLING INFORMATION SUMMARY

41. The deadline for filing claims is customarily ___ from the date of service, unless otherwise specified in the subscriber's or provider's contracts. (Circle the correct answer.)
   a. five years
   b. 90 days
   c. one year
   d. none of the above

42. Most payers currently accept the ___. (Circle the correct answer.)
   a. BCBS form
   b. HCFA-1500 form
   c. HCFA-1450 form
   d. none of the above

43. The most common coinsurance amounts are ___. (Circle the correct answer.)
   a. 20 or 25%
   b. 5 or 10%
   c. 50 or 75%
   d. none of the above

44. The Explanation of Benefits sent to PAR and PPN providers clearly states the patient's ___. (Circle the correct answer.)

 a. coinsurance
 b. deductible
 c. copayment
 d. all of the above

45. Participating providers must accept the allowable rate on all _______________ _______________.

46. NonPARs may collect the _________________ _________________ from the patient. BCBS payments are then sent directly to the _________________.

47. All claims filed by participating providers qualify for an assignment of benefits to the _________________.

48. For each item, enter **T** for a true statement or **F** for a false statement on the line provided.

_______ a. You need to retain a current photocopy of only the front of all patient ID cards.

_______ b. Claims for BlueCard patients with more than one insurance policy must be billed directly to the plan from which the program originated.

_______ c. NonPARs must bill the patient's plan for all nonnational account patients with BlueCards.

_______ d. Rebill claims not paid within 60 days.

_______ e. Some mental health claims are forwarded to a third-party administrator specializing in mental health case management.

Know Your Acronyms

49. Define the following acronyms:

 a. BC ____
 b. BS ____
 c. AHA ____
 d. BCBS ____
 e. BCBSA ____
 f. PAR ____
 g. PPN ____
 h. MM ____
 i. DME ____
 j. PPO ____
 k. POS ____
 l. FEP ____
 m. OPAP ____

n. SSO ______________________________

o. PPA ______________________________

p. EPO ______________________________

q. FEHBP ______________________________

r. OMP ______________________________

s. PCP ______________________________

t. HMO ______________________________

u. UCR ______________________________

v. TPA ______________________________

EXERCISES

50. Complete Case Studies 13-a through 13-h using the blank claim form provided. Follow the step-by-step instructions in the textbook to properly complete the claim form. If a patient has secondary coverage, complete an additional claim form using secondary directions from the textbook. You may choose to use a pencil so corrections can be made.

DATE	REMARKS
01/19/YYYY	

PATIENT		CHART #	SEX	BIRTHDATE
Monty L. Booker	678-22-3434	13-a	M	12/25/1966

MAILING ADDRESS	CITY	STATE	ZIP	HOME PHONE	WORK PHONE
47 Snowflake Road	Anywhere	US	12345	(101) 333 5555	444 5555

EMPLOYER	ADDRESS	PATIENT STATUS
Atlanta Publisher	Anywhere, US	X MARRIED DIVORCED SINGLE STUDENT OTHER

INSURANCE: PRIMARY	ID#	GROUP	SECONDARY POLICY	ID#	GROUP
BCBS US	NXY 678-22-3434	678			

POLICYHOLDER NAME	BIRTHDATE	RELATIONSHIP	POLICYHOLDER NAME	BIRTHDATE	RELATIONSHIP
		Self			

SUPPLEMENTAL PLAN	EMPLOYER

POLICYHOLDER NAME BIRTHDATE RELATIONSHIP

EMPLOYER

REFERRING PHYSICIAN UPIN/SSN

DIAGNOSIS	CODE
1. Abnormal loss of weight	783.21
2. Polydipsia	783.5
3. Polyphagia	783.6
4.	

PLACE OF SERVICE Office

PROCEDURES	CODE	CHARGE
1. New patient OV Level IV	99204	$ 100.00
2. Urinalysis, with microscopy	81001	10.00
3.		
4.		
5.		
6.		

SPECIAL NOTES

TOTAL CHARGES	PAYMENTS	ADJUSTMENTS	BALANCE
$110.00	-0-	-0-	$110.00

RETURN VISIT	PHYSICIAN SIGNATURE
3 weeks	Donald L. Givings, M.D.

MEDICARE D1234 MEDICAID DLG1234 BCBS 12345	**DONALD L. GIVINGS, M.D.** **11350 MEDICAL DRIVE, ANYWHERE US 12345** **PHONE NUMBER (101)111-5555**	EIN 11-123456 SSN 123-12-1234 PIN DG1234 GRP DG12345

PLEASE
DO NOT
STAPLE
IN THIS
AREA

(SAMPLE ONLY - NOT APPROVED FOR USE)

CARRIER

PICA

HEALTH INSURANCE CLAIM FORM

PICA

1. MEDICARE (Medicare #) MEDICAID (Medicaid #) CHAMPUS (Sponsor's SSN) CHAMPVA (VA File #) GROUP HEALTH PLAN (SSN or ID) FECA BLK LUNG (SSN) OTHER (ID)

1a. INSURED'S I.D. NUMBER (FOR PROGRAM IN ITEM 1)

2. PATIENT'S NAME (Last Name, First Name, Middle Initial)

3. PATIENT'S BIRTH DATE MM DD YY SEX M F

4. INSURED'S NAME (Last Name, First Name, Middle Initial)

5. PATIENT'S ADDRESS (No. Street)

6. PATIENT RELATIONSHIP TO INSURED Self Spouse Child Other

7. INSURED'S ADDRESS (No. Street)

CITY STATE

8. PATIENT STATUS Single Married Other

CITY STATE

ZIP CODE TELEPHONE (Include Area Code) ( )

Employed Full-Time Student Part-Time Student

ZIP CODE TELEPHONE (INCLUDE AREA CODE) ( )

9. OTHER INSURED'S NAME (Last Name, First Name, Middle Initial)

10. IS PATIENT'S CONDITION RELATED TO:

11. INSURED'S POLICY GROUP OR FECA NUMBER

a. OTHER INSURED'S POLICY OR GROUP NUMBER

a. EMPLOYMENT? (CURRENT OR PREVIOUS) YES NO

a. INSURED'S DATE OF BIRTH MM DD YY SEX M F

b. OTHER INSURED'S DATE OF BIRTH MM DD YY SEX M F

b. AUTO ACCIDENT? YES NO PLACE (State)

b. EMPLOYER'S NAME OR SCHOOL NAME

c. EMPLOYER'S NAME OR SCHOOL NAME

c. OTHER ACCIDENT? YES NO

c. INSURANCE PLAN NAME OR PROGRAM NAME

d. INSURANCE PLAN NAME OR PROGRAM NAME

10d. RESERVED FOR LOCAL USE

d. IS THERE ANOTHER HEALTH BENEFIT PLAN? YES NO If yes, return to and complete item 9 a – d.

READ BACK OF FORM BEFORE COMPLETING & SIGNING THIS FORM.

12. PATIENT'S OR AUTHORIZED PERSON'S SIGNATURE I authorize the release of any medical or other information necessary to process this claim. I also request payment of government benefits either to myself or to the party who accepts assignment below.

SIGNED DATE

13. INSURED'S OR AUTHORIZED PERSON'S SIGNATURE I authorize payment of medical benefits to the undersigned physician or supplier for services described below.

SIGNED

PATIENT AND INSURED INFORMATION

14. DATE OF CURRENT: MM DD YY ILLNESS (First symptom) OR INJURY (Accident) OR PREGNANCY (LMP)

15. IF PATIENT HAS HAD SAME OR SIMILAR ILLNESS, GIVE FIRST DATE MM DD YY

16. DATES PATIENT UNABLE TO WORK IN CURRENT OCCUPATION FROM MM DD YY TO MM DD YY

17. NAME OF REFERRING PHYSICIAN OR OTHER SOURCE

17a. I.D. NUMBER OF REFERRING PHYSICIAN

18. HOSPITALIZATION DATES RELATED TO CURRENT SERVICES FROM MM DD YY TO MM DD YY

19. RESERVED FOR LOCAL USE

20. OUTSIDE LAB? YES NO $ CHARGES

21. DIAGNOSIS OR NATURE OF ILLNESS OR INJURY. (RELATE ITEMS 1, 2, 3, OR 4 TO ITEM 24E BY LINE)

1. ___ . __
2. ___ . __
3. ___ . __
4. ___ . __

22. MEDICAID RESUBMISSION CODE ORIGINAL REF. NO.

23. PRIOR AUTHORIZATION NUMBER

24. A DATE(S) OF SERVICE From MM DD YY To MM DD YY	B Place of Service	C Type of Service	D PROCEDURES, SERVICES, OR SUPPLIES (Explain Unusual Circumstances) CPT/HCPCS MODIFIER	E DIAGNOSIS CODE	F $ CHARGES	G DAYS OR UNITS	H EPSDT Family Plan	I EMG	J COB	K RESERVED FOR LOCAL USE
1										
2										
3										
4										
5										
6										

25. FEDERAL TAX I.D. NUMBER SSN EIN

26. PATIENT'S ACCOUNT NO.

27. ACCEPT ASSIGNMENT? (For govt. claims, see back) YES NO

28. TOTAL CHARGE $

29. AMOUNT PAID $

30. BALANCE DUE $

31. SIGNATURE OF PHYSICIAN OR SUPPLIER INCLUDING DEGREES OR CREDENTIALS (I certify that the statements on the reverse apply to this bill and are made a part thereof.)

SIGNED DATE

32. NAME AND ADDRESS OF FACILITY WHERE SERVICES WERE RENDERED (If other than home or office)

33. PHYSICIAN'S, SUPPLIER'S BILLING NAME, ADDRESS, ZIP CODE & PHONE #

PIN# GRP#

PHYSICIAN OR SUPPLIER INFORMATION

(SAMPLE ONLY - NOT APPROVED FOR USE)

PLEASE PRINT OR TYPE

SAMPLE FORM 1500
SAMPLE FORM 1500 SAMPLE FORM 1500

Case Study 13-b

DATE	REMARKS
11/07/YYYY	Patient has a $20 copay

PATIENT		CHART #	SEX	BIRTHDATE
Anita B. Strong	214-55-6666	13-b	F	04/25/1959

MAILING ADDRESS	CITY	STATE	ZIP	HOME PHONE	WORK PHONE
124 Prosper Way	Anywhere	US	12345	(101) 333 5555	444 5555

EMPLOYER	ADDRESS	PATIENT STATUS
Self	Anywhere, US	X MARRIED DIVORCED SINGLE STUDENT OTHER

INSURANCE: PRIMARY	ID#	GROUP	SECONDARY POLICY	ID#	GROUP
BCBS US	XWG 214-55-6666	1357			

POLICYHOLDER NAME	BIRTHDATE	RELATIONSHIP	POLICYHOLDER NAME	BIRTHDATE	RELATIONSHIP
		Self			

SUPPLEMENTAL PLAN	EMPLOYER

POLICYHOLDER NAME	BIRTHDATE	RELATIONSHIP	DIAGNOSIS	CODE
			1. Migraine, classical	346.01
EMPLOYER			2.	
			3.	
REFERRING PHYSICIAN UPIN/SSN			4.	

PLACE OF SERVICE Office

PROCEDURES	CODE	CHARGE
1. Est. patient OV Level I	99211	$ 55.00
2.		
3.		
4.		
5.		
6.		

SPECIAL NOTES

TOTAL CHARGES	PAYMENTS	ADJUSTMENTS	BALANCE
$55.00	$20.00	-0-	$35.00

RETURN VISIT	PHYSICIAN SIGNATURE
PRN	Donald L. Givings, M.D.

MEDICARE D1234
MEDICAID DLG1234
BCBS 12345

DONALD L. GIVINGS, M.D.
11350 MEDICAL DRIVE, ANYWHERE US 12345
PHONE NUMBER (101)111-5555

EIN 11-123456
SSN 123-12-1234
PIN DG1234
GRP DG12345

PLEASE
DO NOT
STAPLE
IN THIS
AREA

(SAMPLE ONLY - NOT APPROVED FOR USE)

CARRIER

PICA

HEALTH INSURANCE CLAIM FORM

PICA

1. MEDICARE (Medicare #) MEDICAID (Medicaid #) CHAMPUS (Sponsor's SSN) CHAMPVA (VA File #) GROUP HEALTH PLAN (SSN or ID) FECA BLK LUNG (SSN) OTHER (ID)

1a. INSURED'S I.D. NUMBER (FOR PROGRAM IN ITEM 1)

2. PATIENT'S NAME (Last Name, First Name, Middle Initial)

3. PATIENT'S BIRTH DATE MM DD YY SEX M F

4. INSURED'S NAME (Last Name, First Name, Middle Initial)

5. PATIENT'S ADDRESS (No. Street)

6. PATIENT RELATIONSHIP TO INSURED Self Spouse Child Other

7. INSURED'S ADDRESS (No. Street)

CITY STATE

8. PATIENT STATUS Single Married Other

CITY STATE

ZIP CODE TELEPHONE (Include Area Code) ( )

Employed Full-Time Student Part-Time Student

ZIP CODE TELEPHONE (INCLUDE AREA CODE) ( )

9. OTHER INSURED'S NAME (Last Name, First Name, Middle Initial)

10. IS PATIENT'S CONDITION RELATED TO:

11. INSURED'S POLICY GROUP OR FECA NUMBER

a. OTHER INSURED'S POLICY OR GROUP NUMBER

a. EMPLOYMENT? (CURRENT OR PREVIOUS) YES NO

a. INSURED'S DATE OF BIRTH MM DD YY SEX M F

b. OTHER INSURED'S DATE OF BIRTH MM DD YY SEX M F

b. AUTO ACCIDENT? PLACE (State) YES NO

b. EMPLOYER'S NAME OR SCHOOL NAME

c. EMPLOYER'S NAME OR SCHOOL NAME

c. OTHER ACCIDENT? YES NO

c. INSURANCE PLAN NAME OR PROGRAM NAME

d. INSURANCE PLAN NAME OR PROGRAM NAME

10d. RESERVED FOR LOCAL USE

d. IS THERE ANOTHER HEALTH BENEFIT PLAN? YES NO If yes, return to and complete item 9 a – d.

READ BACK OF FORM BEFORE COMPLETING & SIGNING THIS FORM.

12. PATIENT'S OR AUTHORIZED PERSON'S SIGNATURE I authorize the release of any medical or other information necessary to process this claim. I also request payment of government benefits either to myself or to the party who accepts assignment below.

SIGNED DATE

13. INSURED'S OR AUTHORIZED PERSON'S SIGNATURE I authorize payment of medical benefits to the undersigned physician or supplier for services described below.

SIGNED

PATIENT AND INSURED INFORMATION

14. DATE OF CURRENT: MM DD YY ILLNESS (First symptom) OR INJURY (Accident) OR PREGNANCY (LMP)

15. IF PATIENT HAS HAD SAME OR SIMILAR ILLNESS, GIVE FIRST DATE MM DD YY

16. DATES PATIENT UNABLE TO WORK IN CURRENT OCCUPATION MM DD YY FROM MM DD YY TO

17. NAME OF REFERRING PHYSICIAN OR OTHER SOURCE

17a. I.D. NUMBER OF REFERRING PHYSICIAN

18. HOSPITALIZATION DATES RELATED TO CURRENT SERVICES MM DD YY FROM MM DD YY TO

19. RESERVED FOR LOCAL USE

20. OUTSIDE LAB? YES NO $ CHARGES

21. DIAGNOSIS OR NATURE OF ILLNESS OR INJURY. (RELATE ITEMS 1, 2, 3, OR 4 TO ITEM 24E BY LINE)

1. ___ . __

2. ___ . __

3. ___ . __

4. ___ . __

22. MEDICAID RESUBMISSION CODE ORIGINAL REF. NO.

23. PRIOR AUTHORIZATION NUMBER

24. A DATE(S) OF SERVICE From MM DD YY	To MM DD YY	B Place of Service	C Type of Service	D PROCEDURES, SERVICES, OR SUPPLIES (Explain Unusual Circumstances) CPT/HCPCS MODIFIER	E DIAGNOSIS CODE	F $ CHARGES	G DAYS OR UNITS	H EPSDT Family Plan	I EMG	J COB	K RESERVED FOR LOCAL USE
1											
2											
3											
4											
5											
6											

PHYSICIAN OR SUPPLIER INFORMATION

25. FEDERAL TAX I.D. NUMBER SSN EIN

26. PATIENT'S ACCOUNT NO.

27. ACCEPT ASSIGNMENT? (For govt. claims, see back) YES NO

28. TOTAL CHARGE $

29. AMOUNT PAID $

30. BALANCE DUE $

31. SIGNATURE OF PHYSICIAN OR SUPPLIER INCLUDING DEGREES OR CREDENTIALS (I certify that the statements on the reverse apply to this bill and are made a part thereof.)

SIGNED DATE

32. NAME AND ADDRESS OF FACILITY WHERE SERVICES WERE RENDERED (If other than home or office)

33. PHYSICIAN'S, SUPPLIER'S BILLING NAME, ADDRESS, ZIP CODE & PHONE #

PIN# GRP#

(SAMPLE ONLY - NOT APPROVED FOR USE)

PLEASE PRINT OR TYPE

SAMPLE FORM 1500
SAMPLE FORM 1500 SAMPLE FORM 1500

Case Study 13-c

DATE	REMARKS
07/03/YYYY	

PATIENT		CHART #	SEX	BIRTHDATE
Virginia A. Love	212-44-6161	13-c	F	07/04/1962

MAILING ADDRESS	CITY	STATE	ZIP	HOME PHONE	WORK PHONE
61 Isaiah Circle	Anywhere	US	12345	(101) 333 5555	444 5555

EMPLOYER	ADDRESS	PATIENT STATUS
None		X MARRIED DIVORCED SINGLE STUDENT OTHER

INSURANCE: PRIMARY	ID#	GROUP	SECONDARY POLICY	ID#	GROUP
BCBS POS	XWN 212-56-7972	123			

POLICYHOLDER NAME	BIRTHDATE	RELATIONSHIP	POLICYHOLDER NAME	BIRTHDATE	RELATIONSHIP
Charles L. Love	10/06/60	Spouse			

SUPPLEMENTAL PLAN	EMPLOYER

POLICYHOLDER NAME	BIRTHDATE	RELATIONSHIP

EMPLOYER: Imperial Bayliners

REFERRING PHYSICIAN UPIN/SSN:

DIAGNOSIS	CODE
1. Chronic conjunctivitis	372.10
2. Contact dermatitis	692.9
3.	
4.	

PLACE OF SERVICE: Office

PROCEDURES	CODE	CHARGE
1. Est. patient OV Level I	99211	$ 55.00
2.		
3.		
4.		
5.		
6.		

SPECIAL NOTES

If the conjunctivitis does not clear within one week refer to Dr. Glance

TOTAL CHARGES	PAYMENTS	ADJUSTMENTS	BALANCE
$55.00	-0-	-0-	$55.00

RETURN VISIT	PHYSICIAN SIGNATURE
PRN	Donald L. Givings, M.D.

DONALD L. GIVINGS, M.D.
11350 MEDICAL DRIVE, ANYWHERE US 12345
PHONE NUMBER (101)111-5555

MEDICARE D1234
MEDICAID DLG1234
BCBS 12345

EIN 11-123456
SSN 123-12-1234
PIN DG1234
GRP DG12345

PLEASE
DO NOT
STAPLE
IN THIS
AREA

(SAMPLE ONLY - NOT APPROVED FOR USE)

CARRIER

PICA

HEALTH INSURANCE CLAIM FORM

PICA

1. MEDICARE (Medicare #) MEDICAID (Medicaid #) CHAMPUS (Sponsor's SSN) CHAMPVA (VA File #) GROUP HEALTH PLAN (SSN or ID) FECA BLK LUNG (SSN) OTHER (ID)

1a. INSURED'S I.D. NUMBER (FOR PROGRAM IN ITEM 1)

2. PATIENT'S NAME (Last Name, First Name, Middle Initial)

3. PATIENT'S BIRTH DATE MM DD YY SEX M F

4. INSURED'S NAME (Last Name, First Name, Middle Initial)

5. PATIENT'S ADDRESS (No. Street)

6. PATIENT RELATIONSHIP TO INSURED Self Spouse Child Other

7. INSURED'S ADDRESS (No. Street)

CITY STATE

8. PATIENT STATUS Single Married Other

CITY STATE

ZIP CODE TELEPHONE (Include Area Code) ( )

Employed Full-Time Student Part-Time Student

ZIP CODE TELEPHONE (INCLUDE AREA CODE) ( )

9. OTHER INSURED'S NAME (Last Name, First Name, Middle Initial)

10. IS PATIENT'S CONDITION RELATED TO:

11. INSURED'S POLICY GROUP OR FECA NUMBER

a. OTHER INSURED'S POLICY OR GROUP NUMBER

a. EMPLOYMENT? (CURRENT OR PREVIOUS) YES NO

a. INSURED'S DATE OF BIRTH MM DD YY SEX M F

b. OTHER INSURED'S DATE OF BIRTH MM DD YY SEX M F

b. AUTO ACCIDENT? YES NO PLACE (State)

b. EMPLOYER'S NAME OR SCHOOL NAME

c. EMPLOYER'S NAME OR SCHOOL NAME

c. OTHER ACCIDENT? YES NO

c. INSURANCE PLAN NAME OR PROGRAM NAME

d. INSURANCE PLAN NAME OR PROGRAM NAME

10d. RESERVED FOR LOCAL USE

d. IS THERE ANOTHER HEALTH BENEFIT PLAN? YES NO If yes, return to and complete item 9 a – d.

READ BACK OF FORM BEFORE COMPLETING & SIGNING THIS FORM.

12. PATIENT'S OR AUTHORIZED PERSON'S SIGNATURE I authorize the release of any medical or other information necessary to process this claim. I also request payment of government benefits either to myself or to the party who accepts assignment below.

SIGNED DATE

13. INSURED'S OR AUTHORIZED PERSON'S SIGNATURE I authorize payment of medical benefits to the undersigned physician or supplier for services described below.

SIGNED

PATIENT AND INSURED INFORMATION

14. DATE OF CURRENT: MM DD YY ILLNESS (First symptom) OR INJURY (Accident) OR PREGNANCY (LMP)

15. IF PATIENT HAS HAD SAME OR SIMILAR ILLNESS, GIVE FIRST DATE MM DD YY

16. DATES PATIENT UNABLE TO WORK IN CURRENT OCCUPATION FROM MM DD YY TO MM DD YY

17. NAME OF REFERRING PHYSICIAN OR OTHER SOURCE

17a. I.D. NUMBER OF REFERRING PHYSICIAN

18. HOSPITALIZATION DATES RELATED TO CURRENT SERVICES FROM MM DD YY TO MM DD YY

19. RESERVED FOR LOCAL USE

20. OUTSIDE LAB? YES NO $ CHARGES

21. DIAGNOSIS OR NATURE OF ILLNESS OR INJURY. (RELATE ITEMS 1, 2, 3, OR 4 TO ITEM 24E BY LINE)

1. ___ . __

3. ___ . __

2. ___ . __

4. ___ . __

22. MEDICAID RESUBMISSION CODE ORIGINAL REF. NO.

23. PRIOR AUTHORIZATION NUMBER

24. A DATE(S) OF SERVICE From MM DD YY To MM DD YY	B Place of Service	C Type of Service	D PROCEDURES, SERVICES, OR SUPPLIES (Explain Unusual Circumstances) CPT/HCPCS MODIFIER	E DIAGNOSIS CODE	F $ CHARGES	G DAYS OR UNITS	H EPSDT Family Plan	I EMG	J COB	K RESERVED FOR LOCAL USE
1										
2										
3										
4										
5										
6										

25. FEDERAL TAX I.D. NUMBER SSN EIN

26. PATIENT'S ACCOUNT NO.

27. ACCEPT ASSIGNMENT? (For govt. claims, see back) YES NO

28. TOTAL CHARGE $

29. AMOUNT PAID $

30. BALANCE DUE $

31. SIGNATURE OF PHYSICIAN OR SUPPLIER INCLUDING DEGREES OR CREDENTIALS (I certify that the statements on the reverse apply to this bill and are made a part thereof.)

SIGNED DATE

32. NAME AND ADDRESS OF FACILITY WHERE SERVICES WERE RENDERED (If other than home or office)

33. PHYSICIAN'S, SUPPLIER'S BILLING NAME, ADDRESS, ZIP CODE & PHONE #

PIN# GRP#

PHYSICIAN OR SUPPLIER INFORMATION

(SAMPLE ONLY - NOT APPROVED FOR USE)

PLEASE PRINT OR TYPE

SAMPLE FORM 1500
SAMPLE FORM 1500 SAMPLE FORM 1500

Case Study 13-d

DATE	REMARKS
07/03/YYYY	Prior Authorization #79254

PATIENT		CHART #	SEX	BIRTHDATE
Virginia A. Love	212-44-6161	13-d	F	07/04/1962

MAILING ADDRESS	CITY	STATE	ZIP	HOME PHONE	WORK PHONE
61 Isaiah Circle	Anywhere	US	12345	(101) 333 5555	444 5555

EMPLOYER	ADDRESS	PATIENT STATUS
None		X MARRIED DIVORCED SINGLE STUDENT OTHER

INSURANCE: PRIMARY	ID#	GROUP	SECONDARY POLICY	ID#	GROUP
BCBS POS	XWN 212-56-7972	123			

POLICYHOLDER NAME	BIRTHDATE	RELATIONSHIP	POLICYHOLDER NAME	BIRTHDATE	RELATIONSHIP
Charles L. Love	10/06/60	Spouse			

SUPPLEMENTAL PLAN	EMPLOYER

POLICYHOLDER NAME	BIRTHDATE	RELATIONSHIP

EMPLOYER: Imperial Bayliners

REFERRING PHYSICIAN UPIN/SSN: Donald L. Givings, M.D. 123-12-1234

DIAGNOSIS	CODE
1. Chronic conjunctivitis	372.10
2. Conjunctival degeneration	372.50
3.	
4.	

PLACE OF SERVICE: Office

PROCEDURES	CODE	CHARGE
1. Office consult Level I	99241	$ 65.00
2.		
3.		
4.		
5.		
6.		

SPECIAL NOTES

TOTAL CHARGES	PAYMENTS	ADJUSTMENTS	BALANCE
$65.00	-0-	-0-	$65.00

RETURN VISIT	PHYSICIAN SIGNATURE
	Iris A. Glance, M.D.

MEDICARE I1234
MEDICAID IG1234
BCBS 45678

IRIS A. GLANCE, M.D. OPTHALMOLOGIST
66 GRANITE DRIVE, ANYWHERE US 12345
PHONE NUMBER (101)111-5555

EIN 11616161
SSN 166-12-1234
PIN IG1234
GRP IG12345

PLEASE DO NOT STAPLE IN THIS AREA

(SAMPLE ONLY - NOT APPROVED FOR USE)

CARRIER

PICA

HEALTH INSURANCE CLAIM FORM

PICA

1. MEDICARE (Medicare #) | MEDICAID (Medicaid #) | CHAMPUS (Sponsor's SSN) | CHAMPVA (VA File #) | GROUP HEALTH PLAN (SSN or ID) | FECA BLK LUNG (SSN) | OTHER (ID)

1a. INSURED'S I.D. NUMBER (FOR PROGRAM IN ITEM 1)

2. PATIENT'S NAME (Last Name, First Name, Middle Initial)

3. PATIENT'S BIRTH DATE MM DD YY SEX M F

4. INSURED'S NAME (Last Name, First Name, Middle Initial)

5. PATIENT'S ADDRESS (No. Street)

6. PATIENT RELATIONSHIP TO INSURED Self Spouse Child Other

7. INSURED'S ADDRESS (No. Street)

CITY STATE

8. PATIENT STATUS Single Married Other

CITY STATE

ZIP CODE TELEPHONE (Include Area Code) ( )

Employed Full-Time Student Part-Time Student

ZIP CODE TELEPHONE (INCLUDE AREA CODE) ( )

9. OTHER INSURED'S NAME (Last Name, First Name, Middle Initial)

10. IS PATIENT'S CONDITION RELATED TO:

11. INSURED'S POLICY GROUP OR FECA NUMBER

a. OTHER INSURED'S POLICY OR GROUP NUMBER

a. EMPLOYMENT? (CURRENT OR PREVIOUS) YES NO

a. INSURED'S DATE OF BIRTH MM DD YY SEX M F

b. OTHER INSURED'S DATE OF BIRTH MM DD YY SEX M F

b. AUTO ACCIDENT? PLACE (State) YES NO

b. EMPLOYER'S NAME OR SCHOOL NAME

c. EMPLOYER'S NAME OR SCHOOL NAME

c. OTHER ACCIDENT? YES NO

c. INSURANCE PLAN NAME OR PROGRAM NAME

d. INSURANCE PLAN NAME OR PROGRAM NAME

10d. RESERVED FOR LOCAL USE

d. IS THERE ANOTHER HEALTH BENEFIT PLAN? YES NO If yes, return to and complete item 9 a – d.

READ BACK OF FORM BEFORE COMPLETING & SIGNING THIS FORM.

12. PATIENT'S OR AUTHORIZED PERSON'S SIGNATURE I authorize the release of any medical or other information necessary to process this claim. I also request payment of government benefits either to myself or to the party who accepts assignment below.

SIGNED ______ DATE ______

13. INSURED'S OR AUTHORIZED PERSON'S SIGNATURE I authorize payment of medical benefits to the undersigned physician or supplier for services described below.

SIGNED ______

PATIENT AND INSURED INFORMATION

14. DATE OF CURRENT: MM DD YY ILLNESS (First symptom) OR INJURY (Accident) OR PREGNANCY (LMP)

15. IF PATIENT HAS HAD SAME OR SIMILAR ILLNESS, GIVE FIRST DATE MM DD YY

16. DATES PATIENT UNABLE TO WORK IN CURRENT OCCUPATION FROM MM DD YY TO MM DD YY

17. NAME OF REFERRING PHYSICIAN OR OTHER SOURCE

17a. I.D. NUMBER OF REFERRING PHYSICIAN

18. HOSPITALIZATION DATES RELATED TO CURRENT SERVICES FROM MM DD YY TO MM DD YY

19. RESERVED FOR LOCAL USE

20. OUTSIDE LAB? YES NO $ CHARGES

21. DIAGNOSIS OR NATURE OF ILLNESS OR INJURY. (RELATE ITEMS 1, 2, 3, OR 4 TO ITEM 24E BY LINE)

1. ___ . __ 3. ___ . __

2. ___ . __ 4. ___ . __

22. MEDICAID RESUBMISSION CODE ORIGINAL REF. NO.

23. PRIOR AUTHORIZATION NUMBER

24. A DATE(S) OF SERVICE From MM DD YY To MM DD YY	B Place of Service	C Type of Service	D PROCEDURES, SERVICES, OR SUPPLIES (Explain Unusual Circumstances) CPT/HCPCS MODIFIER	E DIAGNOSIS CODE	F $ CHARGES	G DAYS OR UNITS	H EPSDT Family Plan	I EMG	J COB	K RESERVED FOR LOCAL USE
1										
2										
3										
4										
5										
6										

25. FEDERAL TAX I.D. NUMBER SSN EIN

26. PATIENT'S ACCOUNT NO.

27. ACCEPT ASSIGNMENT? (For govt. claims, see back) YES NO

28. TOTAL CHARGE $

29. AMOUNT PAID $

30. BALANCE DUE $

31. SIGNATURE OF PHYSICIAN OR SUPPLIER INCLUDING DEGREES OR CREDENTIALS (I certify that the statements on the reverse apply to this bill and are made a part thereof.)

SIGNED DATE

32. NAME AND ADDRESS OF FACILITY WHERE SERVICES WERE RENDERED (If other than home or office)

33. PHYSICIAN'S, SUPPLIER'S BILLING NAME, ADDRESS, ZIP CODE & PHONE #

PIN# GRP#

PHYSICIAN OR SUPPLIER INFORMATION

(SAMPLE ONLY - NOT APPROVED FOR USE)

PLEASE PRINT OR TYPE

SAMPLE FORM 1500
SAMPLE FORM 1500 SAMPLE FORM 1500

DATE	REMARKS			
09/03/YYYY				
PATIENT		CHART #	SEX	BIRTHDATE
Keith S. Kutter 313-99-7777		13-e	M	12/01/1955

MAILING ADDRESS	CITY	STATE	ZIP	HOME PHONE	WORK PHONE
22 Pinewood Avenue	Anywhere	US	12345	(101) 333 5555	444 5555

EMPLOYER	ADDRESS	PATIENT STATUS
First League	Anywhere US	X MARRIED DIVORCED SINGLE STUDENT OTHER

INSURANCE: PRIMARY	ID#	GROUP	SECONDARY POLICY	ID#	GROUP
BCBS US	FLX 313-99-7777	567	Aetna	212-44-6868	S234

POLICYHOLDER NAME	BIRTHDATE	RELATIONSHIP	POLICYHOLDER NAME	BIRTHDATE	RELATIONSHIP
		Self	Linda Kutter	05/22/56	Spouse

SUPPLEMENTAL PLAN	EMPLOYER
	Anderson Music & Sound

POLICYHOLDER NAME	BIRTHDATE	RELATIONSHIP	DIAGNOSIS	CODE
			1. Muscle Spasms	728.85
EMPLOYER			2.	
			3.	
REFERRING PHYSICIAN UPIN/SSN			4.	

PLACE OF SERVICE Office

PROCEDURES	CODE	CHARGE
1. Est. patient OV Level II	99212	$ 65.00
2.		
3.		
4.		
5.		
6.		

SPECIAL NOTES

Refer to a chiropractor

TOTAL CHARGES	PAYMENTS	ADJUSTMENTS	BALANCE
$65.00	-0-	-0-	$65.00

RETURN VISIT	PHYSICIAN SIGNATURE
	Donald L. Givings, M.D.

MEDICARE D1234 MEDICAID DLG1234 BCBS 12345	**DONALD L. GIVINGS, M.D.** **11350 MEDICAL DRIVE, ANYWHERE US 12345** **PHONE NUMBER (101)111-5555**	EIN 11-123456 SSN 123-12-1234 PIN DG1234 GRP DG12345

PLEASE
DO NOT
STAPLE
IN THIS
AREA

(SAMPLE ONLY - NOT APPROVED FOR USE)

CARRIER

PICA

HEALTH INSURANCE CLAIM FORM

PICA

1. MEDICARE (Medicare #) MEDICAID (Medicaid #) CHAMPUS (Sponsor's SSN) CHAMPVA (VA File #) GROUP HEALTH PLAN (SSN or ID) FECA BLK LUNG (SSN) OTHER (ID)

1a. INSURED'S I.D. NUMBER (FOR PROGRAM IN ITEM 1)

2. PATIENT'S NAME (Last Name, First Name, Middle Initial)

3. PATIENT'S BIRTH DATE MM DD YY SEX M F

4. INSURED'S NAME (Last Name, First Name, Middle Initial)

5. PATIENT'S ADDRESS (No. Street)

6. PATIENT RELATIONSHIP TO INSURED Self Spouse Child Other

7. INSURED'S ADDRESS (No. Street)

CITY STATE

8. PATIENT STATUS Single Married Other

CITY STATE

ZIP CODE TELEPHONE (Include Area Code) ( )

Employed Full-Time Student Part-Time Student

ZIP CODE TELEPHONE (INCLUDE AREA CODE) ( )

9. OTHER INSURED'S NAME (Last Name, First Name, Middle Initial)

10. IS PATIENT'S CONDITION RELATED TO:

11. INSURED'S POLICY GROUP OR FECA NUMBER

a. OTHER INSURED'S POLICY OR GROUP NUMBER

a. EMPLOYMENT? (CURRENT OR PREVIOUS) YES NO

a. INSURED'S DATE OF BIRTH MM DD YY SEX M F

b. OTHER INSURED'S DATE OF BIRTH MM DD YY SEX M F

b. AUTO ACCIDENT? YES NO PLACE (State)

b. EMPLOYER'S NAME OR SCHOOL NAME

c. EMPLOYER'S NAME OR SCHOOL NAME

c. OTHER ACCIDENT? YES NO

c. INSURANCE PLAN NAME OR PROGRAM NAME

d. INSURANCE PLAN NAME OR PROGRAM NAME

10d. RESERVED FOR LOCAL USE

d. IS THERE ANOTHER HEALTH BENEFIT PLAN? YES NO If yes, return to and complete item 9 a – d.

READ BACK OF FORM BEFORE COMPLETING & SIGNING THIS FORM.

12. PATIENT'S OR AUTHORIZED PERSON'S SIGNATURE I authorize the release of any medical or other information necessary to process this claim. I also request payment of government benefits either to myself or to the party who accepts assignment below.

SIGNED ______ DATE ______

13. INSURED'S OR AUTHORIZED PERSON'S SIGNATURE I authorize payment of medical benefits to the undersigned physician or supplier for services described below.

SIGNED ______

PATIENT AND INSURED INFORMATION

14. DATE OF CURRENT: MM DD YY ◀ ILLNESS (First symptom) OR INJURY (Accident) OR PREGNANCY (LMP)

15. IF PATIENT HAS HAD SAME OR SIMILAR ILLNESS, GIVE FIRST DATE MM DD YY

16. DATES PATIENT UNABLE TO WORK IN CURRENT OCCUPATION FROM MM DD YY TO MM DD YY

17. NAME OF REFERRING PHYSICIAN OR OTHER SOURCE

17a. I.D. NUMBER OF REFERRING PHYSICIAN

18. HOSPITALIZATION DATES RELATED TO CURRENT SERVICES FROM MM DD YY TO MM DD YY

19. RESERVED FOR LOCAL USE

20. OUTSIDE LAB? YES NO $ CHARGES

21. DIAGNOSIS OR NATURE OF ILLNESS OR INJURY. (RELATE ITEMS 1, 2, 3, OR 4 TO ITEM 24E BY LINE)

1. ___ . __ 3. ___ . __

2. ___ . __ 4. ___ . __

22. MEDICAID RESUBMISSION CODE ORIGINAL REF. NO.

23. PRIOR AUTHORIZATION NUMBER

24. A DATE(S) OF SERVICE From MM DD YY To MM DD YY	B Place of Service	C Type of Service	D PROCEDURES, SERVICES, OR SUPPLIES (Explain Unusual Circumstances) CPT/HCPCS MODIFIER	E DIAGNOSIS CODE	F $ CHARGES	G DAYS OR UNITS	H EPSDT Family Plan	I EMG	J COB	K RESERVED FOR LOCAL USE
1										
2										
3										
4										
5										
6										

25. FEDERAL TAX I.D. NUMBER SSN EIN

26. PATIENT'S ACCOUNT NO.

27. ACCEPT ASSIGNMENT? (For govt. claims, see back) YES NO

28. TOTAL CHARGE $

29. AMOUNT PAID $

30. BALANCE DUE $

31. SIGNATURE OF PHYSICIAN OR SUPPLIER INCLUDING DEGREES OR CREDENTIALS (I certify that the statements on the reverse apply to this bill and are made a part thereof.)

SIGNED DATE

32. NAME AND ADDRESS OF FACILITY WHERE SERVICES WERE RENDERED (If other than home or office)

33. PHYSICIAN'S, SUPPLIER'S BILLING NAME, ADDRESS, ZIP CODE & PHONE #

PIN# GRP#

PHYSICIAN OR SUPPLIER INFORMATION

(SAMPLE ONLY - NOT APPROVED FOR USE)

PLEASE PRINT OR TYPE

SAMPLE FORM 1500
SAMPLE FORM 1500 SAMPLE FORM 1500

PLEASE
DO NOT
STAPLE
IN THIS
AREA

(SAMPLE ONLY - NOT APPROVED FOR USE)

CARRIER

PICA

HEALTH INSURANCE CLAIM FORM

PICA

1. MEDICARE (Medicare #) MEDICAID (Medicaid #) CHAMPUS (Sponsor's SSN) CHAMPVA (VA File #) GROUP HEALTH PLAN (SSN or ID) FECA BLK LUNG (SSN) OTHER (ID)

1a. INSURED'S I.D. NUMBER (FOR PROGRAM IN ITEM 1)

2. PATIENT'S NAME (Last Name, First Name, Middle Initial)

3. PATIENT'S BIRTH DATE MM DD YY SEX M F

4. INSURED'S NAME (Last Name, First Name, Middle Initial)

5. PATIENT'S ADDRESS (No. Street)

6. PATIENT RELATIONSHIP TO INSURED Self Spouse Child Other

7. INSURED'S ADDRESS (No. Street)

CITY STATE

8. PATIENT STATUS Single Married Other

CITY STATE

ZIP CODE TELEPHONE (Include Area Code) ( )

Employed Full-Time Student Part-Time Student

ZIP CODE TELEPHONE (INCLUDE AREA CODE) ( )

9. OTHER INSURED'S NAME (Last Name, First Name, Middle Initial)

10. IS PATIENT'S CONDITION RELATED TO:

11. INSURED'S POLICY GROUP OR FECA NUMBER

a. OTHER INSURED'S POLICY OR GROUP NUMBER

a. EMPLOYMENT? (CURRENT OR PREVIOUS) YES NO

a. INSURED'S DATE OF BIRTH MM DD YY SEX M F

b. OTHER INSURED'S DATE OF BIRTH MM DD YY SEX M F

b. AUTO ACCIDENT? PLACE (State) YES NO

b. EMPLOYER'S NAME OR SCHOOL NAME

c. EMPLOYER'S NAME OR SCHOOL NAME

c. OTHER ACCIDENT? YES NO

c. INSURANCE PLAN NAME OR PROGRAM NAME

d. INSURANCE PLAN NAME OR PROGRAM NAME

10d. RESERVED FOR LOCAL USE

d. IS THERE ANOTHER HEALTH BENEFIT PLAN? YES NO If yes, return to and complete item 9 a – d.

READ BACK OF FORM BEFORE COMPLETING & SIGNING THIS FORM.

12. PATIENT'S OR AUTHORIZED PERSON'S SIGNATURE I authorize the release of any medical or other information necessary to process this claim. I also request payment of government benefits either to myself or to the party who accepts assignment below.

SIGNED ______ DATE ______

13. INSURED'S OR AUTHORIZED PERSON'S SIGNATURE I authorize payment of medical benefits to the undersigned physician or supplier for services described below.

SIGNED ______

PATIENT AND INSURED INFORMATION

14. DATE OF CURRENT: MM DD YY ILLNESS (First symptom) OR INJURY (Accident) OR PREGNANCY (LMP)

15. IF PATIENT HAS HAD SAME OR SIMILAR ILLNESS, GIVE FIRST DATE MM DD YY

16. DATES PATIENT UNABLE TO WORK IN CURRENT OCCUPATION FROM MM DD YY TO MM DD YY

17. NAME OF REFERRING PHYSICIAN OR OTHER SOURCE

17a. I.D. NUMBER OF REFERRING PHYSICIAN

18. HOSPITALIZATION DATES RELATED TO CURRENT SERVICES FROM MM DD YY TO MM DD YY

19. RESERVED FOR LOCAL USE

20. OUTSIDE LAB? YES NO $ CHARGES

21. DIAGNOSIS OR NATURE OF ILLNESS OR INJURY. (RELATE ITEMS 1, 2, 3, OR 4 TO ITEM 24E BY LINE)

1. ___ . __
2. ___ . __
3. ___ . __
4. ___ . __

22. MEDICAID RESUBMISSION CODE ORIGINAL REF. NO.

23. PRIOR AUTHORIZATION NUMBER

24. A DATE(S) OF SERVICE From MM DD YY	To MM DD YY	B Place of Service	C Type of Service	D PROCEDURES, SERVICES, OR SUPPLIES (Explain Unusual Circumstances) CPT/HCPCS MODIFIER	E DIAGNOSIS CODE	F $ CHARGES	G DAYS OR UNITS	H EPSDT Family Plan	I EMG	J COB	K RESERVED FOR LOCAL USE
1											
2											
3											
4											
5											
6											

25. FEDERAL TAX I.D. NUMBER SSN EIN

26. PATIENT'S ACCOUNT NO.

27. ACCEPT ASSIGNMENT? (For govt. claims, see back) YES NO

28. TOTAL CHARGE $

29. AMOUNT PAID $

30. BALANCE DUE $

31. SIGNATURE OF PHYSICIAN OR SUPPLIER INCLUDING DEGREES OR CREDENTIALS (I certify that the statements on the reverse apply to this bill and are made a part thereof.)

SIGNED DATE

32. NAME AND ADDRESS OF FACILITY WHERE SERVICES WERE RENDERED (If other than home or office)

33. PHYSICIAN'S, SUPPLIER'S BILLING NAME, ADDRESS, ZIP CODE & PHONE #

PIN# GRP#

PHYSICIAN OR SUPPLIER INFORMATION

(SAMPLE ONLY - NOT APPROVED FOR USE)

PLEASE PRINT OR TYPE

SAMPLE FORM 1500
SAMPLE FORM 1500 SAMPLE FORM 1500

Case Study 13-f

DATE	REMARKS
09/10/YYYY	

PATIENT		CHART #	SEX	BIRTHDATE
Keith S. Kutter	313-99-7777	13-f	M	12/01/1955

MAILING ADDRESS	CITY	STATE	ZIP	HOME PHONE	WORK PHONE
22 Pinewood Avenue	Anywhere	US	12345	(101) 333 5555	444 5555

EMPLOYER	ADDRESS	PATIENT STATUS
First League	Anywhere US	X MARRIED DIVORCED SINGLE STUDENT OTHER

INSURANCE: PRIMARY	ID#	GROUP	SECONDARY POLICY	ID#	GROUP
BCBS US	FLX 313-99-7777	567	Aetna	212-44-6868	S234

POLICYHOLDER NAME	BIRTHDATE	RELATIONSHIP	POLICYHOLDER NAME	BIRTHDATE	RELATIONSHIP
		Self	Linda Kutter	05/22/56	Spouse

SUPPLEMENTAL PLAN	EMPLOYER
	Anderson Music & Sound

POLICYHOLDER NAME	BIRTHDATE	RELATIONSHIP

EMPLOYER

REFERRING PHYSICIAN UPIN/SSN: Donald L. Givings M.D. 123-12-1234

DIAGNOSIS	CODE
1. Cervical lesion	739.1
2. Rib cage lesion	739.8
3. Disorder of soft tissue	729.1
4. Muscle spasms	728.85

PLACE OF SERVICE Office

PROCEDURES	CODE	CHARGE
1. Manipulation, 3-4 regions	98941	$ 55.00
2. Manipulation, extraspinal	98943-51	35.00
3. Massage	97124-51	30.00
4. Mechanical traction	97012-51	27.00
5. Electrical stimulation	97014-51	25.00
6.		

SPECIAL NOTES

TOTAL CHARGES	PAYMENTS	ADJUSTMENTS	BALANCE
$172.00	-0-	-0-	$172.00

RETURN VISIT	PHYSICIAN SIGNATURE
PRN	Robert Strain, D.C.

MEDICARE R1234
MEDICAID RSD1234
BCBS 98765

ROBERT STRAIN, D.C. CHIROPRACTOR
234 WINDING BEND ROAD, ANYWHERE, US 12345
PHONE NUMBER (101)111-5555

EIN 11446688
SSN 222-12-1234
PIN RS1234
GRP RS12345

PLEASE
DO NOT
STAPLE
IN THIS
AREA

(SAMPLE ONLY - NOT APPROVED FOR USE)

CARRIER

PICA

HEALTH INSURANCE CLAIM FORM

PICA

1. MEDICARE (Medicare #) MEDICAID (Medicaid #) CHAMPUS (Sponsor's SSN) CHAMPVA (VA File #) GROUP HEALTH PLAN (SSN or ID) FECA BLK LUNG (SSN) OTHER (ID)

1a. INSURED'S I.D. NUMBER (FOR PROGRAM IN ITEM 1)

2. PATIENT'S NAME (Last Name, First Name, Middle Initial)

3. PATIENT'S BIRTH DATE MM DD YY SEX M F

4. INSURED'S NAME (Last Name, First Name, Middle Initial)

5. PATIENT'S ADDRESS (No. Street)

6. PATIENT RELATIONSHIP TO INSURED Self Spouse Child Other

7. INSURED'S ADDRESS (No. Street)

CITY STATE

8. PATIENT STATUS Single Married Other

CITY STATE

ZIP CODE TELEPHONE (Include Area Code) ( )

Employed Full-Time Student Part-Time Student

ZIP CODE TELEPHONE (INCLUDE AREA CODE) ( )

9. OTHER INSURED'S NAME (Last Name, First Name, Middle Initial)

10. IS PATIENT'S CONDITION RELATED TO:

11. INSURED'S POLICY GROUP OR FECA NUMBER

a. OTHER INSURED'S POLICY OR GROUP NUMBER

a. EMPLOYMENT? (CURRENT OR PREVIOUS) YES NO

a. INSURED'S DATE OF BIRTH MM DD YY SEX M F

b. OTHER INSURED'S DATE OF BIRTH MM DD YY SEX M F

b. AUTO ACCIDENT? PLACE (State) YES NO

b. EMPLOYER'S NAME OR SCHOOL NAME

c. EMPLOYER'S NAME OR SCHOOL NAME

c. OTHER ACCIDENT? YES NO

c. INSURANCE PLAN NAME OR PROGRAM NAME

d. INSURANCE PLAN NAME OR PROGRAM NAME

10d. RESERVED FOR LOCAL USE

d. IS THERE ANOTHER HEALTH BENEFIT PLAN? YES NO If yes, return to and complete item 9 a – d.

READ BACK OF FORM BEFORE COMPLETING & SIGNING THIS FORM.

12. PATIENT'S OR AUTHORIZED PERSON'S SIGNATURE I authorize the release of any medical or other information necessary to process this claim. I also request payment of government benefits either to myself or to the party who accepts assignment below.

SIGNED DATE

13. INSURED'S OR AUTHORIZED PERSON'S SIGNATURE I authorize payment of medical benefits to the undersigned physician or supplier for services described below.

SIGNED

PATIENT AND INSURED INFORMATION

14. DATE OF CURRENT: MM DD YY ILLNESS (First symptom) OR INJURY (Accident) OR PREGNANCY (LMP)

15. IF PATIENT HAS HAD SAME OR SIMILAR ILLNESS, GIVE FIRST DATE MM DD YY

16. DATES PATIENT UNABLE TO WORK IN CURRENT OCCUPATION FROM MM DD YY TO MM DD YY

17. NAME OF REFERRING PHYSICIAN OR OTHER SOURCE

17a. I.D. NUMBER OF REFERRING PHYSICIAN

18. HOSPITALIZATION DATES RELATED TO CURRENT SERVICES FROM MM DD YY TO MM DD YY

19. RESERVED FOR LOCAL USE

20. OUTSIDE LAB? YES NO $ CHARGES

21. DIAGNOSIS OR NATURE OF ILLNESS OR INJURY. (RELATE ITEMS 1, 2, 3, OR 4 TO ITEM 24E BY LINE)

1. ___ . __ 3. ___ . __

2. ___ . __ 4. ___ . __

22. MEDICAID RESUBMISSION CODE ORIGINAL REF. NO.

23. PRIOR AUTHORIZATION NUMBER

24. A DATE(S) OF SERVICE From MM DD YY To MM DD YY	B Place of Service	C Type of Service	D PROCEDURES, SERVICES, OR SUPPLIES (Explain Unusual Circumstances) CPT/HCPCS MODIFIER	E DIAGNOSIS CODE	F $ CHARGES	G DAYS OR UNITS	H EPSDT Family Plan	I EMG	J COB	K RESERVED FOR LOCAL USE
1										
2										
3										
4										
5										
6										

25. FEDERAL TAX I.D. NUMBER SSN EIN

26. PATIENT'S ACCOUNT NO.

27. ACCEPT ASSIGNMENT? (For govt. claims, see back) YES NO

28. TOTAL CHARGE $

29. AMOUNT PAID $

30. BALANCE DUE $

31. SIGNATURE OF PHYSICIAN OR SUPPLIER INCLUDING DEGREES OR CREDENTIALS (I certify that the statements on the reverse apply to this bill and are made a part thereof.)

SIGNED DATE

32. NAME AND ADDRESS OF FACILITY WHERE SERVICES WERE RENDERED (If other than home or office)

33. PHYSICIAN'S, SUPPLIER'S BILLING NAME, ADDRESS, ZIP CODE & PHONE #

PIN# GRP#

PHYSICIAN OR SUPPLIER INFORMATION

(SAMPLE ONLY - NOT APPROVED FOR USE)

PLEASE PRINT OR TYPE

SAMPLE FORM 1500
SAMPLE FORM 1500 SAMPLE FORM 1500

PLEASE
DO NOT
STAPLE
IN THIS
AREA

(SAMPLE ONLY - NOT APPROVED FOR USE)

CARRIER

PICA

HEALTH INSURANCE CLAIM FORM

PICA

1. MEDICARE (Medicare #) MEDICAID (Medicaid #) CHAMPUS (Sponsor's SSN) CHAMPVA (VA File #) GROUP HEALTH PLAN (SSN or ID) FECA BLK LUNG (SSN) OTHER (ID)

1a. INSURED'S I.D. NUMBER (FOR PROGRAM IN ITEM 1)

2. PATIENT'S NAME (Last Name, First Name, Middle Initial)

3. PATIENT'S BIRTH DATE MM DD YY SEX M F

4. INSURED'S NAME (Last Name, First Name, Middle Initial)

5. PATIENT'S ADDRESS (No. Street)

6. PATIENT RELATIONSHIP TO INSURED Self Spouse Child Other

7. INSURED'S ADDRESS (No. Street)

CITY STATE

8. PATIENT STATUS Single Married Other

CITY STATE

ZIP CODE TELEPHONE (Include Area Code) ( )

Employed Full-Time Student Part-Time Student

ZIP CODE TELEPHONE (INCLUDE AREA CODE) ( )

9. OTHER INSURED'S NAME (Last Name, First Name, Middle Initial)

10. IS PATIENT'S CONDITION RELATED TO:

11. INSURED'S POLICY GROUP OR FECA NUMBER

a. OTHER INSURED'S POLICY OR GROUP NUMBER

a. EMPLOYMENT? (CURRENT OR PREVIOUS) YES NO

a. INSURED'S DATE OF BIRTH MM DD YY SEX M F

b. OTHER INSURED'S DATE OF BIRTH MM DD YY SEX M F

b. AUTO ACCIDENT? YES NO PLACE (State)

b. EMPLOYER'S NAME OR SCHOOL NAME

c. EMPLOYER'S NAME OR SCHOOL NAME

c. OTHER ACCIDENT? YES NO

c. INSURANCE PLAN NAME OR PROGRAM NAME

d. INSURANCE PLAN NAME OR PROGRAM NAME

10d. RESERVED FOR LOCAL USE

d. IS THERE ANOTHER HEALTH BENEFIT PLAN? YES NO If yes, return to and complete item 9 a – d.

READ BACK OF FORM BEFORE COMPLETING & SIGNING THIS FORM.

12. PATIENT'S OR AUTHORIZED PERSON'S SIGNATURE I authorize the release of any medical or other information necessary to process this claim. I also request payment of government benefits either to myself or to the party who accepts assignment below.

SIGNED ______ DATE ______

13. INSURED'S OR AUTHORIZED PERSON'S SIGNATURE I authorize payment of medical benefits to the undersigned physician or supplier for services described below.

SIGNED ______

PATIENT AND INSURED INFORMATION

14. DATE OF CURRENT: MM DD YY ILLNESS (First symptom) OR INJURY (Accident) OR PREGNANCY (LMP)

15. IF PATIENT HAS HAD SAME OR SIMILAR ILLNESS, GIVE FIRST DATE MM DD YY

16. DATES PATIENT UNABLE TO WORK IN CURRENT OCCUPATION FROM MM DD YY TO MM DD YY

17. NAME OF REFERRING PHYSICIAN OR OTHER SOURCE

17a. I.D. NUMBER OF REFERRING PHYSICIAN

18. HOSPITALIZATION DATES RELATED TO CURRENT SERVICES FROM MM DD YY TO MM DD YY

19. RESERVED FOR LOCAL USE

20. OUTSIDE LAB? YES NO $ CHARGES

21. DIAGNOSIS OR NATURE OF ILLNESS OR INJURY. (RELATE ITEMS 1, 2, 3, OR 4 TO ITEM 24E BY LINE)

1. ___ . __ 3. ___ . __

2. ___ . __ 4. ___ . __

22. MEDICAID RESUBMISSION CODE ORIGINAL REF. NO.

23. PRIOR AUTHORIZATION NUMBER

24.	A DATE(S) OF SERVICE From MM DD YY	To MM DD YY	B Place of Service	C Type of Service	D PROCEDURES, SERVICES, OR SUPPLIES (Explain Unusual Circumstances) CPT/HCPCS MODIFIER	E DIAGNOSIS CODE	F $ CHARGES	G DAYS OR UNITS	H EPSDT Family Plan	I EMG	J COB	K RESERVED FOR LOCAL USE
1												
2												
3												
4												
5												
6												

25. FEDERAL TAX I.D. NUMBER SSN EIN

26. PATIENT'S ACCOUNT NO.

27. ACCEPT ASSIGNMENT? (For govt. claims, see back) YES NO

28. TOTAL CHARGE $

29. AMOUNT PAID $

30. BALANCE DUE $

31. SIGNATURE OF PHYSICIAN OR SUPPLIER INCLUDING DEGREES OR CREDENTIALS (I certify that the statements on the reverse apply to this bill and are made a part thereof.)

SIGNED DATE

32. NAME AND ADDRESS OF FACILITY WHERE SERVICES WERE RENDERED (If other than home or office)

33. PHYSICIAN'S, SUPPLIER'S BILLING NAME, ADDRESS, ZIP CODE & PHONE #

PIN# GRP#

PHYSICIAN OR SUPPLIER INFORMATION

(SAMPLE ONLY - NOT APPROVED FOR USE)

PLEASE PRINT OR TYPE

SAMPLE FORM 1500
SAMPLE FORM 1500 SAMPLE FORM 1500

Case Study 13-g

DATE	REMARKS
10/23/YYYY	Patient has a $15 copay

PATIENT		CHART #	SEX	BIRTHDATE
Kristen A. Wonder	556-78-7986	13-g	F	04/16/1999

MAILING ADDRESS	CITY	STATE	ZIP	HOME PHONE	WORK PHONE
1654 Willow Tree Dr.	Anywhere	US	12345	(101) 333 5555	444 5555

EMPLOYER	ADDRESS	PATIENT STATUS
None		MARRIED DIVORCED SINGLE (X) STUDENT OTHER

INSURANCE: PRIMARY	ID#	GROUP	SECONDARY POLICY	ID#	GROUP
BCBS US	NYV 415-55-6767	678			

POLICYHOLDER NAME	BIRTHDATE	RELATIONSHIP	POLICYHOLDER NAME	BIRTHDATE	RELATIONSHIP
John F. Wonder	05/22/75	Father			

SUPPLEMENTAL PLAN

EMPLOYER

POLICYHOLDER NAME BIRTHDATE RELATIONSHIP

EMPLOYER: White Water Sales

REFERRING PHYSICIAN UPIN/SSN

DIAGNOSIS	CODE
1. Impacted wax	380.4
2.	
3.	
4.	

PLACE OF SERVICE: Office

PROCEDURES	CODE	CHARGE
1. Est. patient OV Level II	99212	$ 65.00
2. Removal, impacted cerumen	69210	25.00
3.		
4.		
5.		
6.		

SPECIAL NOTES

TOTAL CHARGES	PAYMENTS	ADJUSTMENTS	BALANCE
$90.00	$15.00	-0-	$75.00

RETURN VISIT	PHYSICIAN SIGNATURE
PRN	Donald L. Givings, M.D.

MEDICARE D1234
MEDICAID DLG1234
BCBS 12345

DONALD L. GIVINGS, M.D.
11350 MEDICAL DRIVE, ANYWHERE US 12345
PHONE NUMBER (101)111-5555

EIN 11-123456
SSN 123-12-1234
PIN DG1234
GRP DG12345

PLEASE
DO NOT
STAPLE
IN THIS
AREA

(SAMPLE ONLY - NOT APPROVED FOR USE)

CARRIER

PICA

HEALTH INSURANCE CLAIM FORM

PICA

1. MEDICARE (Medicare #) MEDICAID (Medicaid #) CHAMPUS (Sponsor's SSN) CHAMPVA (VA File #) GROUP HEALTH PLAN (SSN or ID) FECA BLK LUNG (SSN) OTHER (ID)

1a. INSURED'S I.D. NUMBER (FOR PROGRAM IN ITEM 1)

2. PATIENT'S NAME (Last Name, First Name, Middle Initial)

3. PATIENT'S BIRTH DATE MM DD YY SEX M F

4. INSURED'S NAME (Last Name, First Name, Middle Initial)

5. PATIENT'S ADDRESS (No. Street)

6. PATIENT RELATIONSHIP TO INSURED Self Spouse Child Other

7. INSURED'S ADDRESS (No. Street)

CITY STATE

8. PATIENT STATUS Single Married Other

CITY STATE

ZIP CODE TELEPHONE (Include Area Code) ( )

Employed Full-Time Student Part-Time Student

ZIP CODE TELEPHONE (INCLUDE AREA CODE) ( )

9. OTHER INSURED'S NAME (Last Name, First Name, Middle Initial)

10. IS PATIENT'S CONDITION RELATED TO:

11. INSURED'S POLICY GROUP OR FECA NUMBER

a. OTHER INSURED'S POLICY OR GROUP NUMBER

a. EMPLOYMENT? (CURRENT OR PREVIOUS) YES NO

a. INSURED'S DATE OF BIRTH MM DD YY SEX M F

b. OTHER INSURED'S DATE OF BIRTH MM DD YY SEX M F

b. AUTO ACCIDENT? PLACE (State) YES NO

b. EMPLOYER'S NAME OR SCHOOL NAME

c. EMPLOYER'S NAME OR SCHOOL NAME

c. OTHER ACCIDENT? YES NO

c. INSURANCE PLAN NAME OR PROGRAM NAME

d. INSURANCE PLAN NAME OR PROGRAM NAME

10d. RESERVED FOR LOCAL USE

d. IS THERE ANOTHER HEALTH BENEFIT PLAN? YES NO If yes, return to and complete item 9 a – d.

READ BACK OF FORM BEFORE COMPLETING & SIGNING THIS FORM.

12. PATIENT'S OR AUTHORIZED PERSON'S SIGNATURE I authorize the release of any medical or other information necessary to process this claim. I also request payment of government benefits either to myself or to the party who accepts assignment below.

SIGNED ______ DATE ______

13. INSURED'S OR AUTHORIZED PERSON'S SIGNATURE I authorize payment of medical benefits to the undersigned physician or supplier for services described below.

SIGNED ______

PATIENT AND INSURED INFORMATION

14. DATE OF CURRENT: MM DD YY ILLNESS (First symptom) OR INJURY (Accident) OR PREGNANCY (LMP)

15. IF PATIENT HAS HAD SAME OR SIMILAR ILLNESS, GIVE FIRST DATE MM DD YY

16. DATES PATIENT UNABLE TO WORK IN CURRENT OCCUPATION FROM MM DD YY TO MM DD YY

17. NAME OF REFERRING PHYSICIAN OR OTHER SOURCE

17a. I.D. NUMBER OF REFERRING PHYSICIAN

18. HOSPITALIZATION DATES RELATED TO CURRENT SERVICES FROM MM DD YY TO MM DD YY

19. RESERVED FOR LOCAL USE

20. OUTSIDE LAB? YES NO $ CHARGES

21. DIAGNOSIS OR NATURE OF ILLNESS OR INJURY. (RELATE ITEMS 1, 2, 3, OR 4 TO ITEM 24E BY LINE)

1. ___ . ___ 3. ___ . ___

2. ___ . ___ 4. ___ . ___

22. MEDICAID RESUBMISSION CODE ORIGINAL REF. NO.

23. PRIOR AUTHORIZATION NUMBER

24. A DATE(S) OF SERVICE From MM DD YY To MM DD YY	B Place of Service	C Type of Service	D PROCEDURES, SERVICES, OR SUPPLIES (Explain Unusual Circumstances) CPT/HCPCS MODIFIER	E DIAGNOSIS CODE	F $ CHARGES	G DAYS OR UNITS	H EPSDT Family Plan	I EMG	J COB	K RESERVED FOR LOCAL USE
1										
2										
3										
4										
5										
6										

25. FEDERAL TAX I.D. NUMBER SSN EIN

26. PATIENT'S ACCOUNT NO.

27. ACCEPT ASSIGNMENT? (For govt. claims, see back) YES NO

28. TOTAL CHARGE $

29. AMOUNT PAID $

30. BALANCE DUE $

31. SIGNATURE OF PHYSICIAN OR SUPPLIER INCLUDING DEGREES OR CREDENTIALS (I certify that the statements on the reverse apply to this bill and are made a part thereof.)

SIGNED DATE

32. NAME AND ADDRESS OF FACILITY WHERE SERVICES WERE RENDERED (If other than home or office)

33. PHYSICIAN'S, SUPPLIER'S BILLING NAME, ADDRESS, ZIP CODE & PHONE #

PIN# GRP#

PHYSICIAN OR SUPPLIER INFORMATION

(SAMPLE ONLY - NOT APPROVED FOR USE)

PLEASE PRINT OR TYPE

SAMPLE FORM 1500
SAMPLE FORM 1500 SAMPLE FORM 1500

Case Study 13-h

DATE	REMARKS
04/16/YYYY	

PATIENT		CHART #	SEX	BIRTHDATE
Edward R. Turtle	NXG 444-55-2323	13-h	M	09/15/1949

MAILING ADDRESS	CITY	STATE	ZIP	HOME PHONE	WORK PHONE
68 North Street	Anywhere	US	12345	(101) 333 5555	444 5555

EMPLOYER	ADDRESS	PATIENT STATUS
Carpet Pro	Anywhere US	X MARRIED DIVORCED SINGLE STUDENT OTHER

INSURANCE: PRIMARY	ID#	GROUP	SECONDARY POLICY	ID#	GROUP
BCBS Federal	R12345678	105			

POLICYHOLDER NAME	BIRTHDATE	RELATIONSHIP	POLICYHOLDER NAME	BIRTHDATE	RELATIONSHIP
		Self			

SUPPLEMENTAL PLAN	EMPLOYER

POLICYHOLDER NAME	BIRTHDATE	RELATIONSHIP

EMPLOYER: Carpet Pro

REFERRING PHYSICIAN UPIN/SSN:

DIAGNOSIS	CODE
1. Rectal bleeding	569.3
2. Irritable bowel	564.1
3. Abdominal pain	789.00
4.	

PLACE OF SERVICE Mercy Hospital Anywhere Street Anywhere US 12345

PROCEDURES		CODE	CHARGE
1. Init. hospital Level IV	04/14/YYYY	99224	$175.00
2. Subsq. hospital Level III	04/15/YYYY	99233	85.00
3. Hospital discharge 30 min.	04/16/YYYY	99238	75.00
4.			
5.			
6.			

SPECIAL NOTES
Onset 04/07/YYYY

TOTAL CHARGES	PAYMENTS	ADJUSTMENTS	BALANCE
$335.00	-0-	-0-	$335.00

RETURN VISIT	PHYSICIAN SIGNATURE
4 weeks	Donald L. Givings, M.D.

DONALD L. GIVINGS, M.D.
11350 MEDICAL DRIVE, ANYWHERE US 12345
PHONE NUMBER (101)111-5555

MEDICARE D1234
MEDICAID DLG1234
BCBS 12345

EIN 11-123456
SSN 123-12-1234
PIN DG1234
GRP DG12345

PLEASE
DO NOT
STAPLE
IN THIS
AREA

(SAMPLE ONLY - NOT APPROVED FOR USE)

CARRIER

PICA

HEALTH INSURANCE CLAIM FORM

PICA

1. MEDICARE (Medicare #) ☐ MEDICAID (Medicaid #) ☐ CHAMPUS (Sponsor's SSN) ☐ CHAMPVA (VA File #) ☐ GROUP HEALTH PLAN (SSN or ID) ☐ FECA BLK LUNG (SSN) ☐ OTHER (ID) ☐

1a. INSURED'S I.D. NUMBER (FOR PROGRAM IN ITEM 1)

2. PATIENT'S NAME (Last Name, First Name, Middle Initial)

3. PATIENT'S BIRTH DATE MM | DD | YY SEX M ☐ F ☐

4. INSURED'S NAME (Last Name, First Name, Middle Initial)

5. PATIENT'S ADDRESS (No. Street)

6. PATIENT RELATIONSHIP TO INSURED Self ☐ Spouse ☐ Child ☐ Other ☐

7. INSURED'S ADDRESS (No. Street)

CITY | STATE

8. PATIENT STATUS Single ☐ Married ☐ Other ☐

CITY | STATE

ZIP CODE | TELEPHONE (Include Area Code) ( )

Employed ☐ Full-Time Student ☐ Part-Time Student ☐

ZIP CODE | TELEPHONE (INCLUDE AREA CODE) ( )

9. OTHER INSURED'S NAME (Last Name, First Name, Middle Initial)

10. IS PATIENT'S CONDITION RELATED TO:

11. INSURED'S POLICY GROUP OR FECA NUMBER

a. OTHER INSURED'S POLICY OR GROUP NUMBER

a. EMPLOYMENT? (CURRENT OR PREVIOUS) ☐ YES ☐ NO

a. INSURED'S DATE OF BIRTH MM | DD | YY SEX M ☐ F ☐

b. OTHER INSURED'S DATE OF BIRTH MM | DD | YY SEX M ☐ F ☐

b. AUTO ACCIDENT? ☐ YES ☐ NO PLACE (State)

b. EMPLOYER'S NAME OR SCHOOL NAME

c. EMPLOYER'S NAME OR SCHOOL NAME

c. OTHER ACCIDENT? ☐ YES ☐ NO

c. INSURANCE PLAN NAME OR PROGRAM NAME

d. INSURANCE PLAN NAME OR PROGRAM NAME

10d. RESERVED FOR LOCAL USE

d. IS THERE ANOTHER HEALTH BENEFIT PLAN? ☐ YES ☐ NO If yes, return to and complete item 9 a – d.

READ BACK OF FORM BEFORE COMPLETING & SIGNING THIS FORM.

12. PATIENT'S OR AUTHORIZED PERSON'S SIGNATURE I authorize the release of any medical or other information necessary to process this claim. I also request payment of government benefits either to myself or to the party who accepts assignment below.

SIGNED ______________ DATE ______________

13. INSURED'S OR AUTHORIZED PERSON'S SIGNATURE I authorize payment of medical benefits to the undersigned physician or supplier for services described below.

SIGNED ______________

PATIENT AND INSURED INFORMATION

14. DATE OF CURRENT: MM | DD | YY ◀ ILLNESS (First symptom) OR INJURY (Accident) OR PREGNANCY (LMP)

15. IF PATIENT HAS HAD SAME OR SIMILAR ILLNESS, GIVE FIRST DATE MM | DD | YY

16. DATES PATIENT UNABLE TO WORK IN CURRENT OCCUPATION FROM MM | DD | YY TO MM | DD | YY

17. NAME OF REFERRING PHYSICIAN OR OTHER SOURCE

17a. I.D. NUMBER OF REFERRING PHYSICIAN

18. HOSPITALIZATION DATES RELATED TO CURRENT SERVICES FROM MM | DD | YY TO MM | DD | YY

19. RESERVED FOR LOCAL USE

20. OUTSIDE LAB? ☐ YES ☐ NO $ CHARGES

21. DIAGNOSIS OR NATURE OF ILLNESS OR INJURY. (RELATE ITEMS 1, 2, 3, OR 4 TO ITEM 24E BY LINE)

1. ___ . __ 3. ___ . __

2. ___ . __ 4. ___ . __

22. MEDICAID RESUBMISSION CODE | ORIGINAL REF. NO.

23. PRIOR AUTHORIZATION NUMBER

24. A DATE(S) OF SERVICE From MM DD YY	To MM DD YY	B Place of Service	C Type of Service	D PROCEDURES, SERVICES, OR SUPPLIES (Explain Unusual Circumstances) CPT/HCPCS	MODIFIER	E DIAGNOSIS CODE	F $ CHARGES	G DAYS OR UNITS	H EPSDT Family Plan	I EMG	J COB	K RESERVED FOR LOCAL USE
1												
2												
3												
4												
5												
6												

25. FEDERAL TAX I.D. NUMBER SSN ☐ EIN ☐

26. PATIENT'S ACCOUNT NO.

27. ACCEPT ASSIGNMENT? (For govt. claims, see back) ☐ YES ☐ NO

28. TOTAL CHARGE $

29. AMOUNT PAID $

30. BALANCE DUE $

31. SIGNATURE OF PHYSICIAN OR SUPPLIER INCLUDING DEGREES OR CREDENTIALS (I certify that the statements on the reverse apply to this bill and are made a part thereof.)

SIGNED DATE

32. NAME AND ADDRESS OF FACILITY WHERE SERVICES WERE RENDERED (If other than home or office)

33. PHYSICIAN'S, SUPPLIER'S BILLING NAME, ADDRESS, ZIP CODE & PHONE #

PIN# | GRP#

PHYSICIAN OR SUPPLIER INFORMATION

(SAMPLE ONLY - NOT APPROVED FOR USE)

PLEASE PRINT OR TYPE

SAMPLE FORM 1500
SAMPLE FORM 1500 SAMPLE FORM 1500

Medicare

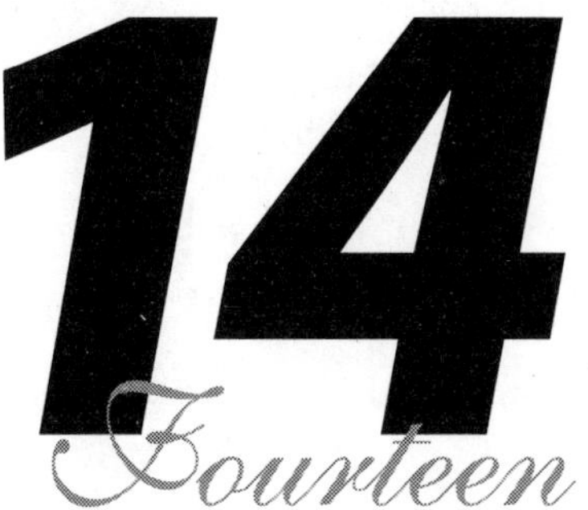

MEDICARE ELIGIBILITY

1. General Medicare eligibility requires individuals or spouses to: (Fill in the blanks.)
   a. have worked at least _______ years in Medicare-covered employment.
   b. be minimum age of _______ years old.
   c. be a citizen or permanent resident of the _______________ _______________.
2. Individuals can also qualify for Medicare coverage if they are younger than 65-years-old and have a _______________ or chronic _______________ disease.

MEDICARE ENROLLMENT

3. Individuals age ___ and over who do not qualify for Social Security benefits may "buy in" to Medicare Part A. (Circle the correct answer.).

   _______ a. 62
   _______ b. 64
   _______ c. 65
   _______ d. none of the above

CRITICAL THINKING

4. Write a paragraph describing the difference between the **Qualified Medicare Beneficiary program** and the **Specified Low-Income Medicare Beneficiary program**.

____

____

____

____

PART A COVERAGE

5. Medicare pays only a portion of a patient's acute care hospitalization expenses, and the patient's out-of-pocket expenses are calculated on a ___ basis. (Circle the correct answer.)
   a. spell-of-illness
   b. benefit period
   c. spell-of-sickness
   d. all of the above

6. A benefit period begins on the first day of hospitalization and ends when the patient has been out of the hospital for ___ consecutive days. (Circle the correct answer.)
   a. 30
   b. 60
   c. 90
   d. none of the above

7. After ninety continuous days of hospitalization, the patient may elect to use his/her ___ lifetime reserve days. (Circle the correct answer.)
   a. ninety-day
   b. thirty-day
   c. sixty-day
   d. none of the above

8. Persons confined to a psychiatric hospital are allowed ___ lifetime reserve days. (Circle the correct answer.)
   a. 190
   b. 160
   c. 90
   d. none of the above

9. Inpatients admitted to a skilled nursing facility after a three-day minimum acute hospital stay, and who meet Medicare's qualified diagnosis and comprehensive treatment plan requirements, pay 2001 rates of: (Fill in the blanks.)
   a. Days 1-20 ______________________
   b. Days 21-100 ______________________
   c. Days 101+ ______________________

10. Match the insurance terms in the first column with the definitions in the second column. Write the correct letter in each blank.

______	Medicare Part A	a. used only once during a patient's lifetime
______	hospice care	b. the temporary hospitalization of a hospice patient
______	ESRD coverage	c. covers institutional care
______	lifetime reserve days	d. all terminally ill patients qualify for this
______	home health services	e. available to patients confined to the home
______	respite care	f. used by persons in need of renal dialysis or transplant

11. Kidney donor coverage includes ___. (Circle the correct answer.)
    a. preoperative testing
    b. surgery
    c. postoperative services
    d. all of the above

12. All payments for medical expenses incurred by a kidney donor are made directly to the ___. (Circle the correct answer.)
    a. health care providers
    b. kidney donor
    c. kidney recipient
    d. any of the above

13. Heart and heart-lung transplants are now covered if the person is Medicare-eligible and the transplant takes place in a Medicare-certified regional ___. (Circle the correct answer.)
    a. hospital
    b. medical center
    c. transplant center
    d. any of the above

14. Liver transplants for adults are covered if the person is Medicare-eligible and does not have ___. (Circle the correct answer.)
    a. hepatitis B
    b. a malignancy
    c. surgery
    d. all of the above

PART B COVERAGE

15. Medicare Part B does not cover ___. (Circle the correct answer.)
    a. diagnostic testing
    b. routine physicals
    c. ambulance services
    d. physician services

16. Which of the following statements about Medicare Part B is NOT true? (Circle the correct answer.)
    a. Medicare pays for therapeutic shoes for hypertensive patients.
    b. Medicare pays for influenza, hepatitis B, and pneumonococcal vaccines.
    c. Medicare pays for drugs that are not self-administered.
    d. none of the above

17. The following preventive screening services were added to the benefits under the Balanced Budget Act of 1997: (Fill in the blanks.)
    a. annual ____________________ screening for women over age 39
    b. annual colorectal screening/fecal-occult blood for patients age ____________________ and older
    c. colorectal screening/flexible sigmoidoscopies every ____________________ ____________________ for patients age 50 and over

d. colorectal screening/colonoscopies every two years if the patient is at high risk for

______________________ ______________________

e. screening ______________ and clinical ______________ examinations every three years

18. The patient is required to pay a $ ______________ annual deductible and ______________ percent of the Medicare allowed charges on all covered benefits, except in the outpatient setting.

19. Describe the possible consequences for providers who are in violation of Medicare regulations by routinely refraining from collecting the patient's deductible and coinsurance.

____

20. The coinsurance for outpatient mental health treatments is ___ of allowed charges. (Circle the correct answer.)

a. 20%

b. 50%

c. 75%

d. There is no coinsurance.

PARTICIPATING/NONPARTICIPATING PROVIDERS

21. Indicate whether each of the following applies to **PAR** or **NonPAR** providers on the line provided.

a. __________ providers must accept assignment on clinical laboratory charges

b. __________ bonuses are provided to carriers for recruitment and enrollment of these providers

c. __________ direct payment is made of all claims

d. __________ balance billing of the patient is forbidden

e. __________ faster processing of assigned claims occurs

f. __________ patient must sign a Surgical Disclosure form for all nonassigned surgical fees over $500

g. __________ provider fees are restricted to no more than the "limiting charge" on nonassigned claims

h. __________ providers use a 5% high fee schedule

i. __________ provider collections are restricted to only the deductible and coinsurance due at the time of service on an assigned claim

22. Calculate each example using the charges provided.

NonPAR charges "limiting fee"	$95
NonPAR Medicare allowed charge	$80
The patient owes NonPAR provider	$_______
Total payment to NonPAR provider	$_______

23. Calculate each example using the charges provided.

PAR charges usual fee	$100
PARMedicare allowed charge	$ 75
PAR adjustment	$_______
Patient payment to PAR provider	$_______
Total payment to PAR provider	$_______

24. If a NonPAR provider does not heed the carrier's warnings to desist from flagrant abuse of the "limiting charge" rules, the potential fine has been increased to ___. (Circle the correct answer.)

a. $2,000

b. $5,000

c. $10,000

d. $20,000

25. When is a NonPAR not restricted to billing the "limiting fee" on a specific claim?

____

CRITICAL THINKING

26. Write a paragraph describing the use of the Surgery Disclosure form and the penalties for not using this form.

____

____

____

____

____

____

27. Federal law requires that all providers submit claims to Medicare if they provide a Medicare-covered service to a patient enrolled in Medicare Part B. This regulation does not apply if ___. (Circle the correct answer.)

a. the patient disenrolled before the service was furnished

b. the patient has not enrolled in Part B

c. the patient or the patient's legal representative refuses to sign an authorization for release of medical information

d. all of the above

28. The Privacy Act of 1979 forbids the regional carrier from disclosing the status of any unassigned claim beyond the ___. (Circle the correct answer.)

a. date the claim was received by the carrier

b. date the claim was paid, denied, or suspended

c. general reason the claim was suspended

d. all of the above

29. Which of the following Medicare-covered services are paid only on an assigned basis? (Circle the correct answer.)

a. Ambulatory Surgery Center facility fees

b. clinical diagnostic laboratory services

c. physician services provided to BCBS eligible recipients

d. physician services provided to Medicaid eligible recipients

30. Which of the following statements about Medicare Part B is NOT true? (Circle the correct answer.)
    a. Medicare requires that assignment be accepted on all claims for services performed in an outpatient setting by physicians.
    b. Medicare requires that assignment be accepted on all claims for services performed in an outpatient setting by nurse practitioners.
    c. Medicare requires that assignment be accepted on all claims for services performed in an outpatient setting by physician assistants.
    d. Medicare requires that assignment be accepted on all claims for services performed in an outpatient setting by clinical social workers.

31. Define *balance billing.* ______________________________

____

MEDICARE FEE SCHEDULE (MFS)

32. List the three relative value units for each procedure/service code.
    a. ______________________________
    b. ______________________________
    c. ______________________________

33. For each item, enter **T** for a true statement or **F** for a false statement on the line provided.

_______ a. Medicare law requires payment only for services or supplies that are considered reasonable and necessary for the stated diagnosis.

_______ b. Medicare may cover procedures deemed to be unproved, experimental, or investigational in nature.

_______ c. The patient must pay the full cost of the procedures denied by Medicare as not medically necessary.

_______ d. The patient must agree in writing, after receiving the services, to personally pay for services denied by Medicare as not medically necessary.

_______ e. The provider must refund any payment received from a patient for a service denied by Medicare as not medically necessary unless the patient agreed verbally to personally pay for such services.

_______ f. A refund is not required if the provider could not have known a specific treatment would be ruled unnecessary.

MEDICARE AS A SECONDARY PAYER

34. What should a provider do to prevent fines and penalties for routinely billing Medicare as primary payer when it is the secondary payer? ______________________________

____

35. The following statements apply to Medicare Secondary Payer fee schedule rules. (Fill in the blanks.)
    a. The primary insurance fee schedule overrules the Medicare schedule on ______________ claims only.

b. NonPARs who do not accept assignment are ________________ from collecting amounts above the applicable limiting charge.

c. Providers are not required to file Medicare secondary claims unless the ________________ specifically requests it.

36. If a primary payer pays a claim after Medicare has already paid the claim as a "conditional primary payer" what action must the provider take? ________________________________.

MEDICARE PLANS

37. List two forms of additional insurance persons who are eligible for Medicare often purchase.
    a. ________________________________
    b. ________________________________

38. Which of the following statements about a Medigap policy is NOT true? (Circle the correct answer.)
    a. A Medigap policy is a private, commercial plan that collects the premiums directly from the patient.
    b. Medigap premiums can widely vary even within the same geographic area.
    c. NonPAR providers are required to include Medigap information on the claim form.
    d. The NonPAR provider does not receive an EOB directly from Medicare for nonassigned claims.

39. For each question, enter **Y** for yes or **N** for no on the line provided.
    _______ a. Is an Employer-Sponsored Retirement Plan regulated by the federal government?
    _______ b. Are premiums for an Employer-Sponsored Retirement Plan paid by the employer?
    _______ c. Are health care providers required to file Employer-Sponsored Retirement Plan claims?
    _______ d. If the employer-sponsored retirement claim is not forwarded electronically, will the patient need to file for benefits after the Medicare EOB is received?

40. The Medicare-Medicaid Crossover program is: (Fill in the blanks.)
    a. a combination of the ________________ / ________________ programs.
    b. available to Medicare-eligible persons with incomes below the federal ________________ level.

41. List five advantages of joining a Medicare HMO.
    a. ________________________________
    b. ________________________________
    c. ________________________________
    d. ________________________________
    e. ________________________________

42. List three disadvantages of joining a Medicare HMO.
    a. ________________________________
    b. ________________________________
    c. ________________________________

43. All Medicare patients should be asked, at each visit, if they are currently enrolled in a(n) ________________________ program.

44. For HMO-authorized fee-for-service specialty care, the claim is sent directly to ___. (Circle the correct answer.)
   a. the HMO
   b. the patient
   c. Medicare
   d. none of the above

45. What is the deadline for filing Medicare-HMO claims? (Circle the correct answer.)
   a. 45 days
   b. 90 days
   c. one year
   d. HMO specific

CRITICAL THINKING

46. Why is it important that a practice's billing department be aware of each HMO's timely filing restrictions?

____

____

MANAGED CARE ORGANIZATIONS

47. Provider Sponsored Organizations are managed care organizations owned and operated by a network of ______________ and ______________ rather than by an insurance company.

48. Preferred Provider Organizations provide care through a network of ____________ and ____________.

49. Medicare MSA is a special savings account that is used by the ______________ to pay medical bills.

BILLING NOTES

50. Explain how the regional carrier for traditional Medicare claims is selected by HCFA.

____

51. Complete the following sentences.
   a. The words that appear on a Railroad Retirement Medicare card are ____________________ ____________________.
   b. On the Railroad Retirement Medicare card, the nine-digit identification number has a(n) ____.
   c. Coal miners' claims are sent to the ____.
   d. The claim filing deadline for both regular Medicare and Railroad Retirement claims is ____.
   e. A claim for services performed in late November 2000 must be postmarked on or before ____.
   f. The claim form that must be completed for all paper claims is the ______________________.
   g. All providers are required to file Medicare claims for their ______________________.
   h. When Medicare is the secondary payer, the ______________________________ must be attached to the Medicare claim.

Know Your Acronyms

52. Define the following acronyms:

    a. SSA __________

    b. FI __________

    c. ESRD __________

    d. IEP __________

    e. QMB __________

    f. SLMB __________

    g. NonPAR __________

    h. LLP __________

    i. MFS __________

    j. RBRVS __________

    k. MSP __________

    l. GEP __________

    m. PSO __________

    n. MSA __________

    o. DMERC __________

    p. UPIN __________

    q. PAR __________

    r. PIN __________

    s. PAYERID __________

    t. CLIA __________

    u. LC __________

    v. ABN __________

    w. MSN __________

    x. MSP __________

    y. SCID __________

    z. RUV __________

    aa. GAF __________

    bb. CF __________

    cc. PPO __________

    dd. PFFS __________

EXERCISES

1. Complete Case Studies 14-a through 14-l using the blank claim form provided. Follow the step-by-step instructions given in the textbook to properly complete the claim form. If a patient has secondary coverage, complete an additional claim form using secondary directions from the textbook. You may choose to use a pencil so corrections can be made.

DATE	REMARKS			
07/12/YYYY				

PATIENT		CHART #	SEX	BIRTHDATE
Alice E. Worthington	444-22-3333	14-a	F	02/16/1926

MAILING ADDRESS	CITY	STATE	ZIP	HOME PHONE	WORK PHONE
3301 Sunny Day Dr.	Anywhere	US	12345	(101) 333-5555	

EMPLOYER	ADDRESS	PATIENT STATUS
	Anywhere US	MARRIED DIVORCED SINGLE (X) STUDENT OTHER

INSURANCE: PRIMARY	ID#	GROUP	SECONDARY POLICY
Medicare	444-22-3333A		

POLICYHOLDER NAME	BIRTHDATE	RELATIONSHIP	POLICYHOLDER NAME	BIRTHDATE	RELATIONSHIP
		Self			

SUPPLEMENTAL PLAN	EMPLOYER

POLICYHOLDER NAME	BIRTHDATE	RELATIONSHIP

EMPLOYER

REFERRING PHYSICIAN UPIN/SSN

DIAGNOSIS	CODE
1. Breast lump	611.72
2. Breast pain	611.71
3. Family history breast cancer	V16.3
4.	

PLACE OF SERVICE Office

PROCEDURES	CODE	CHARGE
1. Ext. patient OV Level II	99212	$65.00
2.		
3.		
4.		
5.		
6.		

SPECIAL NOTES

Refer to Dr. Kutter

TOTAL CHARGES	PAYMENTS	ADJUSTMENTS	BALANCE
$65.00	-0-	-0-	$65.00

RETURN VISIT	PHYSICIAN SIGNATURE
	Donald L. Givings, M.D.

MEDICARE # D1234
MEDICAID # DLG1234
BCBS # 12345

DONALD L. GIVINGS, M.D.
11350 MEDICAL DRIVE, ANYWHERE, US 12345
PHONE NUMBER (101)111-5555

EIN # 11123456
SSN # 123-12-1234
UPIN # DG1234

PLEASE
DO NOT
STAPLE
IN THIS
AREA

(SAMPLE ONLY - NOT APPROVED FOR USE)

CARRIER

PICA

HEALTH INSURANCE CLAIM FORM

PICA

1. MEDICARE (Medicare #) | MEDICAID (Medicaid #) | CHAMPUS (Sponsor's SSN) | CHAMPVA (VA File #) | GROUP HEALTH PLAN (SSN or ID) | FECA BLK LUNG (SSN) | OTHER (ID)

1a. INSURED'S I.D. NUMBER (FOR PROGRAM IN ITEM 1)

2. PATIENT'S NAME (Last Name, First Name, Middle Initial)

3. PATIENT'S BIRTH DATE MM DD YY — SEX M F

4. INSURED'S NAME (Last Name, First Name, Middle Initial)

5. PATIENT'S ADDRESS (No. Street)

6. PATIENT RELATIONSHIP TO INSURED — Self Spouse Child Other

7. INSURED'S ADDRESS (No. Street)

CITY — STATE

8. PATIENT STATUS — Single Married Other; Employed Full-Time Student Part-Time Student

CITY — STATE

ZIP CODE — TELEPHONE (Include Area Code) ( )

ZIP CODE — TELEPHONE (INCLUDE AREA CODE) ( )

9. OTHER INSURED'S NAME (Last Name, First Name, Middle Initial)

10. IS PATIENT'S CONDITION RELATED TO:

11. INSURED'S POLICY GROUP OR FECA NUMBER

a. OTHER INSURED'S POLICY OR GROUP NUMBER

a. EMPLOYMENT? (CURRENT OR PREVIOUS) — YES NO

a. INSURED'S DATE OF BIRTH MM DD YY — SEX M F

b. OTHER INSURED'S DATE OF BIRTH MM DD YY — SEX M F

b. AUTO ACCIDENT? — YES NO — PLACE (State)

b. EMPLOYER'S NAME OR SCHOOL NAME

c. EMPLOYER'S NAME OR SCHOOL NAME

c. OTHER ACCIDENT? — YES NO

c. INSURANCE PLAN NAME OR PROGRAM NAME

d. INSURANCE PLAN NAME OR PROGRAM NAME

10d. RESERVED FOR LOCAL USE

d. IS THERE ANOTHER HEALTH BENEFIT PLAN? — YES NO — If yes, return to and complete item 9 a – d.

READ BACK OF FORM BEFORE COMPLETING & SIGNING THIS FORM.

12. PATIENT'S OR AUTHORIZED PERSON'S SIGNATURE I authorize the release of any medical or other information necessary to process this claim. I also request payment of government benefits either to myself or to the party who accepts assignment below.

SIGNED ______ DATE ______

13. INSURED'S OR AUTHORIZED PERSON'S SIGNATURE I authorize payment of medical benefits to the undersigned physician or supplier for services described below.

SIGNED ______

PATIENT AND INSURED INFORMATION

14. DATE OF CURRENT: MM DD YY — ILLNESS (First symptom) OR INJURY (Accident) OR PREGNANCY (LMP)

15. IF PATIENT HAS HAD SAME OR SIMILAR ILLNESS, GIVE FIRST DATE MM DD YY

16. DATES PATIENT UNABLE TO WORK IN CURRENT OCCUPATION — FROM MM DD YY TO MM DD YY

17. NAME OF REFERRING PHYSICIAN OR OTHER SOURCE

17a. I.D. NUMBER OF REFERRING PHYSICIAN

18. HOSPITALIZATION DATES RELATED TO CURRENT SERVICES — FROM MM DD YY TO MM DD YY

19. RESERVED FOR LOCAL USE

20. OUTSIDE LAB? — YES NO — $ CHARGES

21. DIAGNOSIS OR NATURE OF ILLNESS OR INJURY. (RELATE ITEMS 1, 2, 3, OR 4 TO ITEM 24E BY LINE)

1. ___ . __
2. ___ . __
3. ___ . __
4. ___ . __

22. MEDICAID RESUBMISSION CODE — ORIGINAL REF. NO.

23. PRIOR AUTHORIZATION NUMBER

24. A DATE(S) OF SERVICE From MM DD YY To MM DD YY	B Place of Service	C Type of Service	D PROCEDURES, SERVICES, OR SUPPLIES (Explain Unusual Circumstances) CPT/HCPCS MODIFIER	E DIAGNOSIS CODE	F $ CHARGES	G DAYS OR UNITS	H EPSDT Family Plan	I EMG	J COB	K RESERVED FOR LOCAL USE
1										
2										
3										
4										
5										
6										

25. FEDERAL TAX I.D. NUMBER — SSN EIN

26. PATIENT'S ACCOUNT NO.

27. ACCEPT ASSIGNMENT? (For govt. claims, see back) — YES NO

28. TOTAL CHARGE $

29. AMOUNT PAID $

30. BALANCE DUE $

31. SIGNATURE OF PHYSICIAN OR SUPPLIER INCLUDING DEGREES OR CREDENTIALS (I certify that the statements on the reverse apply to this bill and are made a part thereof.)

SIGNED DATE

32. NAME AND ADDRESS OF FACILITY WHERE SERVICES WERE RENDERED (If other than home or office)

33. PHYSICIAN'S, SUPPLIER'S BILLING NAME, ADDRESS, ZIP CODE & PHONE #

PIN# — GRP#

PHYSICIAN OR SUPPLIER INFORMATION

(SAMPLE ONLY - NOT APPROVED FOR USE)

PLEASE PRINT OR TYPE

SAMPLE FORM 1500
SAMPLE FORM 1500 SAMPLE FORM 1500

Case Study 14-b

DATE	REMARKS
07/15/YYYY	

PATIENT		CHART #	SEX	BIRTHDATE
Alice E. Worthington	444-22-3333	14-b	F	02/16/1926

MAILING ADDRESS	CITY	STATE	ZIP	HOME PHONE	WORK PHONE
3301 Sunny Day Dr.	Anywhere	US	12345	(101) 333-5555	

EMPLOYER	ADDRESS	PATIENT STATUS
		MARRIED DIVORCED SINGLE (X) STUDENT OTHER

INSURANCE: PRIMARY	ID#	GROUP	SECONDARY POLICY
Medicare	444-22-3333A		

POLICYHOLDER NAME	BIRTHDATE	RELATIONSHIP	POLICYHOLDER NAME	BIRTHDATE	RELATIONSHIP
		Self			

SUPPLEMENTAL PLAN	EMPLOYER

POLICYHOLDER NAME	BIRTHDATE	RELATIONSHIP

EMPLOYER

REFERRING PHYSICIAN UPIN/SSN: Donald L. Givings, M.D. 123-12-1234

DIAGNOSIS	CODE
1. Breast lump	611.72
2. Breast pain	611.71
3. Family history breast cancer	V16.3
4.	

PLACE OF SERVICE Office

PROCEDURES	CODE	CHARGE
1. Office Consult Level II	99242	$75.00
2.		
3.		
4.		
5.		
6.		

SPECIAL NOTES

TOTAL CHARGES	PAYMENTS	ADJUSTMENTS	BALANCE
$75.00	-0-	-0-	$75.00

RETURN VISIT	PHYSICIAN SIGNATURE
	Jonathan B. Kutter, M.D.

MEDICARE # J1234
MEDICAID # JBK1234
BCBS # 12885

JONATHAN B. KUTTER, M.D. SURGERY
339 WOODLAND PLACE, ANYWHERE, US 12345
PHONE NUMBER (101)111-5555

EIN # 11556677
SSN # 245-12-1234
UPIN # JK1234

PLEASE DO NOT STAPLE IN THIS AREA

(SAMPLE ONLY - NOT APPROVED FOR USE)

PICA

HEALTH INSURANCE CLAIM FORM

PICA

CARRIER

1. MEDICARE (Medicare #) MEDICAID (Medicaid #) CHAMPUS (Sponsor's SSN) CHAMPVA (VA File #) GROUP HEALTH PLAN (SSN or ID) FECA BLK LUNG (SSN) OTHER (ID)

1a. INSURED'S I.D. NUMBER (FOR PROGRAM IN ITEM 1)

2. PATIENT'S NAME (Last Name, First Name, Middle Initial)

3. PATIENT'S BIRTH DATE MM DD YY SEX M F

4. INSURED'S NAME (Last Name, First Name, Middle Initial)

5. PATIENT'S ADDRESS (No. Street)

6. PATIENT RELATIONSHIP TO INSURED Self Spouse Child Other

7. INSURED'S ADDRESS (No. Street)

CITY STATE

8. PATIENT STATUS Single Married Other

CITY STATE

ZIP CODE TELEPHONE (Include Area Code) ( )

Employed Full-Time Student Part-Time Student

ZIP CODE TELEPHONE (INCLUDE AREA CODE) ( )

9. OTHER INSURED'S NAME (Last Name, First Name, Middle Initial)

10. IS PATIENT'S CONDITION RELATED TO:

11. INSURED'S POLICY GROUP OR FECA NUMBER

a. OTHER INSURED'S POLICY OR GROUP NUMBER

a. EMPLOYMENT? (CURRENT OR PREVIOUS) YES NO

a. INSURED'S DATE OF BIRTH MM DD YY SEX M F

b. OTHER INSURED'S DATE OF BIRTH MM DD YY SEX M F

b. AUTO ACCIDENT? PLACE (State) YES NO

b. EMPLOYER'S NAME OR SCHOOL NAME

c. EMPLOYER'S NAME OR SCHOOL NAME

c. OTHER ACCIDENT? YES NO

c. INSURANCE PLAN NAME OR PROGRAM NAME

d. INSURANCE PLAN NAME OR PROGRAM NAME

10d. RESERVED FOR LOCAL USE

d. IS THERE ANOTHER HEALTH BENEFIT PLAN? YES NO If yes, return to and complete item 9 a – d.

READ BACK OF FORM BEFORE COMPLETING & SIGNING THIS FORM.

12. PATIENT'S OR AUTHORIZED PERSON'S SIGNATURE I authorize the release of any medical or other information necessary to process this claim. I also request payment of government benefits either to myself or to the party who accepts assignment below.

SIGNED ____ DATE ____

13. INSURED'S OR AUTHORIZED PERSON'S SIGNATURE I authorize payment of medical benefits to the undersigned physician or supplier for services described below.

SIGNED ____

PATIENT AND INSURED INFORMATION

14. DATE OF CURRENT: MM DD YY ILLNESS (First symptom) OR INJURY (Accident) OR PREGNANCY (LMP)

15. IF PATIENT HAS HAD SAME OR SIMILAR ILLNESS, GIVE FIRST DATE MM DD YY

16. DATES PATIENT UNABLE TO WORK IN CURRENT OCCUPATION FROM MM DD YY TO MM DD YY

17. NAME OF REFERRING PHYSICIAN OR OTHER SOURCE

17a. I.D. NUMBER OF REFERRING PHYSICIAN

18. HOSPITALIZATION DATES RELATED TO CURRENT SERVICES FROM MM DD YY TO MM DD YY

19. RESERVED FOR LOCAL USE

20. OUTSIDE LAB? YES NO $ CHARGES

21. DIAGNOSIS OR NATURE OF ILLNESS OR INJURY. (RELATE ITEMS 1, 2, 3, OR 4 TO ITEM 24E BY LINE)

1. ___ . __ 3. ___ . __

2. ___ . __ 4. ___ . __

22. MEDICAID RESUBMISSION CODE ORIGINAL REF. NO.

23. PRIOR AUTHORIZATION NUMBER

24. A DATE(S) OF SERVICE From MM DD YY To MM DD YY	B Place of Service	C Type of Service	D PROCEDURES, SERVICES, OR SUPPLIES (Explain Unusual Circumstances) CPT/HCPCS MODIFIER	E DIAGNOSIS CODE	F $ CHARGES	G DAYS OR UNITS	H EPSDT Family Plan	I EMG	J COB	K RESERVED FOR LOCAL USE
1										
2										
3										
4										
5										
6										

25. FEDERAL TAX I.D. NUMBER SSN EIN

26. PATIENT'S ACCOUNT NO.

27. ACCEPT ASSIGNMENT? (For govt. claims, see back) YES NO

28. TOTAL CHARGE $

29. AMOUNT PAID $

30. BALANCE DUE $

31. SIGNATURE OF PHYSICIAN OR SUPPLIER INCLUDING DEGREES OR CREDENTIALS (I certify that the statements on the reverse apply to this bill and are made a part thereof.)

SIGNED DATE

32. NAME AND ADDRESS OF FACILITY WHERE SERVICES WERE RENDERED (If other than home or office)

33. PHYSICIAN'S, SUPPLIER'S BILLING NAME, ADDRESS, ZIP CODE & PHONE #

PIN# GRP#

PHYSICIAN OR SUPPLIER INFORMATION

(SAMPLE ONLY - NOT APPROVED FOR USE)

PLEASE PRINT OR TYPE

SAMPLE FORM 1500
SAMPLE FORM 1500 SAMPLE FORM 1500

Case Study 14-c

DATE	REMARKS
07/22/YYYY	Alice was in the hospital from July 22 through July 25

PATIENT		CHART #	SEX	BIRTHDATE
Alice E. Worthington	444-22-3333	14-c	F	02/16/1926

MAILING ADDRESS	CITY	STATE	ZIP	HOME PHONE	WORK PHONE
3301 Sunny Day Dr.	Anywhere	US	12345	(101) 333-5555	

EMPLOYER	ADDRESS	PATIENT STATUS
	Anywhere US	MARRIED DIVORCED SINGLE (X) STUDENT OTHER

INSURANCE: PRIMARY	ID#	GROUP	SECONDARY POLICY
Medicare	444-22-3333A		

POLICYHOLDER NAME	BIRTHDATE	RELATIONSHIP	POLICYHOLDER NAME	BIRTHDATE	RELATIONSHIP
		Self			

SUPPLEMENTAL PLAN	EMPLOYER

POLICYHOLDER NAME | BIRTHDATE | RELATIONSHIP

EMPLOYER

REFERRING PHYSICIAN UPIN/SSN: Donald L. Givings, M.D. 123-12-1234

DIAGNOSIS	CODE
1. Breast cancer	174.8
2.	
3.	
4.	

PLACE OF SERVICE Mercy Hospital, Anywhere St., Anywhere, US 12345 PIN# M1234

PROCEDURES	CODE	CHARGE
1. Mastectomy, Simple, Complete 07/22/YYYY	19180	$1,200.00
2.		
3.		
4.		
5.		
6.		

SPECIAL NOTES

TOTAL CHARGES	PAYMENTS	ADJUSTMENTS	BALANCE
$1,200.00	-0-	-0-	$1,200.00

RETURN VISIT	PHYSICIAN SIGNATURE
	Jonathan B. Kutter, M.D.

MEDICARE # J1234
MEDICAID # JBK1234
BCBS # 12885

JONATHAN B. KUTTER, M.D. SURGERY
339 WOODLAND PLACE, ANYWHERE, US 12345
PHONE NUMBER (101)111-5555

EIN # 11556677
SSN # 245-12-1234
UPIN # JK1234

PLEASE DO NOT STAPLE IN THIS AREA

(SAMPLE ONLY - NOT APPROVED FOR USE)

CARRIER

PICA

HEALTH INSURANCE CLAIM FORM

PICA

1. MEDICARE (Medicare #) MEDICAID (Medicaid #) CHAMPUS (Sponsor's SSN) CHAMPVA (VA File #) GROUP HEALTH PLAN (SSN or ID) FECA BLK LUNG (SSN) OTHER (ID)

1a. INSURED'S I.D. NUMBER (FOR PROGRAM IN ITEM 1)

2. PATIENT'S NAME (Last Name, First Name, Middle Initial)

3. PATIENT'S BIRTH DATE MM DD YY SEX M F

4. INSURED'S NAME (Last Name, First Name, Middle Initial)

5. PATIENT'S ADDRESS (No. Street)

6. PATIENT RELATIONSHIP TO INSURED Self Spouse Child Other

7. INSURED'S ADDRESS (No. Street)

CITY STATE

8. PATIENT STATUS Single Married Other

CITY STATE

ZIP CODE TELEPHONE (Include Area Code) ( )

Employed Full-Time Student Part-Time Student

ZIP CODE TELEPHONE (INCLUDE AREA CODE) ( )

9. OTHER INSURED'S NAME (Last Name, First Name, Middle Initial)

10. IS PATIENT'S CONDITION RELATED TO:

11. INSURED'S POLICY GROUP OR FECA NUMBER

a. OTHER INSURED'S POLICY OR GROUP NUMBER

a. EMPLOYMENT? (CURRENT OR PREVIOUS) YES NO

a. INSURED'S DATE OF BIRTH MM DD YY SEX M F

b. OTHER INSURED'S DATE OF BIRTH MM DD YY SEX M F

b. AUTO ACCIDENT? PLACE (State) YES NO

b. EMPLOYER'S NAME OR SCHOOL NAME

c. EMPLOYER'S NAME OR SCHOOL NAME

c. OTHER ACCIDENT? YES NO

c. INSURANCE PLAN NAME OR PROGRAM NAME

d. INSURANCE PLAN NAME OR PROGRAM NAME

10d. RESERVED FOR LOCAL USE

d. IS THERE ANOTHER HEALTH BENEFIT PLAN? YES NO If yes, return to and complete item 9 a – d.

READ BACK OF FORM BEFORE COMPLETING & SIGNING THIS FORM.

12. PATIENT'S OR AUTHORIZED PERSON'S SIGNATURE I authorize the release of any medical or other information necessary to process this claim. I also request payment of government benefits either to myself or to the party who accepts assignment below.

SIGNED DATE

13. INSURED'S OR AUTHORIZED PERSON'S SIGNATURE I authorize payment of medical benefits to the undersigned physician or supplier for services described below.

SIGNED

PATIENT AND INSURED INFORMATION

14. DATE OF CURRENT: MM DD YY ILLNESS (First symptom) OR INJURY (Accident) OR PREGNANCY (LMP)

15. IF PATIENT HAS HAD SAME OR SIMILAR ILLNESS, GIVE FIRST DATE MM DD YY

16. DATES PATIENT UNABLE TO WORK IN CURRENT OCCUPATION FROM MM DD YY TO MM DD YY

17. NAME OF REFERRING PHYSICIAN OR OTHER SOURCE

17a. I.D. NUMBER OF REFERRING PHYSICIAN

18. HOSPITALIZATION DATES RELATED TO CURRENT SERVICES FROM MM DD YY TO MM DD YY

19. RESERVED FOR LOCAL USE

20. OUTSIDE LAB? YES NO $ CHARGES

21. DIAGNOSIS OR NATURE OF ILLNESS OR INJURY. (RELATE ITEMS 1, 2, 3, OR 4 TO ITEM 24E BY LINE)

1. ___ . __

3. ___ . __

2. ___ . __

4. ___ . __

22. MEDICAID RESUBMISSION CODE ORIGINAL REF. NO.

23. PRIOR AUTHORIZATION NUMBER

24.	A DATE(S) OF SERVICE From MM DD YY To MM DD YY	B Place of Service	C Type of Service	D PROCEDURES, SERVICES, OR SUPPLIES (Explain Unusual Circumstances) CPT/HCPCS MODIFIER	E DIAGNOSIS CODE	F $ CHARGES	G DAYS OR UNITS	H EPSDT Family Plan	I EMG	J COB	K RESERVED FOR LOCAL USE
1											
2											
3											
4											
5											
6											

25. FEDERAL TAX I.D. NUMBER SSN EIN

26. PATIENT'S ACCOUNT NO.

27. ACCEPT ASSIGNMENT? (For govt. claims, see back) YES NO

28. TOTAL CHARGE $

29. AMOUNT PAID $

30. BALANCE DUE $

31. SIGNATURE OF PHYSICIAN OR SUPPLIER INCLUDING DEGREES OR CREDENTIALS (I certify that the statements on the reverse apply to this bill and are made a part thereof.)

SIGNED DATE

32. NAME AND ADDRESS OF FACILITY WHERE SERVICES WERE RENDERED (If other than home or office)

33. PHYSICIAN'S, SUPPLIER'S BILLING NAME, ADDRESS, ZIP CODE & PHONE #

PIN# GRP#

PHYSICIAN OR SUPPLIER INFORMATION

(SAMPLE ONLY - NOT APPROVED FOR USE)

PLEASE PRINT OR TYPE

SAMPLE FORM 1500
SAMPLE FORM 1500 SAMPLE FORM 1500

Case Study 14-d

DATE	REMARKS			
08/25/YYYY	Today's visit is included in global surgery			

PATIENT		CHART #	SEX	BIRTHDATE
Alice E. Worthington	444-22-3333	14-d	F	02/16/1926

MAILING ADDRESS	CITY	STATE	ZIP	HOME PHONE	WORK PHONE
3301 Sunny Day Dr.	Anywhere	US	12345	(101) 333-5555	

EMPLOYER	ADDRESS	PATIENT STATUS
	Anywhere US	MARRIED DIVORCED SINGLE (X) STUDENT OTHER

INSURANCE: PRIMARY	ID#	GROUP	SECONDARY POLICY
Medicare	444-22-3333A		

POLICYHOLDER NAME	BIRTHDATE	RELATIONSHIP	POLICYHOLDER NAME	BIRTHDATE	RELATIONSHIP
		Self			

SUPPLEMENTAL PLAN	EMPLOYER

POLICYHOLDER NAME	BIRTHDATE	RELATIONSHIP

EMPLOYER

REFERRING PHYSICIAN UPIN/SSN	
Donald L. Givings, M.D.	123-12-1234

DIAGNOSIS	CODE
1. Breast cancer	174.8
2.	
3.	
4.	

PLACE OF SERVICE Office

PROCEDURES	CODE	CHARGE
1. Postoperative follow-up visit	99024	$0.00
2.		
3.		
4.		
5.		
6.		

SPECIAL NOTES

TOTAL CHARGES	PAYMENTS	ADJUSTMENTS	BALANCE
$0.00	-0-	-0-	$0.00

RETURN VISIT	PHYSICIAN SIGNATURE
	Jonathan B. Kutter, M.D.

MEDICARE # J1234
MEDICAID # JBK1234
BCBS # 12885

JONATHAN B. KUTTER, M.D. SURGERY
339 WOODLAND PLACE, ANYWHERE, US 12345
PHONE NUMBER (101)111-5555

EIN # 11556677
SSN # 245-12-1234
UPIN # JK1234

PLEASE DO NOT STAPLE IN THIS AREA

(SAMPLE ONLY - NOT APPROVED FOR USE)

CARRIER

PICA

HEALTH INSURANCE CLAIM FORM

PICA

1. MEDICARE (Medicare #) | MEDICAID (Medicaid #) | CHAMPUS (Sponsor's SSN) | CHAMPVA (VA File #) | GROUP HEALTH PLAN (SSN or ID) | FECA BLK LUNG (SSN) | OTHER (ID)

1a. INSURED'S I.D. NUMBER (FOR PROGRAM IN ITEM 1)

2. PATIENT'S NAME (Last Name, First Name, Middle Initial)

3. PATIENT'S BIRTH DATE MM DD YY SEX M F

4. INSURED'S NAME (Last Name, First Name, Middle Initial)

5. PATIENT'S ADDRESS (No. Street)

6. PATIENT RELATIONSHIP TO INSURED Self Spouse Child Other

7. INSURED'S ADDRESS (No. Street)

CITY STATE

8. PATIENT STATUS Single Married Other

CITY STATE

ZIP CODE TELEPHONE (Include Area Code) ( )

Employed Full-Time Student Part-Time Student

ZIP CODE TELEPHONE (INCLUDE AREA CODE) ( )

9. OTHER INSURED'S NAME (Last Name, First Name, Middle Initial)

10. IS PATIENT'S CONDITION RELATED TO:

11. INSURED'S POLICY GROUP OR FECA NUMBER

a. OTHER INSURED'S POLICY OR GROUP NUMBER

a. EMPLOYMENT? (CURRENT OR PREVIOUS) YES NO

a. INSURED'S DATE OF BIRTH MM DD YY SEX M F

b. OTHER INSURED'S DATE OF BIRTH MM DD YY SEX M F

b. AUTO ACCIDENT? PLACE (State) YES NO

b. EMPLOYER'S NAME OR SCHOOL NAME

c. EMPLOYER'S NAME OR SCHOOL NAME

c. OTHER ACCIDENT? YES NO

c. INSURANCE PLAN NAME OR PROGRAM NAME

d. INSURANCE PLAN NAME OR PROGRAM NAME

10d. RESERVED FOR LOCAL USE

d. IS THERE ANOTHER HEALTH BENEFIT PLAN? YES NO If yes, return to and complete item 9 a – d.

READ BACK OF FORM BEFORE COMPLETING & SIGNING THIS FORM.

12. PATIENT'S OR AUTHORIZED PERSON'S SIGNATURE I authorize the release of any medical or other information necessary to process this claim. I also request payment of government benefits either to myself or to the party who accepts assignment below.

SIGNED ____________ DATE ____________

13. INSURED'S OR AUTHORIZED PERSON'S SIGNATURE I authorize payment of medical benefits to the undersigned physician or supplier for services described below.

SIGNED ____________

PATIENT AND INSURED INFORMATION

14. DATE OF CURRENT: MM DD YY ILLNESS (First symptom) OR INJURY (Accident) OR PREGNANCY (LMP)

15. IF PATIENT HAS HAD SAME OR SIMILAR ILLNESS, GIVE FIRST DATE MM DD YY

16. DATES PATIENT UNABLE TO WORK IN CURRENT OCCUPATION FROM MM DD YY TO MM DD YY

17. NAME OF REFERRING PHYSICIAN OR OTHER SOURCE

17a. I.D. NUMBER OF REFERRING PHYSICIAN

18. HOSPITALIZATION DATES RELATED TO CURRENT SERVICES FROM MM DD YY TO MM DD YY

19. RESERVED FOR LOCAL USE

20. OUTSIDE LAB? YES NO $ CHARGES

21. DIAGNOSIS OR NATURE OF ILLNESS OR INJURY. (RELATE ITEMS 1, 2, 3, OR 4 TO ITEM 24E BY LINE)

1. ___ . __

2. ___ . __

3. ___ . __

4. ___ . __

22. MEDICAID RESUBMISSION CODE ORIGINAL REF. NO.

23. PRIOR AUTHORIZATION NUMBER

24. A DATE(S) OF SERVICE From MM DD YY	To MM DD YY	B Place of Service	C Type of Service	D PROCEDURES, SERVICES, OR SUPPLIES (Explain Unusual Circumstances) CPT/HCPCS MODIFIER	E DIAGNOSIS CODE	F $ CHARGES	G DAYS OR UNITS	H EPSDT Family Plan	I EMG	J COB	K RESERVED FOR LOCAL USE
1											
2											
3											
4											
5											
6											

25. FEDERAL TAX I.D. NUMBER SSN EIN

26. PATIENT'S ACCOUNT NO.

27. ACCEPT ASSIGNMENT? (For govt. claims, see back) YES NO

28. TOTAL CHARGE $

29. AMOUNT PAID $

30. BALANCE DUE $

31. SIGNATURE OF PHYSICIAN OR SUPPLIER INCLUDING DEGREES OR CREDENTIALS (I certify that the statements on the reverse apply to this bill and are made a part thereof.)

SIGNED DATE

32. NAME AND ADDRESS OF FACILITY WHERE SERVICES WERE RENDERED (If other than home or office)

33. PHYSICIAN'S, SUPPLIER'S BILLING NAME, ADDRESS, ZIP CODE & PHONE #

PIN# GRP#

PHYSICIAN OR SUPPLIER INFORMATION

(SAMPLE ONLY - NOT APPROVED FOR USE)

PLEASE PRINT OR TYPE

SAMPLE FORM 1500
SAMPLE FORM 1500 SAMPLE FORM 1500

DATE	REMARKS
08/10/YYYY	

PATIENT	CHART #	SEX	BIRTHDATE
Rebecca Nichols 667-14-3344	14-e	F	10/12/1925

MAILING ADDRESS	CITY	STATE	ZIP	HOME PHONE	WORK PHONE
384 Dean Street	Anywhere	US	12345	(101) 333-5555	

EMPLOYER	ADDRESS	PATIENT STATUS
	Anywhere US	MARRIED DIVORCED SINGLE (X) STUDENT OTHER

INSURANCE: PRIMARY	ID#	GROUP	SECONDARY POLICY
Medicare	667-14-3344A		

POLICYHOLDER NAME	BIRTHDATE	RELATIONSHIP	POLICYHOLDER NAME	BIRTHDATE	RELATIONSHIP
		Self			

SUPPLEMENTAL PLAN	EMPLOYER

POLICYHOLDER NAME | BIRTHDATE | RELATIONSHIP

EMPLOYER

REFERRING PHYSICIAN UPIN/SSN

DIAGNOSIS	CODE
1. Rectal bleeding	569.3
2. Diarrhea	787.91
3. Abnormal loss of weight	783.21
4.	

PLACE OF SERVICE Mercy Hospital, Anywhere St., Anywhere, US 12345 PIN# M1234

PROCEDURES		CODE	CHARGE
1. Initial Hosp. Level IV	08/06/YYYY	99224	$175.00
2. Subsq. Hosp. Level III	08/07/YYYY	99233	$85.00
3. Subsq. Hosp. Level III	08/08/YYYY	99233	$85.00
4. Subsq. Hosp. Level II	08/09/YYYY	99232	$75.00
5. Hosp. Discharge 30 min.	08/10/YYYY	99238	$75.00
6.			

SPECIAL NOTES

Dr. Gestive saw the patient for a consult on August 7 & August 8

TOTAL CHARGES	PAYMENTS	ADJUSTMENTS	BALANCE
$495.00	-0-	-0-	$495.00

RETURN VISIT	PHYSICIAN SIGNATURE
	Donald L. Givings, M.D.

DONALD L. GIVINGS, M.D.
11350 MEDICAL DRIVE, ANYWHERE, US 12345
PHONE NUMBER (101)111-5555

MEDICARE # D1234
MEDICAID # DLG1234
BCBS # 12345

EIN # 11123456
SSN # 123-12-1234
UPIN # DG1234

PLEASE
DO NOT
STAPLE
IN THIS
AREA

(SAMPLE ONLY - NOT APPROVED FOR USE)

CARRIER

PICA

HEALTH INSURANCE CLAIM FORM

PICA

1. MEDICARE (Medicare #) MEDICAID (Medicaid #) CHAMPUS (Sponsor's SSN) CHAMPVA (VA File #) GROUP HEALTH PLAN (SSN or ID) FECA BLK LUNG (SSN) OTHER (ID)

1a. INSURED'S I.D. NUMBER (FOR PROGRAM IN ITEM 1)

2. PATIENT'S NAME (Last Name, First Name, Middle Initial)

3. PATIENT'S BIRTH DATE MM DD YY SEX M F

4. INSURED'S NAME (Last Name, First Name, Middle Initial)

5. PATIENT'S ADDRESS (No. Street)

6. PATIENT RELATIONSHIP TO INSURED Self Spouse Child Other

7. INSURED'S ADDRESS (No. Street)

CITY STATE

8. PATIENT STATUS Single Married Other

CITY STATE

ZIP CODE TELEPHONE (Include Area Code) ( )

Employed Full-Time Student Part-Time Student

ZIP CODE TELEPHONE (INCLUDE AREA CODE) ( )

9. OTHER INSURED'S NAME (Last Name, First Name, Middle Initial)

10. IS PATIENT'S CONDITION RELATED TO:

11. INSURED'S POLICY GROUP OR FECA NUMBER

a. OTHER INSURED'S POLICY OR GROUP NUMBER

a. EMPLOYMENT? (CURRENT OR PREVIOUS) YES NO

a. INSURED'S DATE OF BIRTH MM DD YY SEX M F

b. OTHER INSURED'S DATE OF BIRTH MM DD YY SEX M F

b. AUTO ACCIDENT? YES NO PLACE (State)

b. EMPLOYER'S NAME OR SCHOOL NAME

c. EMPLOYER'S NAME OR SCHOOL NAME

c. OTHER ACCIDENT? YES NO

c. INSURANCE PLAN NAME OR PROGRAM NAME

d. INSURANCE PLAN NAME OR PROGRAM NAME

10d. RESERVED FOR LOCAL USE

d. IS THERE ANOTHER HEALTH BENEFIT PLAN? YES NO If yes, return to and complete item 9 a – d.

READ BACK OF FORM BEFORE COMPLETING & SIGNING THIS FORM.

12. PATIENT'S OR AUTHORIZED PERSON'S SIGNATURE I authorize the release of any medical or other information necessary to process this claim. I also request payment of government benefits either to myself or to the party who accepts assignment below.

SIGNED ____ DATE ____

13. INSURED'S OR AUTHORIZED PERSON'S SIGNATURE I authorize payment of medical benefits to the undersigned physician or supplier for services described below.

SIGNED ____

PATIENT AND INSURED INFORMATION

14. DATE OF CURRENT: MM DD YY ILLNESS (First symptom) OR INJURY (Accident) OR PREGNANCY (LMP)

15. IF PATIENT HAS HAD SAME OR SIMILAR ILLNESS, GIVE FIRST DATE MM DD YY

16. DATES PATIENT UNABLE TO WORK IN CURRENT OCCUPATION FROM MM DD YY TO MM DD YY

17. NAME OF REFERRING PHYSICIAN OR OTHER SOURCE

17a. I.D. NUMBER OF REFERRING PHYSICIAN

18. HOSPITALIZATION DATES RELATED TO CURRENT SERVICES FROM MM DD YY TO MM DD YY

19. RESERVED FOR LOCAL USE

20. OUTSIDE LAB? YES NO $ CHARGES

21. DIAGNOSIS OR NATURE OF ILLNESS OR INJURY. (RELATE ITEMS 1, 2, 3, OR 4 TO ITEM 24E BY LINE)

1. ___ . __ 3. ___ . __

2. ___ . __ 4. ___ . __

22. MEDICAID RESUBMISSION CODE ORIGINAL REF. NO.

23. PRIOR AUTHORIZATION NUMBER

24.	A DATE(S) OF SERVICE From MM DD YY	To MM DD YY	B Place of Service	C Type of Service	D PROCEDURES, SERVICES, OR SUPPLIES (Explain Unusual Circumstances) CPT/HCPCS MODIFIER	E DIAGNOSIS CODE	F $ CHARGES	G DAYS OR UNITS	H EPSDT Family Plan	I EMG	J COB	K RESERVED FOR LOCAL USE
1												
2												
3												
4												
5												
6												

25. FEDERAL TAX I.D. NUMBER SSN EIN

26. PATIENT'S ACCOUNT NO.

27. ACCEPT ASSIGNMENT? (For govt. claims, see back) YES NO

28. TOTAL CHARGE $

29. AMOUNT PAID $

30. BALANCE DUE $

31. SIGNATURE OF PHYSICIAN OR SUPPLIER INCLUDING DEGREES OR CREDENTIALS (I certify that the statements on the reverse apply to this bill and are made a part thereof.)

SIGNED DATE

32. NAME AND ADDRESS OF FACILITY WHERE SERVICES WERE RENDERED (If other than home or office)

33. PHYSICIAN'S, SUPPLIER'S BILLING NAME, ADDRESS, ZIP CODE & PHONE #

PIN# GRP#

PHYSICIAN OR SUPPLIER INFORMATION

(SAMPLE ONLY - NOT APPROVED FOR USE)

PLEASE PRINT OR TYPE

SAMPLE FORM 1500
SAMPLE FORM 1500 SAMPLE FORM 1500

Case Study 14-f

DATE	REMARKS
08/07/YYYY	Miss Nichols was in the hospital from August 6 through August 10

PATIENT		CHART #	SEX	BIRTHDATE
Rebecca Nichols	667-14-3344	14-f	F	10/12/1925

MAILING ADDRESS	CITY	STATE	ZIP	HOME PHONE	WORK PHONE
384 Dean Street	Anywhere	US	12345	(101) 333-5555	

EMPLOYER	ADDRESS	PATIENT STATUS
	Anywhere US	MARRIED DIVORCED SINGLE (X) STUDENT OTHER

INSURANCE: PRIMARY	ID#	GROUP	SECONDARY POLICY
Medicare	667-14-3344A		

POLICYHOLDER NAME	BIRTHDATE	RELATIONSHIP	POLICYHOLDER NAME	BIRTHDATE	RELATIONSHIP
		Self			

SUPPLEMENTAL PLAN	EMPLOYER

POLICYHOLDER NAME	BIRTHDATE	RELATIONSHIP

EMPLOYER

REFERRING PHYSICIAN UPIN/SSN: Donald L. Givings, M.D. 123-12-1234

DIAGNOSIS	CODE
1. Diverticulitis of the colon with hemorrhage	562.13
2.	
3.	
4.	

PLACE OF SERVICE Mercy Hospital, Anywhere St., Anywhere, US 12345 PIN# M1234

PROCEDURES		CODE	CHARGE
1. Initial Inpatient Consult Level IV	08/07/YYYY	99254	$220.00
2. Follow-up Inpatient Consult Level III	08/08/YYYY	99263	$80.00
3.			
4.			
5.			
6.			

SPECIAL NOTES

TOTAL CHARGES	PAYMENTS	ADJUSTMENTS	BALANCE
$300.00	-0-	-0-	$300.00

RETURN VISIT	PHYSICIAN SIGNATURE
	Colin D. Gestive, M.D.

MEDICARE # C1234
MEDICAID # CGD1234
BCBS # 44345

COLIN D. GESTIVE, M.D. GASTROENTEROLOGY
35 ULCER PLACE, ANYWHERE, US 12345
PHONE NUMBER (101)111-5555

EIN # 11-447766
SSN # 321-12-1234
UPIN # CD1234

PLEASE
DO NOT
STAPLE
IN THIS
AREA

(SAMPLE ONLY - NOT APPROVED FOR USE)

CARRIER

PICA

HEALTH INSURANCE CLAIM FORM

PICA

1. MEDICARE (Medicare #) MEDICAID (Medicaid #) CHAMPUS (Sponsor's SSN) CHAMPVA (VA File #) GROUP HEALTH PLAN (SSN or ID) FECA BLK LUNG (SSN) OTHER (ID)

1a. INSURED'S I.D. NUMBER (FOR PROGRAM IN ITEM 1)

2. PATIENT'S NAME (Last Name, First Name, Middle Initial)

3. PATIENT'S BIRTH DATE MM DD YY SEX M F

4. INSURED'S NAME (Last Name, First Name, Middle Initial)

5. PATIENT'S ADDRESS (No. Street)

6. PATIENT RELATIONSHIP TO INSURED Self Spouse Child Other

7. INSURED'S ADDRESS (No. Street)

CITY STATE

8. PATIENT STATUS Single Married Other

CITY STATE

ZIP CODE TELEPHONE (Include Area Code) ( )

Employed Full-Time Student Part-Time Student

ZIP CODE TELEPHONE (INCLUDE AREA CODE) ( )

9. OTHER INSURED'S NAME (Last Name, First Name, Middle Initial)

10. IS PATIENT'S CONDITION RELATED TO:

11. INSURED'S POLICY GROUP OR FECA NUMBER

a. OTHER INSURED'S POLICY OR GROUP NUMBER

a. EMPLOYMENT? (CURRENT OR PREVIOUS) YES NO

a. INSURED'S DATE OF BIRTH MM DD YY SEX M F

b. OTHER INSURED'S DATE OF BIRTH MM DD YY SEX M F

b. AUTO ACCIDENT? PLACE (State) YES NO

b. EMPLOYER'S NAME OR SCHOOL NAME

c. EMPLOYER'S NAME OR SCHOOL NAME

c. OTHER ACCIDENT? YES NO

c. INSURANCE PLAN NAME OR PROGRAM NAME

d. INSURANCE PLAN NAME OR PROGRAM NAME

10d. RESERVED FOR LOCAL USE

d. IS THERE ANOTHER HEALTH BENEFIT PLAN? YES NO If yes, return to and complete item 9 a – d.

READ BACK OF FORM BEFORE COMPLETING & SIGNING THIS FORM.

12. PATIENT'S OR AUTHORIZED PERSON'S SIGNATURE I authorize the release of any medical or other information necessary to process this claim. I also request payment of government benefits either to myself or to the party who accepts assignment below.

SIGNED DATE

13. INSURED'S OR AUTHORIZED PERSON'S SIGNATURE I authorize payment of medical benefits to the undersigned physician or supplier for services described below.

SIGNED

PATIENT AND INSURED INFORMATION

14. DATE OF CURRENT: MM DD YY ILLNESS (First symptom) OR INJURY (Accident) OR PREGNANCY (LMP)

15. IF PATIENT HAS HAD SAME OR SIMILAR ILLNESS, GIVE FIRST DATE MM DD YY

16. DATES PATIENT UNABLE TO WORK IN CURRENT OCCUPATION FROM MM DD YY TO MM DD YY

17. NAME OF REFERRING PHYSICIAN OR OTHER SOURCE

17a. I.D. NUMBER OF REFERRING PHYSICIAN

18. HOSPITALIZATION DATES RELATED TO CURRENT SERVICES FROM MM DD YY TO MM DD YY

19. RESERVED FOR LOCAL USE

20. OUTSIDE LAB? YES NO $ CHARGES

21. DIAGNOSIS OR NATURE OF ILLNESS OR INJURY. (RELATE ITEMS 1, 2, 3, OR 4 TO ITEM 24E BY LINE)

1. ___ . __
2. ___ . __
3. ___ . __
4. ___ . __

22. MEDICAID RESUBMISSION CODE ORIGINAL REF. NO.

23. PRIOR AUTHORIZATION NUMBER

24.	A DATE(S) OF SERVICE From MM DD YY To MM DD YY	B Place of Service	C Type of Service	D PROCEDURES, SERVICES, OR SUPPLIES (Explain Unusual Circumstances) CPT/HCPCS MODIFIER	E DIAGNOSIS CODE	F $ CHARGES	G DAYS OR UNITS	H EPSDT Family Plan	I EMG	J COB	K RESERVED FOR LOCAL USE
1											
2											
3											
4											
5											
6											

25. FEDERAL TAX I.D. NUMBER SSN EIN

26. PATIENT'S ACCOUNT NO.

27. ACCEPT ASSIGNMENT? (For govt. claims, see back) YES NO

28. TOTAL CHARGE $

29. AMOUNT PAID $

30. BALANCE DUE $

31. SIGNATURE OF PHYSICIAN OR SUPPLIER INCLUDING DEGREES OR CREDENTIALS (I certify that the statements on the reverse apply to this bill and are made a part thereof.)

SIGNED DATE

32. NAME AND ADDRESS OF FACILITY WHERE SERVICES WERE RENDERED (If other than home or office)

33. PHYSICIAN'S, SUPPLIER'S BILLING NAME, ADDRESS, ZIP CODE & PHONE #

PIN# GRP#

PHYSICIAN OR SUPPLIER INFORMATION

(SAMPLE ONLY - NOT APPROVED FOR USE)

PLEASE PRINT OR TYPE

SAMPLE FORM 1500
SAMPLE FORM 1500 SAMPLE FORM 1500

Case Study 14-g

DATE	REMARKS
10/03/YYYY	Dr. Mason is NonPAR with Medicare

PATIENT		CHART #	SEX	BIRTHDATE
Samual T. Mahoney Jr.	312-78-5894	14-g	M	09/04/1930

MAILING ADDRESS	CITY	STATE	ZIP	HOME PHONE	WORK PHONE
498 Meadow Lane	Anywhere	US	12345	(101) 333-5555	

EMPLOYER	ADDRESS	PATIENT STATUS
	Anywhere US	X MARRIED DIVORCED SINGLE STUDENT OTHER

INSURANCE: PRIMARY	ID#	GROUP	SECONDARY POLICY
Medicare	312-78-5894A		

POLICYHOLDER NAME	BIRTHDATE	RELATIONSHIP	POLICYHOLDER NAME	BIRTHDATE	RELATIONSHIP
		Self			

SUPPLEMENTAL PLAN	EMPLOYER

POLICYHOLDER NAME	BIRTHDATE	RELATIONSHIP

EMPLOYER

REFERRING PHYSICIAN UPIN/SSN

DIAGNOSIS	CODE
1. Asthma, unspecified	493.90
2. URI	465.9
3.	
4.	

PLACE OF SERVICE Office

PROCEDURES	CODE	CHARGE
1. Est. Patient OV Level II	99212	$25.16
2.		
3.		
4.		
5.		
6.		

SPECIAL NOTES

TOTAL CHARGES	PAYMENTS	ADJUSTMENTS	BALANCE
$25.16	$25.16	-0-	$0.00

RETURN VISIT	PHYSICIAN SIGNATURE
	Lisa M. Mason, M.D.

MEDICARE # L1234
MEDICAID # LMM1234
BCBS # 39994

LISA M. MASON, M.D. FAMILY PRACTICE
547 ANTIGUA ROAD, ANYWHERE, US 12345
PHONE NUMBER (101)111-5555

EIN # 11495867
SSN # 333-12-9484
UPIN # LM4234

PLEASE
DO NOT
STAPLE
IN THIS
AREA

(SAMPLE ONLY - NOT APPROVED FOR USE)

CARRIER

PICA

HEALTH INSURANCE CLAIM FORM

PICA

1. MEDICARE (Medicare #) MEDICAID (Medicaid #) CHAMPUS (Sponsor's SSN) CHAMPVA (VA File #) GROUP HEALTH PLAN (SSN or ID) FECA BLK LUNG (SSN) OTHER (ID)

1a. INSURED'S I.D. NUMBER (FOR PROGRAM IN ITEM 1)

2. PATIENT'S NAME (Last Name, First Name, Middle Initial)

3. PATIENT'S BIRTH DATE MM DD YY SEX M F

4. INSURED'S NAME (Last Name, First Name, Middle Initial)

5. PATIENT'S ADDRESS (No. Street)

6. PATIENT RELATIONSHIP TO INSURED Self Spouse Child Other

7. INSURED'S ADDRESS (No. Street)

CITY STATE

8. PATIENT STATUS Single Married Other

CITY STATE

ZIP CODE TELEPHONE (Include Area Code) ( )

Employed Full-Time Student Part-Time Student

ZIP CODE TELEPHONE (INCLUDE AREA CODE) ( )

9. OTHER INSURED'S NAME (Last Name, First Name, Middle Initial)

10. IS PATIENT'S CONDITION RELATED TO:

11. INSURED'S POLICY GROUP OR FECA NUMBER

a. OTHER INSURED'S POLICY OR GROUP NUMBER

a. EMPLOYMENT? (CURRENT OR PREVIOUS) YES NO

a. INSURED'S DATE OF BIRTH MM DD YY SEX M F

b. OTHER INSURED'S DATE OF BIRTH MM DD YY SEX M F

b. AUTO ACCIDENT? YES NO PLACE (State)

b. EMPLOYER'S NAME OR SCHOOL NAME

c. EMPLOYER'S NAME OR SCHOOL NAME

c. OTHER ACCIDENT? YES NO

c. INSURANCE PLAN NAME OR PROGRAM NAME

d. INSURANCE PLAN NAME OR PROGRAM NAME

10d. RESERVED FOR LOCAL USE

d. IS THERE ANOTHER HEALTH BENEFIT PLAN? YES NO If yes, return to and complete item 9 a – d.

READ BACK OF FORM BEFORE COMPLETING & SIGNING THIS FORM.

12. PATIENT'S OR AUTHORIZED PERSON'S SIGNATURE I authorize the release of any medical or other information necessary to process this claim. I also request payment of government benefits either to myself or to the party who accepts assignment below.

SIGNED DATE

13. INSURED'S OR AUTHORIZED PERSON'S SIGNATURE I authorize payment of medical benefits to the undersigned physician or supplier for services described below.

SIGNED

PATIENT AND INSURED INFORMATION

14. DATE OF CURRENT: MM DD YY ILLNESS (First symptom) OR INJURY (Accident) OR PREGNANCY (LMP)

15. IF PATIENT HAS HAD SAME OR SIMILAR ILLNESS, GIVE FIRST DATE MM DD YY

16. DATES PATIENT UNABLE TO WORK IN CURRENT OCCUPATION FROM MM DD YY TO MM DD YY

17. NAME OF REFERRING PHYSICIAN OR OTHER SOURCE

17a. I.D. NUMBER OF REFERRING PHYSICIAN

18. HOSPITALIZATION DATES RELATED TO CURRENT SERVICES FROM MM DD YY TO MM DD YY

19. RESERVED FOR LOCAL USE

20. OUTSIDE LAB? YES NO $ CHARGES

21. DIAGNOSIS OR NATURE OF ILLNESS OR INJURY. (RELATE ITEMS 1, 2, 3, OR 4 TO ITEM 24E BY LINE)

1. ___ . __

2. ___ . __

3. ___ . __

4. ___ . __

22. MEDICAID RESUBMISSION CODE ORIGINAL REF. NO.

23. PRIOR AUTHORIZATION NUMBER

24. A DATE(S) OF SERVICE From MM DD YY To MM DD YY	B Place of Service	C Type of Service	D PROCEDURES, SERVICES, OR SUPPLIES (Explain Unusual Circumstances) CPT/HCPCS MODIFIER	E DIAGNOSIS CODE	F $ CHARGES	G DAYS OR UNITS	H EPSDT Family Plan	I EMG	J COB	K RESERVED FOR LOCAL USE
1										
2										
3										
4										
5										
6										

25. FEDERAL TAX I.D. NUMBER SSN EIN

26. PATIENT'S ACCOUNT NO.

27. ACCEPT ASSIGNMENT? (For govt. claims, see back) YES NO

28. TOTAL CHARGE $

29. AMOUNT PAID $

30. BALANCE DUE $

31. SIGNATURE OF PHYSICIAN OR SUPPLIER INCLUDING DEGREES OR CREDENTIALS (I certify that the statements on the reverse apply to this bill and are made a part thereof.)

SIGNED DATE

32. NAME AND ADDRESS OF FACILITY WHERE SERVICES WERE RENDERED (If other than home or office)

33. PHYSICIAN'S, SUPPLIER'S BILLING NAME, ADDRESS, ZIP CODE & PHONE #

PIN# GRP#

PHYSICIAN OR SUPPLIER INFORMATION

(SAMPLE ONLY - NOT APPROVED FOR USE)

PLEASE PRINT OR TYPE

SAMPLE FORM 1500
SAMPLE FORM 1500 SAMPLE FORM 1500

Case Study 14-h

DATE	REMARKS
03/07/YYYY	Medigap Payer Identification Number 123456994

PATIENT	CHART #	SEX	BIRTHDATE
Abraham N. Freed 645-45-4545	14-h	M	10/03/1922

MAILING ADDRESS	CITY	STATE	ZIP	HOME PHONE	WORK PHONE
12 Nottingham Circle	Anywhere	US	12345	(101) 333-5555	

EMPLOYER	ADDRESS	PATIENT STATUS
	Anywhere US	X MARRIED DIVORCED SINGLE STUDENT OTHER

INSURANCE: PRIMARY	ID#	GROUP	SECONDARY POLICY
Medicare	645-45-4545A		

POLICYHOLDER NAME	BIRTHDATE	RELATIONSHIP	POLICYHOLDER NAME	BIRTHDATE	RELATIONSHIP
		Self			

SUPPLEMENTAL PLAN	EMPLOYER
BCBS Medigap NXY645-45-4545 987	

POLICYHOLDER NAME	BIRTHDATE	RELATIONSHIP
		Self

EMPLOYER
Retired Johnson Steel

REFERRING PHYSICIAN UPIN/SSN

DIAGNOSIS	CODE
1. Hypertension, malignant	401.0
2. Dizziness	780.2
3.	
4.	

PLACE OF SERVICE Office

PROCEDURES	CODE	CHARGE
1. New patient OV Level IV	99204	$100.00
2. EKG	93000	$50.00
3. Venipuncture	36415	$8.00
4.		
5.		
6.		

SPECIAL NOTES

TOTAL CHARGES	PAYMENTS	ADJUSTMENTS	BALANCE
$158.00	-0-	-0-	$158.00

RETURN VISIT	PHYSICIAN SIGNATURE
2 Weeks	Donald L. Givings, M.D.

DONALD L. GIVINGS, M.D.
11350 MEDICAL DRIVE, ANYWHERE, US 12345
PHONE NUMBER (101)111-5555

MEDICARE # D1234
MEDICAID # DLG1234
BCBS # 12345

EIN # 11123456
SSN # 123-12-1234
UPIN # DG1234

PLEASE
DO NOT
STAPLE
IN THIS
AREA

(SAMPLE ONLY - NOT APPROVED FOR USE)

CARRIER

PICA

HEALTH INSURANCE CLAIM FORM

PICA

1. MEDICARE (Medicare #) MEDICAID (Medicaid #) CHAMPUS (Sponsor's SSN) CHAMPVA (VA File #) GROUP HEALTH PLAN (SSN or ID) FECA BLK LUNG (SSN) OTHER (ID)

1a. INSURED'S I.D. NUMBER (FOR PROGRAM IN ITEM 1)

2. PATIENT'S NAME (Last Name, First Name, Middle Initial)

3. PATIENT'S BIRTH DATE MM DD YY SEX M F

4. INSURED'S NAME (Last Name, First Name, Middle Initial)

5. PATIENT'S ADDRESS (No. Street)

6. PATIENT RELATIONSHIP TO INSURED Self Spouse Child Other

7. INSURED'S ADDRESS (No. Street)

CITY STATE

8. PATIENT STATUS Single Married Other

CITY STATE

ZIP CODE TELEPHONE (Include Area Code) ( )

Employed Full-Time Student Part-Time Student

ZIP CODE TELEPHONE (INCLUDE AREA CODE) ( )

9. OTHER INSURED'S NAME (Last Name, First Name, Middle Initial)

10. IS PATIENT'S CONDITION RELATED TO:

11. INSURED'S POLICY GROUP OR FECA NUMBER

a. OTHER INSURED'S POLICY OR GROUP NUMBER

a. EMPLOYMENT? (CURRENT OR PREVIOUS) YES NO

a. INSURED'S DATE OF BIRTH MM DD YY SEX M F

b. OTHER INSURED'S DATE OF BIRTH MM DD YY SEX M F

b. AUTO ACCIDENT? PLACE (State) YES NO

b. EMPLOYER'S NAME OR SCHOOL NAME

c. EMPLOYER'S NAME OR SCHOOL NAME

c. OTHER ACCIDENT? YES NO

c. INSURANCE PLAN NAME OR PROGRAM NAME

d. INSURANCE PLAN NAME OR PROGRAM NAME

10d. RESERVED FOR LOCAL USE

d. IS THERE ANOTHER HEALTH BENEFIT PLAN? YES NO If yes, return to and complete item 9 a – d.

READ BACK OF FORM BEFORE COMPLETING & SIGNING THIS FORM.

12. PATIENT'S OR AUTHORIZED PERSON'S SIGNATURE I authorize the release of any medical or other information necessary to process this claim. I also request payment of government benefits either to myself or to the party who accepts assignment below.

SIGNED ______ DATE ______

13. INSURED'S OR AUTHORIZED PERSON'S SIGNATURE I authorize payment of medical benefits to the undersigned physician or supplier for services described below.

SIGNED ______

PATIENT AND INSURED INFORMATION

14. DATE OF CURRENT: MM DD YY ILLNESS (First symptom) OR INJURY (Accident) OR PREGNANCY (LMP)

15. IF PATIENT HAS HAD SAME OR SIMILAR ILLNESS, GIVE FIRST DATE MM DD YY

16. DATES PATIENT UNABLE TO WORK IN CURRENT OCCUPATION MM DD YY FROM TO

17. NAME OF REFERRING PHYSICIAN OR OTHER SOURCE

17a. I.D. NUMBER OF REFERRING PHYSICIAN

18. HOSPITALIZATION DATES RELATED TO CURRENT SERVICES MM DD YY FROM TO

19. RESERVED FOR LOCAL USE

20. OUTSIDE LAB? YES NO $ CHARGES

21. DIAGNOSIS OR NATURE OF ILLNESS OR INJURY. (RELATE ITEMS 1, 2, 3, OR 4 TO ITEM 24E BY LINE)

1. ___ . __ 3. ___ . __

2. ___ . __ 4. ___ . __

22. MEDICAID RESUBMISSION CODE ORIGINAL REF. NO.

23. PRIOR AUTHORIZATION NUMBER

24. A DATE(S) OF SERVICE From MM DD YY To MM DD YY	B Place of Service	C Type of Service	D PROCEDURES, SERVICES, OR SUPPLIES (Explain Unusual Circumstances) CPT/HCPCS MODIFIER	E DIAGNOSIS CODE	F $ CHARGES	G DAYS OR UNITS	H EPSDT Family Plan	I EMG	J COB	K RESERVED FOR LOCAL USE
1										
2										
3										
4										
5										
6										

25. FEDERAL TAX I.D. NUMBER SSN EIN

26. PATIENT'S ACCOUNT NO.

27. ACCEPT ASSIGNMENT? (For govt. claims, see back) YES NO

28. TOTAL CHARGE $

29. AMOUNT PAID $

30. BALANCE DUE $

31. SIGNATURE OF PHYSICIAN OR SUPPLIER INCLUDING DEGREES OR CREDENTIALS (I certify that the statements on the reverse apply to this bill and are made a part thereof.)

SIGNED DATE

32. NAME AND ADDRESS OF FACILITY WHERE SERVICES WERE RENDERED (If other than home or office)

33. PHYSICIAN'S, SUPPLIER'S BILLING NAME, ADDRESS, ZIP CODE & PHONE #

PIN# GRP#

PHYSICIAN OR SUPPLIER INFORMATION

(SAMPLE ONLY - NOT APPROVED FOR USE)

PLEASE PRINT OR TYPE

SAMPLE FORM 1500
SAMPLE FORM 1500 SAMPLE FORM 1500

PLEASE
DO NOT
STAPLE
IN THIS
AREA

(SAMPLE ONLY - NOT APPROVED FOR USE)

CARRIER

PICA

HEALTH INSURANCE CLAIM FORM

PICA

1. MEDICARE (Medicare #) MEDICAID (Medicaid #) CHAMPUS (Sponsor's SSN) CHAMPVA (VA File #) GROUP HEALTH PLAN (SSN or ID) FECA BLK LUNG (SSN) OTHER (ID)

1a. INSURED'S I.D. NUMBER (FOR PROGRAM IN ITEM 1)

2. PATIENT'S NAME (Last Name, First Name, Middle Initial)

3. PATIENT'S BIRTH DATE MM DD YY SEX M F

4. INSURED'S NAME (Last Name, First Name, Middle Initial)

5. PATIENT'S ADDRESS (No. Street)

6. PATIENT RELATIONSHIP TO INSURED Self Spouse Child Other

7. INSURED'S ADDRESS (No. Street)

CITY STATE

8. PATIENT STATUS Single Married Other

CITY STATE

ZIP CODE TELEPHONE (Include Area Code) ( )

Employed Full-Time Student Part-Time Student

ZIP CODE TELEPHONE (INCLUDE AREA CODE) ( )

9. OTHER INSURED'S NAME (Last Name, First Name, Middle Initial)

10. IS PATIENT'S CONDITION RELATED TO:

11. INSURED'S POLICY GROUP OR FECA NUMBER

a. OTHER INSURED'S POLICY OR GROUP NUMBER

a. EMPLOYMENT? (CURRENT OR PREVIOUS) YES NO

a. INSURED'S DATE OF BIRTH MM DD YY SEX M F

b. OTHER INSURED'S DATE OF BIRTH MM DD YY SEX M F

b. AUTO ACCIDENT? PLACE (State) YES NO

b. EMPLOYER'S NAME OR SCHOOL NAME

c. EMPLOYER'S NAME OR SCHOOL NAME

c. OTHER ACCIDENT? YES NO

c. INSURANCE PLAN NAME OR PROGRAM NAME

d. INSURANCE PLAN NAME OR PROGRAM NAME

10d. RESERVED FOR LOCAL USE

d. IS THERE ANOTHER HEALTH BENEFIT PLAN? YES NO If yes, return to and complete item 9 a – d.

READ BACK OF FORM BEFORE COMPLETING & SIGNING THIS FORM.

12. PATIENT'S OR AUTHORIZED PERSON'S SIGNATURE I authorize the release of any medical or other information necessary to process this claim. I also request payment of government benefits either to myself or to the party who accepts assignment below.

SIGNED ______ DATE ______

13. INSURED'S OR AUTHORIZED PERSON'S SIGNATURE I authorize payment of medical benefits to the undersigned physician or supplier for services described below.

SIGNED ______

PATIENT AND INSURED INFORMATION

14. DATE OF CURRENT: MM DD YY ILLNESS (First symptom) OR INJURY (Accident) OR PREGNANCY (LMP)

15. IF PATIENT HAS HAD SAME OR SIMILAR ILLNESS, GIVE FIRST DATE MM DD YY

16. DATES PATIENT UNABLE TO WORK IN CURRENT OCCUPATION FROM MM DD YY TO MM DD YY

17. NAME OF REFERRING PHYSICIAN OR OTHER SOURCE

17a. I.D. NUMBER OF REFERRING PHYSICIAN

18. HOSPITALIZATION DATES RELATED TO CURRENT SERVICES FROM MM DD YY TO MM DD YY

19. RESERVED FOR LOCAL USE

20. OUTSIDE LAB? YES NO $ CHARGES

21. DIAGNOSIS OR NATURE OF ILLNESS OR INJURY. (RELATE ITEMS 1, 2, 3, OR 4 TO ITEM 24E BY LINE)

1. ___ . __
2. ___ . __
3. ___ . __
4. ___ . __

22. MEDICAID RESUBMISSION CODE ORIGINAL REF. NO.

23. PRIOR AUTHORIZATION NUMBER

24. A DATE(S) OF SERVICE From MM DD YY To MM DD YY	B Place of Service	C Type of Service	D PROCEDURES, SERVICES, OR SUPPLIES (Explain Unusual Circumstances) CPT/HCPCS MODIFIER	E DIAGNOSIS CODE	F $ CHARGES	G DAYS OR UNITS	H EPSDT Family Plan	I EMG	J COB	K RESERVED FOR LOCAL USE
1										
2										
3										
4										
5										
6										

25. FEDERAL TAX I.D. NUMBER SSN EIN

26. PATIENT'S ACCOUNT NO.

27. ACCEPT ASSIGNMENT? (For govt. claims, see back) YES NO

28. TOTAL CHARGE $

29. AMOUNT PAID $

30. BALANCE DUE $

31. SIGNATURE OF PHYSICIAN OR SUPPLIER INCLUDING DEGREES OR CREDENTIALS (I certify that the statements on the reverse apply to this bill and are made a part thereof.)

SIGNED DATE

32. NAME AND ADDRESS OF FACILITY WHERE SERVICES WERE RENDERED (If other than home or office)

33. PHYSICIAN'S, SUPPLIER'S BILLING NAME, ADDRESS, ZIP CODE & PHONE #

PIN# GRP#

PHYSICIAN OR SUPPLIER INFORMATION

(SAMPLE ONLY - NOT APPROVED FOR USE)

PLEASE PRINT OR TYPE

SAMPLE FORM 1500
SAMPLE FORM 1500 SAMPLE FORM 1500

Case Study 14-i

DATE	REMARKS
03/07/YYYY	Medigap Payer Identification Number 123456994

PATIENT		CHART #	SEX	BIRTHDATE
Esther K. Freed	777-66-4444	14-i	F	03/26/1925

MAILING ADDRESS	CITY	STATE	ZIP	HOME PHONE	WORK PHONE
12 Nottingham Circle	Anywhere	US	12345	(101) 333-5555	

EMPLOYER	ADDRESS	PATIENT STATUS
	Anywhere US	X MARRIED DIVORCED SINGLE STUDENT OTHER

INSURANCE: PRIMARY	ID#	GROUP	SECONDARY POLICY
Medicare	777-66-4444A		

POLICYHOLDER NAME	BIRTHDATE	RELATIONSHIP	POLICYHOLDER NAME	BIRTHDATE	RELATIONSHIP
		Self			

SUPPLEMENTAL PLAN	EMPLOYER
BCBS Medigap NXY645-45-4545 987	

POLICYHOLDER NAME	BIRTHDATE	RELATIONSHIP
Abraham N. Freed	10/03/22	Spouse

EMPLOYER

Retired Johnson Steel

REFERRING PHYSICIAN UPIN/SSN

DIAGNOSIS	CODE
1. Bronchopneumonia	485
2. Hemoptysis	786.3
3. Hematuria	599.7
4.	

PLACE OF SERVICE Office

PROCEDURES	CODE	CHARGE
1. New patient OV Level IV	99204	$100.00
2. Chest Xray 2 views	71020	$50.00
3. Urinalysis, with microscopy	81001	$10.00
4.		
5.		
6.		

SPECIAL NOTES

TOTAL CHARGES	PAYMENTS	ADJUSTMENTS	BALANCE
$160.00	-0-	-0-	$160.00

RETURN VISIT	PHYSICIAN SIGNATURE
2 Weeks	Donald L. Givings, M.D.

MEDICARE # D1234
MEDICAID # DLG1234
BCBS # 12345

DONALD L. GIVINGS, M.D.
11350 MEDICAL DRIVE, ANYWHERE, US 12345
PHONE NUMBER (101)111-5555

EIN # 11123456
SSN # 123-12-1234
UPIN # DG1234

PLEASE
DO NOT
STAPLE
IN THIS
AREA

(SAMPLE ONLY - NOT APPROVED FOR USE)

CARRIER

PICA

HEALTH INSURANCE CLAIM FORM

PICA

1. MEDICARE (Medicare #) MEDICAID (Medicaid #) CHAMPUS (Sponsor's SSN) CHAMPVA (VA File #) GROUP HEALTH PLAN (SSN or ID) FECA BLK LUNG (SSN) OTHER (ID)

1a. INSURED'S I.D. NUMBER (FOR PROGRAM IN ITEM 1)

2. PATIENT'S NAME (Last Name, First Name, Middle Initial)

3. PATIENT'S BIRTH DATE MM DD YY SEX M F

4. INSURED'S NAME (Last Name, First Name, Middle Initial)

5. PATIENT'S ADDRESS (No. Street)

6. PATIENT RELATIONSHIP TO INSURED Self Spouse Child Other

7. INSURED'S ADDRESS (No. Street)

CITY STATE

8. PATIENT STATUS Single Married Other

CITY STATE

ZIP CODE TELEPHONE (Include Area Code) ( )

Employed Full-Time Student Part-Time Student

ZIP CODE TELEPHONE (INCLUDE AREA CODE) ( )

9. OTHER INSURED'S NAME (Last Name, First Name, Middle Initial)

10. IS PATIENT'S CONDITION RELATED TO:

11. INSURED'S POLICY GROUP OR FECA NUMBER

a. OTHER INSURED'S POLICY OR GROUP NUMBER

a. EMPLOYMENT? (CURRENT OR PREVIOUS) YES NO

a. INSURED'S DATE OF BIRTH MM DD YY SEX M F

b. OTHER INSURED'S DATE OF BIRTH MM DD YY SEX M F

b. AUTO ACCIDENT? PLACE (State) YES NO

b. EMPLOYER'S NAME OR SCHOOL NAME

c. EMPLOYER'S NAME OR SCHOOL NAME

c. OTHER ACCIDENT? YES NO

c. INSURANCE PLAN NAME OR PROGRAM NAME

d. INSURANCE PLAN NAME OR PROGRAM NAME

10d. RESERVED FOR LOCAL USE

d. IS THERE ANOTHER HEALTH BENEFIT PLAN? YES NO If yes, return to and complete item 9 a – d.

READ BACK OF FORM BEFORE COMPLETING & SIGNING THIS FORM.

12. PATIENT'S OR AUTHORIZED PERSON'S SIGNATURE I authorize the release of any medical or other information necessary to process this claim. I also request payment of government benefits either to myself or to the party who accepts assignment below.

SIGNED ____________ DATE ____________

13. INSURED'S OR AUTHORIZED PERSON'S SIGNATURE I authorize payment of medical benefits to the undersigned physician or supplier for services described below.

SIGNED ____________

PATIENT AND INSURED INFORMATION

14. DATE OF CURRENT: MM DD YY ILLNESS (First symptom) OR INJURY (Accident) OR PREGNANCY (LMP)

15. IF PATIENT HAS HAD SAME OR SIMILAR ILLNESS, GIVE FIRST DATE MM DD YY

16. DATES PATIENT UNABLE TO WORK IN CURRENT OCCUPATION FROM MM DD YY TO MM DD YY

17. NAME OF REFERRING PHYSICIAN OR OTHER SOURCE

17a. I.D. NUMBER OF REFERRING PHYSICIAN

18. HOSPITALIZATION DATES RELATED TO CURRENT SERVICES FROM MM DD YY TO MM DD YY

19. RESERVED FOR LOCAL USE

20. OUTSIDE LAB? YES NO $ CHARGES

21. DIAGNOSIS OR NATURE OF ILLNESS OR INJURY. (RELATE ITEMS 1, 2, 3, OR 4 TO ITEM 24E BY LINE)

1. ____ . __
2. ____ . __
3. ____ . __
4. ____ . __

22. MEDICAID RESUBMISSION CODE ORIGINAL REF. NO.

23. PRIOR AUTHORIZATION NUMBER

24. A DATE(S) OF SERVICE From MM DD YY	To MM DD YY	B Place of Service	C Type of Service	D PROCEDURES, SERVICES, OR SUPPLIES (Explain Unusual Circumstances) CPT/HCPCS | MODIFIER	E DIAGNOSIS CODE	F $ CHARGES	G DAYS OR UNITS	H EPSDT Family Plan	I EMG	J COB	K RESERVED FOR LOCAL USE
1											
2											
3											
4											
5											
6											

25. FEDERAL TAX I.D. NUMBER SSN EIN

26. PATIENT'S ACCOUNT NO.

27. ACCEPT ASSIGNMENT? (For govt. claims, see back) YES NO

28. TOTAL CHARGE $

29. AMOUNT PAID $

30. BALANCE DUE $

31. SIGNATURE OF PHYSICIAN OR SUPPLIER INCLUDING DEGREES OR CREDENTIALS (I certify that the statements on the reverse apply to this bill and are made a part thereof.)

SIGNED DATE

32. NAME AND ADDRESS OF FACILITY WHERE SERVICES WERE RENDERED (If other than home or office)

33. PHYSICIAN'S, SUPPLIER'S BILLING NAME, ADDRESS, ZIP CODE & PHONE #

PIN# GRP#

PHYSICIAN OR SUPPLIER INFORMATION

(SAMPLE ONLY - NOT APPROVED FOR USE)

PLEASE PRINT OR TYPE

SAMPLE FORM 1500
SAMPLE FORM 1500 SAMPLE FORM 1500

PLEASE
DO NOT
STAPLE
IN THIS
AREA

(SAMPLE ONLY - NOT APPROVED FOR USE)

CARRIER

PICA

HEALTH INSURANCE CLAIM FORM

PICA

1. MEDICARE (Medicare #) MEDICAID (Medicaid #) CHAMPUS (Sponsor's SSN) CHAMPVA (VA File #) GROUP HEALTH PLAN (SSN or ID) FECA BLK LUNG (SSN) OTHER (ID)

1a. INSURED'S I.D. NUMBER (FOR PROGRAM IN ITEM 1)

2. PATIENT'S NAME (Last Name, First Name, Middle Initial)

3. PATIENT'S BIRTH DATE MM DD YY SEX M F

4. INSURED'S NAME (Last Name, First Name, Middle Initial)

5. PATIENT'S ADDRESS (No. Street)

6. PATIENT RELATIONSHIP TO INSURED Self Spouse Child Other

7. INSURED'S ADDRESS (No. Street)

CITY STATE

8. PATIENT STATUS Single Married Other

CITY STATE

ZIP CODE TELEPHONE (Include Area Code) ( )

Employed Full-Time Student Part-Time Student

ZIP CODE TELEPHONE (INCLUDE AREA CODE) ( )

9. OTHER INSURED'S NAME (Last Name, First Name, Middle Initial)

10. IS PATIENT'S CONDITION RELATED TO:

11. INSURED'S POLICY GROUP OR FECA NUMBER

a. OTHER INSURED'S POLICY OR GROUP NUMBER

a. EMPLOYMENT? (CURRENT OR PREVIOUS) YES NO

a. INSURED'S DATE OF BIRTH MM DD YY SEX M F

b. OTHER INSURED'S DATE OF BIRTH MM DD YY SEX M F

b. AUTO ACCIDENT? YES NO PLACE (State)

b. EMPLOYER'S NAME OR SCHOOL NAME

c. EMPLOYER'S NAME OR SCHOOL NAME

c. OTHER ACCIDENT? YES NO

c. INSURANCE PLAN NAME OR PROGRAM NAME

d. INSURANCE PLAN NAME OR PROGRAM NAME

10d. RESERVED FOR LOCAL USE

d. IS THERE ANOTHER HEALTH BENEFIT PLAN? YES NO If yes, return to and complete item 9 a – d.

READ BACK OF FORM BEFORE COMPLETING & SIGNING THIS FORM.

12. PATIENT'S OR AUTHORIZED PERSON'S SIGNATURE I authorize the release of any medical or other information necessary to process this claim. I also request payment of government benefits either to myself or to the party who accepts assignment below.

SIGNED DATE

13. INSURED'S OR AUTHORIZED PERSON'S SIGNATURE I authorize payment of medical benefits to the undersigned physician or supplier for services described below.

SIGNED

PATIENT AND INSURED INFORMATION

14. DATE OF CURRENT: MM DD YY ILLNESS (First symptom) OR INJURY (Accident) OR PREGNANCY (LMP)

15. IF PATIENT HAS HAD SAME OR SIMILAR ILLNESS, GIVE FIRST DATE MM DD YY

16. DATES PATIENT UNABLE TO WORK IN CURRENT OCCUPATION FROM MM DD YY TO MM DD YY

17. NAME OF REFERRING PHYSICIAN OR OTHER SOURCE

17a. I.D. NUMBER OF REFERRING PHYSICIAN

18. HOSPITALIZATION DATES RELATED TO CURRENT SERVICES FROM MM DD YY TO MM DD YY

19. RESERVED FOR LOCAL USE

20. OUTSIDE LAB? YES NO $ CHARGES

21. DIAGNOSIS OR NATURE OF ILLNESS OR INJURY. (RELATE ITEMS 1, 2, 3, OR 4 TO ITEM 24E BY LINE)

1. ___ . __
2. ___ . __
3. ___ . __
4. ___ . __

22. MEDICAID RESUBMISSION CODE ORIGINAL REF. NO.

23. PRIOR AUTHORIZATION NUMBER

24. A DATE(S) OF SERVICE From MM DD YY To MM DD YY	B Place of Service	C Type of Service	D PROCEDURES, SERVICES, OR SUPPLIES (Explain Unusual Circumstances) CPT/HCPCS MODIFIER	E DIAGNOSIS CODE	F $ CHARGES	G DAYS OR UNITS	H EPSDT Family Plan	I EMG	J COB	K RESERVED FOR LOCAL USE
1										
2										
3										
4										
5										
6										

25. FEDERAL TAX I.D. NUMBER SSN EIN

26. PATIENT'S ACCOUNT NO.

27. ACCEPT ASSIGNMENT? (For govt. claims, see back) YES NO

28. TOTAL CHARGE $

29. AMOUNT PAID $

30. BALANCE DUE $

31. SIGNATURE OF PHYSICIAN OR SUPPLIER INCLUDING DEGREES OR CREDENTIALS (I certify that the statements on the reverse apply to this bill and are made a part thereof.)

SIGNED DATE

32. NAME AND ADDRESS OF FACILITY WHERE SERVICES WERE RENDERED (If other than home or office)

33. PHYSICIAN'S, SUPPLIER'S BILLING NAME, ADDRESS, ZIP CODE & PHONE #

PIN# GRP#

PHYSICIAN OR SUPPLIER INFORMATION

(SAMPLE ONLY - NOT APPROVED FOR USE)

PLEASE PRINT OR TYPE

SAMPLE FORM 1500
SAMPLE FORM 1500 SAMPLE FORM 1500

Case Study 14-j

DATE	REMARKS				
03/17/YYYY	Medigap Payer Identification Number 334455993				

PATIENT		CHART #	SEX	BIRTHDATE
Mary R. Booth	212-77-4444	14-j	F	10/14/1933

MAILING ADDRESS	CITY	STATE	ZIP	HOME PHONE	WORK PHONE
1007 Bond Avenue	Anywhere	US	12345	(101) 333-5555	X

EMPLOYER	ADDRESS	PATIENT STATUS
	Anywhere US	MARRIED DIVORCED SINGLE (X) STUDENT OTHER

INSURANCE: PRIMARY	ID#	GROUP	SECONDARY POLICY
Medicare	212-77-4444A		

POLICYHOLDER NAME	BIRTHDATE	RELATIONSHIP	POLICYHOLDER NAME	BIRTHDATE	RELATIONSHIP
		Self			

SUPPLEMENTAL PLAN		EMPLOYER
AARP Medigap	212-77-4444	

POLICYHOLDER NAME	BIRTHDATE	RELATIONSHIP

EMPLOYER: Retired Mt. Royal Drugs

REFERRING PHYSICIAN UPIN/SSN:

DIAGNOSIS	CODE
1. Hypertension, benign	401.1
2.	
3.	
4.	

PLACE OF SERVICE Office

PROCEDURES	CODE	CHARGE
1. Est. patient OV Level I	99211	$55.00
2.		
3.		
4.		
5.		
6.		

SPECIAL NOTES

TOTAL CHARGES	PAYMENTS	ADJUSTMENTS	BALANCE
$55.00	-0-	-0-	$55.00

RETURN VISIT	PHYSICIAN SIGNATURE
3 Months	Donald L. Givings, M.D.

MEDICARE # D1234
MEDICAID # DLG1234
BCBS # 12345

DONALD L. GIVINGS, M.D.
11350 MEDICAL DRIVE, ANYWHERE, US 12345
PHONE NUMBER (101)111-5555

EIN # 11123456
SSN # 123-12-1234
UPIN # DG1234

PLEASE DO NOT STAPLE IN THIS AREA

(SAMPLE ONLY - NOT APPROVED FOR USE)

CARRIER

PICA

HEALTH INSURANCE CLAIM FORM

PICA

1. MEDICARE (Medicare #) MEDICAID (Medicaid #) CHAMPUS (Sponsor's SSN) CHAMPVA (VA File #) GROUP HEALTH PLAN (SSN or ID) FECA BLK LUNG (SSN) OTHER (ID)

1a. INSURED'S I.D. NUMBER (FOR PROGRAM IN ITEM 1)

2. PATIENT'S NAME (Last Name, First Name, Middle Initial)

3. PATIENT'S BIRTH DATE MM DD YY SEX M F

4. INSURED'S NAME (Last Name, First Name, Middle Initial)

5. PATIENT'S ADDRESS (No. Street)

6. PATIENT RELATIONSHIP TO INSURED Self Spouse Child Other

7. INSURED'S ADDRESS (No. Street)

CITY STATE

8. PATIENT STATUS Single Married Other

CITY STATE

ZIP CODE TELEPHONE (Include Area Code) ( )

Employed Full-Time Student Part-Time Student

ZIP CODE TELEPHONE (INCLUDE AREA CODE) ( )

9. OTHER INSURED'S NAME (Last Name, First Name, Middle Initial)

10. IS PATIENT'S CONDITION RELATED TO:

11. INSURED'S POLICY GROUP OR FECA NUMBER

a. OTHER INSURED'S POLICY OR GROUP NUMBER

a. EMPLOYMENT? (CURRENT OR PREVIOUS) YES NO

a. INSURED'S DATE OF BIRTH MM DD YY SEX M F

b. OTHER INSURED'S DATE OF BIRTH MM DD YY SEX M F

b. AUTO ACCIDENT? PLACE (State) YES NO

b. EMPLOYER'S NAME OR SCHOOL NAME

c. EMPLOYER'S NAME OR SCHOOL NAME

c. OTHER ACCIDENT? YES NO

c. INSURANCE PLAN NAME OR PROGRAM NAME

d. INSURANCE PLAN NAME OR PROGRAM NAME

10d. RESERVED FOR LOCAL USE

d. IS THERE ANOTHER HEALTH BENEFIT PLAN? YES NO If yes, return to and complete item 9 a – d.

READ BACK OF FORM BEFORE COMPLETING & SIGNING THIS FORM.

12. PATIENT'S OR AUTHORIZED PERSON'S SIGNATURE I authorize the release of any medical or other information necessary to process this claim. I also request payment of government benefits either to myself or to the party who accepts assignment below.

SIGNED ______ DATE ______

13. INSURED'S OR AUTHORIZED PERSON'S SIGNATURE I authorize payment of medical benefits to the undersigned physician or supplier for services described below.

SIGNED ______

PATIENT AND INSURED INFORMATION

14. DATE OF CURRENT: MM DD YY ILLNESS (First symptom) OR INJURY (Accident) OR PREGNANCY (LMP)

15. IF PATIENT HAS HAD SAME OR SIMILAR ILLNESS, GIVE FIRST DATE MM DD YY

16. DATES PATIENT UNABLE TO WORK IN CURRENT OCCUPATION FROM MM DD YY TO MM DD YY

17. NAME OF REFERRING PHYSICIAN OR OTHER SOURCE

17a. I.D. NUMBER OF REFERRING PHYSICIAN

18. HOSPITALIZATION DATES RELATED TO CURRENT SERVICES FROM MM DD YY TO MM DD YY

19. RESERVED FOR LOCAL USE

20. OUTSIDE LAB? YES NO $ CHARGES

21. DIAGNOSIS OR NATURE OF ILLNESS OR INJURY. (RELATE ITEMS 1, 2, 3, OR 4 TO ITEM 24E BY LINE)

1. ___ . __ 3. ___ . __

2. ___ . __ 4. ___ . __

22. MEDICAID RESUBMISSION CODE ORIGINAL REF. NO.

23. PRIOR AUTHORIZATION NUMBER

24. A DATE(S) OF SERVICE From MM DD YY	To MM DD YY	B Place of Service	C Type of Service	D PROCEDURES, SERVICES, OR SUPPLIES (Explain Unusual Circumstances) CPT/HCPCS MODIFIER	E DIAGNOSIS CODE	F $ CHARGES	G DAYS OR UNITS	H EPSDT Family Plan	I EMG	J COB	K RESERVED FOR LOCAL USE
1											
2											
3											
4											
5											
6											

25. FEDERAL TAX I.D. NUMBER SSN EIN

26. PATIENT'S ACCOUNT NO.

27. ACCEPT ASSIGNMENT? (For govt. claims, see back) YES NO

28. TOTAL CHARGE $

29. AMOUNT PAID $

30. BALANCE DUE $

31. SIGNATURE OF PHYSICIAN OR SUPPLIER INCLUDING DEGREES OR CREDENTIALS (I certify that the statements on the reverse apply to this bill and are made a part thereof.)

SIGNED DATE

32. NAME AND ADDRESS OF FACILITY WHERE SERVICES WERE RENDERED (If other than home or office)

33. PHYSICIAN'S, SUPPLIER'S BILLING NAME, ADDRESS, ZIP CODE & PHONE #

PIN# GRP#

PHYSICIAN OR SUPPLIER INFORMATION

(SAMPLE ONLY - NOT APPROVED FOR USE)

PLEASE PRINT OR TYPE

SAMPLE FORM 1500
SAMPLE FORM 1500 SAMPLE FORM 1500

PLEASE
DO NOT
STAPLE
IN THIS
AREA

(SAMPLE ONLY - NOT APPROVED FOR USE)

CARRIER

PICA

HEALTH INSURANCE CLAIM FORM

PICA

1. MEDICARE (Medicare #) MEDICAID (Medicaid #) CHAMPUS (Sponsor's SSN) CHAMPVA (VA File #) GROUP HEALTH PLAN (SSN or ID) FECA BLK LUNG (SSN) OTHER (ID)

1a. INSURED'S I.D. NUMBER (FOR PROGRAM IN ITEM 1)

2. PATIENT'S NAME (Last Name, First Name, Middle Initial)

3. PATIENT'S BIRTH DATE MM DD YY SEX M F

4. INSURED'S NAME (Last Name, First Name, Middle Initial)

5. PATIENT'S ADDRESS (No. Street)

6. PATIENT RELATIONSHIP TO INSURED Self Spouse Child Other

7. INSURED'S ADDRESS (No. Street)

CITY STATE

8. PATIENT STATUS Single Married Other

CITY STATE

ZIP CODE TELEPHONE (Include Area Code) ( )

Employed Full-Time Student Part-Time Student

ZIP CODE TELEPHONE (INCLUDE AREA CODE) ( )

9. OTHER INSURED'S NAME (Last Name, First Name, Middle Initial)

10. IS PATIENT'S CONDITION RELATED TO:

11. INSURED'S POLICY GROUP OR FECA NUMBER

a. OTHER INSURED'S POLICY OR GROUP NUMBER

a. EMPLOYMENT? (CURRENT OR PREVIOUS) YES NO

a. INSURED'S DATE OF BIRTH MM DD YY SEX M F

b. OTHER INSURED'S DATE OF BIRTH MM DD YY SEX M F

b. AUTO ACCIDENT? PLACE (State) YES NO

b. EMPLOYER'S NAME OR SCHOOL NAME

c. EMPLOYER'S NAME OR SCHOOL NAME

c. OTHER ACCIDENT? YES NO

c. INSURANCE PLAN NAME OR PROGRAM NAME

d. INSURANCE PLAN NAME OR PROGRAM NAME

10d. RESERVED FOR LOCAL USE

d. IS THERE ANOTHER HEALTH BENEFIT PLAN? YES NO If yes, return to and complete item 9 a – d.

READ BACK OF FORM BEFORE COMPLETING & SIGNING THIS FORM.

12. PATIENT'S OR AUTHORIZED PERSON'S SIGNATURE I authorize the release of any medical or other information necessary to process this claim. I also request payment of government benefits either to myself or to the party who accepts assignment below.

SIGNED ____ DATE ____

13. INSURED'S OR AUTHORIZED PERSON'S SIGNATURE I authorize payment of medical benefits to the undersigned physician or supplier for services described below.

SIGNED ____

PATIENT AND INSURED INFORMATION

14. DATE OF CURRENT: MM DD YY ◀ ILLNESS (First symptom) OR INJURY (Accident) OR PREGNANCY (LMP)

15. IF PATIENT HAS HAD SAME OR SIMILAR ILLNESS, GIVE FIRST DATE MM DD YY

16. DATES PATIENT UNABLE TO WORK IN CURRENT OCCUPATION FROM MM DD YY TO MM DD YY

17. NAME OF REFERRING PHYSICIAN OR OTHER SOURCE

17a. I.D. NUMBER OF REFERRING PHYSICIAN

18. HOSPITALIZATION DATES RELATED TO CURRENT SERVICES FROM MM DD YY TO MM DD YY

19. RESERVED FOR LOCAL USE

20. OUTSIDE LAB? YES NO $ CHARGES

21. DIAGNOSIS OR NATURE OF ILLNESS OR INJURY. (RELATE ITEMS 1, 2, 3, OR 4 TO ITEM 24E BY LINE)

1. ___ . __
2. ___ . __
3. ___ . __
4. ___ . __

22. MEDICAID RESUBMISSION CODE ORIGINAL REF. NO.

23. PRIOR AUTHORIZATION NUMBER

24. A DATE(S) OF SERVICE From MM DD YY To MM DD YY	B Place of Service	C Type of Service	D PROCEDURES, SERVICES, OR SUPPLIES (Explain Unusual Circumstances) CPT/HCPCS MODIFIER	E DIAGNOSIS CODE	F $ CHARGES	G DAYS OR UNITS	H EPSDT Family Plan	I EMG	J COB	K RESERVED FOR LOCAL USE
1										
2										
3										
4										
5										
6										

25. FEDERAL TAX I.D. NUMBER SSN EIN

26. PATIENT'S ACCOUNT NO.

27. ACCEPT ASSIGNMENT? (For govt. claims, see back) YES NO

28. TOTAL CHARGE $

29. AMOUNT PAID $

30. BALANCE DUE $

31. SIGNATURE OF PHYSICIAN OR SUPPLIER INCLUDING DEGREES OR CREDENTIALS (I certify that the statements on the reverse apply to this bill and are made a part thereof.)

SIGNED DATE

32. NAME AND ADDRESS OF FACILITY WHERE SERVICES WERE RENDERED (If other than home or office)

33. PHYSICIAN'S, SUPPLIER'S BILLING NAME, ADDRESS, ZIP CODE & PHONE #

PIN# GRP#

PHYSICIAN OR SUPPLIER INFORMATION

(SAMPLE ONLY - NOT APPROVED FOR USE)

PLEASE PRINT OR TYPE

SAMPLE FORM 1500
SAMPLE FORM 1500 SAMPLE FORM 1500

Case Study 14-k

DATE	REMARKS				
12/15/YYYY					
PATIENT		CHART #	SEX	BIRTHDATE	
Patricia S. Delaney 485375869		14-k	F	04/12/1931	
MAILING ADDRESS	CITY	STATE	ZIP	HOME PHONE	WORK PHONE
485 Garden Lane	Anywhere	US	12345	(101) 333-5555	
EMPLOYER	ADDRESS	PATIENT STATUS			
	Anywhere US	MARRIED DIVORCED SINGLE (X) STUDENT OTHER			
INSURANCE: PRIMARY	ID#	GROUP	SECONDARY POLICY		
Medicare	485375869A				
POLICYHOLDER NAME	BIRTHDATE	RELATIONSHIP	POLICYHOLDER NAME	BIRTHDATE	RELATIONSHIP
		Self			
SUPPLEMENTAL PLAN			EMPLOYER		
Medicaid		22886644XT			
POLICYHOLDER NAME	BIRTHDATE	RELATIONSHIP	DIAGNOSIS		CODE
		Self	1. Rosacea		695.3
EMPLOYER			2.		
			3.		
REFERRING PHYSICIAN UPIN/SSN			4.		
PLACE OF SERVICE Office					

PROCEDURES	CODE	CHARGE
1. Est. patient OV Level I	99211	$55.00
2.		
3.		
4.		
5.		
6.		

SPECIAL NOTES

Refer patient to a Dermatologist

TOTAL CHARGES	PAYMENTS	ADJUSTMENTS	BALANCE
$55.00	-0-	-0-	$55.00

RETURN VISIT	PHYSICIAN SIGNATURE
PRN	Donald L. Givings, M.D.

MEDICARE # D1234
MEDICAID # DLG1234
BCBS # 12345

DONALD L. GIVINGS, M.D.
11350 MEDICAL DRIVE, ANYWHERE, US 12345
PHONE NUMBER (101)111-5555

EIN # 11123456
SSN # 123-12-1234
UPIN # DG1234

PLEASE
DO NOT
STAPLE
IN THIS
AREA

(SAMPLE ONLY - NOT APPROVED FOR USE)

CARRIER

PICA

HEALTH INSURANCE CLAIM FORM

PICA

1. MEDICARE (Medicare #) MEDICAID (Medicaid #) CHAMPUS (Sponsor's SSN) CHAMPVA (VA File #) GROUP HEALTH PLAN (SSN or ID) FECA BLK LUNG (SSN) OTHER (ID)

1a. INSURED'S I.D. NUMBER (FOR PROGRAM IN ITEM 1)

2. PATIENT'S NAME (Last Name, First Name, Middle Initial)

3. PATIENT'S BIRTH DATE MM DD YY SEX M F

4. INSURED'S NAME (Last Name, First Name, Middle Initial)

5. PATIENT'S ADDRESS (No. Street)

6. PATIENT RELATIONSHIP TO INSURED Self Spouse Child Other

7. INSURED'S ADDRESS (No. Street)

CITY STATE

8. PATIENT STATUS Single Married Other

CITY STATE

ZIP CODE TELEPHONE (Include Area Code) ( )

Employed Full-Time Student Part-Time Student

ZIP CODE TELEPHONE (INCLUDE AREA CODE) ( )

9. OTHER INSURED'S NAME (Last Name, First Name, Middle Initial)

10. IS PATIENT'S CONDITION RELATED TO:

11. INSURED'S POLICY GROUP OR FECA NUMBER

a. OTHER INSURED'S POLICY OR GROUP NUMBER

a. EMPLOYMENT? (CURRENT OR PREVIOUS) YES NO

a. INSURED'S DATE OF BIRTH MM DD YY SEX M F

b. OTHER INSURED'S DATE OF BIRTH MM DD YY SEX M F

b. AUTO ACCIDENT? PLACE (State) YES NO

b. EMPLOYER'S NAME OR SCHOOL NAME

c. EMPLOYER'S NAME OR SCHOOL NAME

c. OTHER ACCIDENT? YES NO

c. INSURANCE PLAN NAME OR PROGRAM NAME

d. INSURANCE PLAN NAME OR PROGRAM NAME

10d. RESERVED FOR LOCAL USE

d. IS THERE ANOTHER HEALTH BENEFIT PLAN? YES NO If yes, return to and complete item 9 a – d.

READ BACK OF FORM BEFORE COMPLETING & SIGNING THIS FORM.

12. PATIENT'S OR AUTHORIZED PERSON'S SIGNATURE I authorize the release of any medical or other information necessary to process this claim. I also request payment of government benefits either to myself or to the party who accepts assignment below.

SIGNED DATE

13. INSURED'S OR AUTHORIZED PERSON'S SIGNATURE I authorize payment of medical benefits to the undersigned physician or supplier for services described below.

SIGNED

PATIENT AND INSURED INFORMATION

14. DATE OF CURRENT: MM DD YY ILLNESS (First symptom) OR INJURY (Accident) OR PREGNANCY (LMP)

15. IF PATIENT HAS HAD SAME OR SIMILAR ILLNESS, GIVE FIRST DATE MM DD YY

16. DATES PATIENT UNABLE TO WORK IN CURRENT OCCUPATION FROM MM DD YY TO MM DD YY

17. NAME OF REFERRING PHYSICIAN OR OTHER SOURCE

17a. I.D. NUMBER OF REFERRING PHYSICIAN

18. HOSPITALIZATION DATES RELATED TO CURRENT SERVICES FROM MM DD YY TO MM DD YY

19. RESERVED FOR LOCAL USE

20. OUTSIDE LAB? YES NO $ CHARGES

21. DIAGNOSIS OR NATURE OF ILLNESS OR INJURY. (RELATE ITEMS 1, 2, 3, OR 4 TO ITEM 24E BY LINE)

1. ___ . __ 3. ___ . __

2. ___ . __ 4. ___ . __

22. MEDICAID RESUBMISSION CODE ORIGINAL REF. NO.

23. PRIOR AUTHORIZATION NUMBER

24. A DATE(S) OF SERVICE From MM DD YY To MM DD YY	B Place of Service	C Type of Service	D PROCEDURES, SERVICES, OR SUPPLIES (Explain Unusual Circumstances) CPT/HCPCS MODIFIER	E DIAGNOSIS CODE	F $ CHARGES	G DAYS OR UNITS	H EPSDT Family Plan	I EMG	J COB	K RESERVED FOR LOCAL USE
1										
2										
3										
4										
5										
6										

25. FEDERAL TAX I.D. NUMBER SSN EIN

26. PATIENT'S ACCOUNT NO.

27. ACCEPT ASSIGNMENT? (For govt. claims, see back) YES NO

28. TOTAL CHARGE $

29. AMOUNT PAID $

30. BALANCE DUE $

31. SIGNATURE OF PHYSICIAN OR SUPPLIER INCLUDING DEGREES OR CREDENTIALS (I certify that the statements on the reverse apply to this bill and are made a part thereof.)

SIGNED DATE

32. NAME AND ADDRESS OF FACILITY WHERE SERVICES WERE RENDERED (If other than home or office)

33. PHYSICIAN'S, SUPPLIER'S BILLING NAME, ADDRESS, ZIP CODE & PHONE #

PIN# GRP#

PHYSICIAN OR SUPPLIER INFORMATION

(SAMPLE ONLY - NOT APPROVED FOR USE)

PLEASE PRINT OR TYPE

SAMPLE FORM 1500
SAMPLE FORM 1500 SAMPLE FORM 1500

Case Study 14-I

DATE	REMARKS
12/15/YYYY	

PATIENT	CHART #	SEX	BIRTHDATE
Patricia S. Delaney 485375869	14-I	F	04/12/1931

MAILING ADDRESS	CITY	STATE	ZIP	HOME PHONE	WORK PHONE
485 Garden Lane	Anywhere	US	12345	(101) 333-5555	

EMPLOYER	ADDRESS	PATIENT STATUS
	Anywhere US	MARRIED DIVORCED SINGLE (X) STUDENT OTHER

INSURANCE: PRIMARY	ID#	GROUP	SECONDARY POLICY
Medicare	485375869A		

POLICYHOLDER NAME	BIRTHDATE	RELATIONSHIP	POLICYHOLDER NAME	BIRTHDATE	RELATIONSHIP
		Self			

SUPPLEMENTAL PLAN	EMPLOYER
Medicaid 22886644XT	

POLICYHOLDER NAME	BIRTHDATE	RELATIONSHIP
		Self

EMPLOYER

REFERRING PHYSICIAN UPIN/SSN: Donald L. Givings, M.D. 123-12-1234

DIAGNOSIS	CODE
1. Rosacea	695.3
2.	
3.	
4.	

PLACE OF SERVICE Office

PROCEDURES	CODE	CHARGE
1. Office Consult Level III	99243	$85.00
2.		
3.		
4.		
5.		
6.		

SPECIAL NOTES

TOTAL CHARGES	PAYMENTS	ADJUSTMENTS	BALANCE
$85.00	-0-	-0-	$85.00

RETURN VISIT	PHYSICIAN SIGNATURE
PRN	Claire M. Skinner, M.D.

MEDICARE # C1234
MEDICAID # CMS1234
BCBS # 94949

CLAIRE M. SKINNER, M.D. DERMATOLOGY
50 CLEAR VIEW DRIVE, ANYWHERE, US 12345
PHONE NUMBER (101)111-5555

EIN # 11555555
SSN # 333-44-1234
UPIN # CS1234

PLEASE
DO NOT
STAPLE
IN THIS
AREA

(SAMPLE ONLY - NOT APPROVED FOR USE)

CARRIER

PICA

HEALTH INSURANCE CLAIM FORM

PICA

1. MEDICARE (Medicare #) MEDICAID (Medicaid #) CHAMPUS (Sponsor's SSN) CHAMPVA (VA File #) GROUP HEALTH PLAN (SSN or ID) FECA BLK LUNG (SSN) OTHER (ID)

1a. INSURED'S I.D. NUMBER (FOR PROGRAM IN ITEM 1)

2. PATIENT'S NAME (Last Name, First Name, Middle Initial)

3. PATIENT'S BIRTH DATE MM DD YY SEX M F

4. INSURED'S NAME (Last Name, First Name, Middle Initial)

5. PATIENT'S ADDRESS (No. Street)

6. PATIENT RELATIONSHIP TO INSURED Self Spouse Child Other

7. INSURED'S ADDRESS (No. Street)

CITY STATE

8. PATIENT STATUS Single Married Other

CITY STATE

ZIP CODE TELEPHONE (Include Area Code) ( )

Employed Full-Time Student Part-Time Student

ZIP CODE TELEPHONE (INCLUDE AREA CODE) ( )

9. OTHER INSURED'S NAME (Last Name, First Name, Middle Initial)

10. IS PATIENT'S CONDITION RELATED TO:

11. INSURED'S POLICY GROUP OR FECA NUMBER

a. OTHER INSURED'S POLICY OR GROUP NUMBER

a. EMPLOYMENT? (CURRENT OR PREVIOUS) YES NO

a. INSURED'S DATE OF BIRTH MM DD YY SEX M F

b. OTHER INSURED'S DATE OF BIRTH MM DD YY SEX M F

b. AUTO ACCIDENT? PLACE (State) YES NO

b. EMPLOYER'S NAME OR SCHOOL NAME

c. EMPLOYER'S NAME OR SCHOOL NAME

c. OTHER ACCIDENT? YES NO

c. INSURANCE PLAN NAME OR PROGRAM NAME

d. INSURANCE PLAN NAME OR PROGRAM NAME

10d. RESERVED FOR LOCAL USE

d. IS THERE ANOTHER HEALTH BENEFIT PLAN? YES NO If yes, return to and complete item 9 a – d.

READ BACK OF FORM BEFORE COMPLETING & SIGNING THIS FORM.

12. PATIENT'S OR AUTHORIZED PERSON'S SIGNATURE I authorize the release of any medical or other information necessary to process this claim. I also request payment of government benefits either to myself or to the party who accepts assignment below.

SIGNED DATE

13. INSURED'S OR AUTHORIZED PERSON'S SIGNATURE I authorize payment of medical benefits to the undersigned physician or supplier for services described below.

SIGNED

PATIENT AND INSURED INFORMATION

14. DATE OF CURRENT: MM DD YY ILLNESS (First symptom) OR INJURY (Accident) OR PREGNANCY (LMP)

15. IF PATIENT HAS HAD SAME OR SIMILAR ILLNESS, GIVE FIRST DATE MM DD YY

16. DATES PATIENT UNABLE TO WORK IN CURRENT OCCUPATION FROM MM DD YY TO MM DD YY

17. NAME OF REFERRING PHYSICIAN OR OTHER SOURCE

17a. I.D. NUMBER OF REFERRING PHYSICIAN

18. HOSPITALIZATION DATES RELATED TO CURRENT SERVICES FROM MM DD YY TO MM DD YY

19. RESERVED FOR LOCAL USE

20. OUTSIDE LAB? YES NO $ CHARGES

21. DIAGNOSIS OR NATURE OF ILLNESS OR INJURY. (RELATE ITEMS 1, 2, 3, OR 4 TO ITEM 24E BY LINE)

1. ___ . __ 3. ___ . __

2. ___ . __ 4. ___ . __

22. MEDICAID RESUBMISSION CODE ORIGINAL REF. NO.

23. PRIOR AUTHORIZATION NUMBER

24.	A DATE(S) OF SERVICE From MM DD YY To MM DD YY	B Place of Service	C Type of Service	D PROCEDURES, SERVICES, OR SUPPLIES (Explain Unusual Circumstances) CPT/HCPCS MODIFIER	E DIAGNOSIS CODE	F $ CHARGES	G DAYS OR UNITS	H EPSDT Family Plan	I EMG	J COB	K RESERVED FOR LOCAL USE
1											
2											
3											
4											
5											
6											

25. FEDERAL TAX I.D. NUMBER SSN EIN

26. PATIENT'S ACCOUNT NO.

27. ACCEPT ASSIGNMENT? (For govt. claims, see back) YES NO

28. TOTAL CHARGE $

29. AMOUNT PAID $

30. BALANCE DUE $

31. SIGNATURE OF PHYSICIAN OR SUPPLIER INCLUDING DEGREES OR CREDENTIALS (I certify that the statements on the reverse apply to this bill and are made a part thereof.)

SIGNED DATE

32. NAME AND ADDRESS OF FACILITY WHERE SERVICES WERE RENDERED (If other than home or office)

33. PHYSICIAN'S, SUPPLIER'S BILLING NAME, ADDRESS, ZIP CODE & PHONE #

PIN# GRP#

PHYSICIAN OR SUPPLIER INFORMATION

(SAMPLE ONLY - NOT APPROVED FOR USE)

PLEASE PRINT OR TYPE

SAMPLE FORM 1500
SAMPLE FORM 1500 SAMPLE FORM 1500

Complete the Medical Necessity Statement for Danielle H. Ford, Case Study 14-m.

Practice Letterhead

To My Medicare Patients:

My primary concern as your physician is to provide you with the best possible care. Medicare does not pay for all services and will only allow those which it determines, under the guidelines spelled out in the Omnibus Reconciliation Act of 1986 Section 1862(a)(1), to be reasonable and necessary. Under this law, a procedure or service deemed to be medically unreasonable or unnecessary will be denied. Since I believe each scheduled visit or planned procedure is both reasonable and necessary, I am required to notify you in advance that the following procedures or services listed below, which we have mutually agreed on, may be denied by Medicare.

Date of Service ______________________

Description of Service	Charge
______________________________________	______
______________________________________	______
______________________________________	______

Denial may be for the following reasons:

1. Medicare does not usually pay for this many visits or treatments,
2. Medicare does not usually pay for this many services within this period of time, and/or
3. Medicare does not usually pay for this type of service for your condition.

I, however, believe these procedures/services to be both reasonable and necessary for your condition, and will assist you in collecting payment from Medicare. In order for me to assist you in this matter, the law requires that you read the following agreement and sign it.

I have been informed by ______________________________ that he/she believes, in my case, Medicare is likely to deny payment for the services and reasons stated above. If Medicare denies payment, I agree to be personally and fully responsible for payment.

Beneficiary's Name: ___________________________ Medicare ID # ___________________ or

Beneficiary's Signature ____

or

Authorized Representative's Signature ____________________________________

Case Study 14-m

DATE	REMARKS
08/09/YYYY	Have the patient sign a Medicare Medical Necessity form

PATIENT		CHART #	SEX	BIRTHDATE
Danielle H. Ford	756-66-7878	14-m	F	12/10/1922

MAILING ADDRESS	CITY	STATE	ZIP	HOME PHONE	WORK PHONE
28 Delightful Drive	Anywhere	US	12345	(101) 333-5555	

EMPLOYER	ADDRESS	PATIENT STATUS
	Anywhere US	MARRIED DIVORCED SINGLE (X) STUDENT OTHER

INSURANCE: PRIMARY	ID#	GROUP	SECONDARY POLICY
Medicare	756-66-7878W		

POLICYHOLDER NAME	BIRTHDATE	RELATIONSHIP	POLICYHOLDER NAME	BIRTHDATE	RELATIONSHIP

SUPPLEMENTAL PLAN	EMPLOYER

POLICYHOLDER NAME	BIRTHDATE	RELATIONSHIP

EMPLOYER

REFERRING PHYSICIAN UPIN/SSN

DIAGNOSIS	CODE
1. Routine examination	V70.0
2.	
3.	
4.	

PLACE OF SERVICE Office

PROCEDURES	CODE	CHARGE
1. Preventive medicine, 65 years and over	9939	$65.00
2.		
3.		
4.		
5.		
6.		

SPECIAL NOTES

TOTAL CHARGES	PAYMENTS	ADJUSTMENTS	BALANCE
$65.00	$65.00	-0-	$0.00

RETURN VISIT	PHYSICIAN SIGNATURE
PRN	Donald L. Givings, M.D.

DONALD L. GIVINGS, M.D.
11350 MEDICAL DRIVE, ANYWHERE, US 12345
PHONE NUMBER (101)111-5555

MEDICARE # D1234
MEDICAID # DLG1234
BCBS # 12345

EIN # 11123456
SSN # 123-12-1234
UPIN # DG1234

PLEASE DO NOT STAPLE IN THIS AREA

(SAMPLE ONLY - NOT APPROVED FOR USE)

CARRIER

PICA

HEALTH INSURANCE CLAIM FORM

PICA

1. MEDICARE (Medicare #) MEDICAID (Medicaid #) CHAMPUS (Sponsor's SSN) CHAMPVA (VA File #) GROUP HEALTH PLAN (SSN or ID) FECA BLK LUNG (SSN) OTHER (ID)

1a. INSURED'S I.D. NUMBER (FOR PROGRAM IN ITEM 1)

2. PATIENT'S NAME (Last Name, First Name, Middle Initial)

3. PATIENT'S BIRTH DATE MM DD YY SEX M F

4. INSURED'S NAME (Last Name, First Name, Middle Initial)

5. PATIENT'S ADDRESS (No. Street)

6. PATIENT RELATIONSHIP TO INSURED Self Spouse Child Other

7. INSURED'S ADDRESS (No. Street)

CITY STATE

8. PATIENT STATUS Single Married Other

CITY STATE

ZIP CODE TELEPHONE (Include Area Code) ( )

Employed Full-Time Student Part-Time Student

ZIP CODE TELEPHONE (INCLUDE AREA CODE) ( )

9. OTHER INSURED'S NAME (Last Name, First Name, Middle Initial)

10. IS PATIENT'S CONDITION RELATED TO:

11. INSURED'S POLICY GROUP OR FECA NUMBER

a. OTHER INSURED'S POLICY OR GROUP NUMBER

a. EMPLOYMENT? (CURRENT OR PREVIOUS) YES NO

a. INSURED'S DATE OF BIRTH MM DD YY SEX M F

b. OTHER INSURED'S DATE OF BIRTH MM DD YY SEX M F

b. AUTO ACCIDENT? PLACE (State) YES NO

b. EMPLOYER'S NAME OR SCHOOL NAME

c. EMPLOYER'S NAME OR SCHOOL NAME

c. OTHER ACCIDENT? YES NO

c. INSURANCE PLAN NAME OR PROGRAM NAME

d. INSURANCE PLAN NAME OR PROGRAM NAME

10d. RESERVED FOR LOCAL USE

d. IS THERE ANOTHER HEALTH BENEFIT PLAN? YES NO If yes, return to and complete item 9 a – d.

READ BACK OF FORM BEFORE COMPLETING & SIGNING THIS FORM.

12. PATIENT'S OR AUTHORIZED PERSON'S SIGNATURE I authorize the release of any medical or other information necessary to process this claim. I also request payment of government benefits either to myself or to the party who accepts assignment below.

SIGNED ____________ DATE ____________

13. INSURED'S OR AUTHORIZED PERSON'S SIGNATURE I authorize payment of medical benefits to the undersigned physician or supplier for services described below.

SIGNED ____________

PATIENT AND INSURED INFORMATION

14. DATE OF CURRENT: MM DD YY ILLNESS (First symptom) OR INJURY (Accident) OR PREGNANCY (LMP)

15. IF PATIENT HAS HAD SAME OR SIMILAR ILLNESS, GIVE FIRST DATE MM DD YY

16. DATES PATIENT UNABLE TO WORK IN CURRENT OCCUPATION FROM MM DD YY TO MM DD YY

17. NAME OF REFERRING PHYSICIAN OR OTHER SOURCE

17a. I.D. NUMBER OF REFERRING PHYSICIAN

18. HOSPITALIZATION DATES RELATED TO CURRENT SERVICES FROM MM DD YY TO MM DD YY

19. RESERVED FOR LOCAL USE

20. OUTSIDE LAB? YES NO $ CHARGES

21. DIAGNOSIS OR NATURE OF ILLNESS OR INJURY. (RELATE ITEMS 1, 2, 3, OR 4 TO ITEM 24E BY LINE)

1. ___ . __ 3. ___ . __

2. ___ . __ 4. ___ . __

22. MEDICAID RESUBMISSION CODE ORIGINAL REF. NO.

23. PRIOR AUTHORIZATION NUMBER

24. A DATE(S) OF SERVICE From MM DD YY To MM DD YY	B Place of Service	C Type of Service	D PROCEDURES, SERVICES, OR SUPPLIES (Explain Unusual Circumstances) CPT/HCPCS MODIFIER	E DIAGNOSIS CODE	F $ CHARGES	G DAYS OR UNITS	H EPSDT Family Plan	I EMG	J COB	K RESERVED FOR LOCAL USE
1										
2										
3										
4										
5										
6										

25. FEDERAL TAX I.D. NUMBER SSN EIN

26. PATIENT'S ACCOUNT NO.

27. ACCEPT ASSIGNMENT? (For govt. claims, see back) YES NO

28. TOTAL CHARGE $

29. AMOUNT PAID $

30. BALANCE DUE $

31. SIGNATURE OF PHYSICIAN OR SUPPLIER INCLUDING DEGREES OR CREDENTIALS (I certify that the statements on the reverse apply to this bill and are made a part thereof.)

SIGNED DATE

32. NAME AND ADDRESS OF FACILITY WHERE SERVICES WERE RENDERED (If other than home or office)

33. PHYSICIAN'S, SUPPLIER'S BILLING NAME, ADDRESS, ZIP CODE & PHONE #

PIN# GRP#

PHYSICIAN OR SUPPLIER INFORMATION

(SAMPLE ONLY - NOT APPROVED FOR USE)

PLEASE PRINT OR TYPE

SAMPLE FORM 1500
SAMPLE FORM 1500 SAMPLE FORM 1500

Medicaid

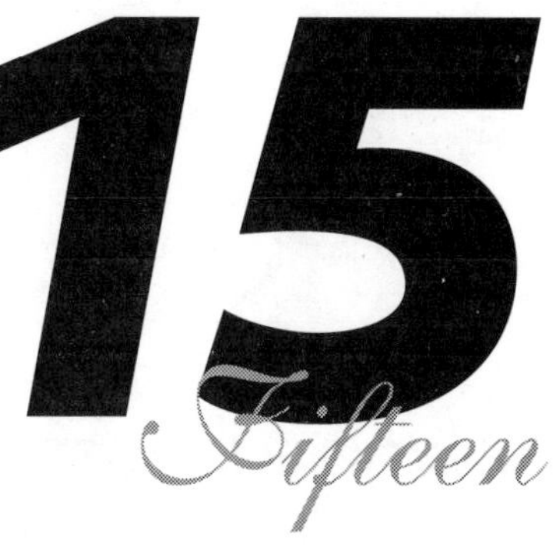

FEDERAL ELIGIBILITY REQUIREMENTS

1. When a patient claims to be eligible for Medicaid benefits, what must be presented as proof? ________

____

2. In many cases, what does Medicaid eligibility depend on? ____________________

3. What do most states use for verification of Medicaid eligibility? ____________________

MEDICAID SERVICES

4. What does the EPSDT legislation mandate? ____________________

____

5. Many states have implemented a ________________ ________________ to track over-utilization of services.

6. List six medical situations that require preauthorization from Medicaid.

   a. ____________________
   b. ____________________
   c. ____________________
   d. ____________________
   e. ____________________
   f. ____________________

7. Medicaid makes payment directly to ___. (Circle the correct answer.)

   a. Medicare
   b. patients
   c. providers
   d. all of the above

8. Emergency services and family planning services are exempt from ___.

9. Medicaid recipients excluded from copayments include ___. (Circle the correct answer.)
   a. children over the age of 18
   b. hypertensive adults
   c. pregnant women
   d. all of the above

10. The portion of the Medicaid program paid by the federal government is known as the
    _______________ _______________ _______________ _______________.

RELATIONSHIP BETWEEN MEDICAID-MEDICARE

11. Define *dual eligibles.* ____
    ____
    ____

12. Services covered by both programs are paid first by __________ and the difference by __________.

MEDICAID AS A SECONDARY PAYER

13. Medicaid is always the ___. (Circle the correct answer.)
    a. primary insurance
    b. secondary insurance
    c. payer of last resort
    d. none of the above

14. Medicaid is billed only ___. (Circle the correct answer.)
    a. if other coverage denies responsibility for payment
    b. if other coverage pays less than the Medicaid fee schedule
    c. if Medicaid covers procedures not covered by another policy
    d. all of the above

PARTICIPATING PROVIDERS

15. If a patient has Medicaid and a service was performed that is a Medicaid-covered benefit, can the provider balance bill the patient? ____________

16. Can a Medicaid patient be billed for a service that is not a Medicaid-covered benefit? ____________

MEDICAID AND MANAGED CARE

17. Many states have requested federal permission to enroll Medicaid beneficiaries into ___ programs. (Circle the correct answer.)
    a. HMO
    b. PPO
    c. POS
    d. all of the above

18. Most Medicaid HMO programs offer capitated services to ___. (Circle the correct answer.)
    a. chronically ill members
    b. healthier members
    c. members in rural communities
    d. any of the above

19. All Medicaid HMO patients have a ___. (Circle the correct answer.)
    a. primary care physician
    b. case manager
    c. gatekeeper
    d. any of the above

BILLING INFORMATION NOTES

20. In most states, the required form for submitting Medicaid claims is the ___. (Circle the correct answer.)
    a. UB-92
    b. HCFA-1450
    c. HCFA-1500
    d. none of the above

21. The deadline for filing claims for Medicaid patients ___. (Circle the correct answer.)
    a. varies from state to state
    b. is 30 days
    c. is 60 days
    d. is 90 days

22. Medicaid crossover claims follow the ___ deadlines for claims. (Circle the correct answer.)
    a. Medicaid
    b. secondary
    c. Medicare
    d. none of the above

23. State why collection of fees for uncovered services is difficult. ______________________________

____

____

24. If the assignment of benefits is not marked on the HCFA-1500 claim form, what can happen to reimbursement?

____

____

25. For each question, enter **Y** for yes or **N** for no on the line provided.

_______ a. Can a provider attempt to collect the difference between the Medicaid payment and the fee charged if the patient did not reveal that he/she was a Medicaid recipient at the time of service?

_______ b. Can there be a deductible for persons in the medically indigent classification?

_______ c. Are copayments required for some categories of Medicaid recipients?

_______ d. Does the Medicaid recipient pay a premium for medical coverage?

_______ e. If the patient's condition warrants extension of authorized inpatient days, should the hospital seek authorization for additional inpatient days?

_______ f. Can Medicaid patients be eligible for Medicaid benefits one month and not the next?

_______ g. Are cards issued for the "Unborn child of..." valid for services as soon as the child is born?

Know Your Acronyms

26. Define the following acronyms:

a. SSI _______________________________________

b. AFDC _______________________________________

c. EPSDT _______________________________________

d. TANF _______________________________________

e. SCHIP _______________________________________

f. ADA _______________________________________

g. FPL _______________________________________

h. MN _______________________________________

i. FMAP _______________________________________

j. QMB _______________________________________

k. SLMB _______________________________________

l. QI _______________________________________

m. ODWI _______________________________________

EXERCISES

1. Complete the Case Studies, 15-a through 15-f, using the blank claim form provided. Follow the step-by-step instructions from the textbook to properly complete the claim form. You may choose to use a pencil so corrections can be made.

Case Study 15-a

DATE	REMARKS		
11/13/YYYY			

PATIENT	CHART #	SEX	BIRTHDATE
Sharon W. Casey 333-55-7979	15-a	F	10/06/1970

MAILING ADDRESS	CITY	STATE	ZIP	HOME PHONE	WORK PHONE
483 Oakdale Avenue	Anywhere	US	12345	(101) 333-5555	

EMPLOYER	ADDRESS	PATIENT STATUS
		MARRIED DIVORCED SINGLE (X) STUDENT OTHER

INSURANCE: PRIMARY	ID#	GROUP	SECONDARY POLICY
Medicaid	22334455		

POLICYHOLDER NAME	BIRTHDATE	RELATIONSHIP	POLICYHOLDER NAME	BIRTHDATE	RELATIONSHIP

SUPPLEMENTAL PLAN	EMPLOYER

POLICYHOLDER NAME BIRTHDATE RELATIONSHIP

EMPLOYER

REFERRING PHYSICIAN UPIN/SSN

DIAGNOSIS	CODE
1. Excessive menstruation	626.2
2. Irregular menstrual cycle	626.4
3.	
4.	

PLACE OF SERVICE Office

PROCEDURES	CODE	CHARGE
1. Est. patient Ov Level III	99213	$75.00
2.		
3.		
4.		
5.		
6.		

SPECIAL NOTES

Refer patient to GYN

TOTAL CHARGES	PAYMENTS	ADJUSTMENTS	BALANCE
$75.00	-0-	-0-	$75.00

RETURN VISIT	PHYSICIAN SIGNATURE
PRN	Donald L. Givings, M.D.

MEDICARE # D1234
MEDICAID # DLG1234
BCBS # 12345

DONALD L. GIVINGS, M.D.
11350 MEDICAL DRIVE, ANYWHERE, US 12345
PHONE NUMBER (101)111-5555

EIN # 11123456
SSN # 123-12-1234
UPIN # DG1234

PLEASE
DO NOT
STAPLE
IN THIS
AREA

(SAMPLE ONLY - NOT APPROVED FOR USE)

CARRIER

PICA

HEALTH INSURANCE CLAIM FORM

PICA

1. MEDICARE (Medicare #) MEDICAID (Medicaid #) CHAMPUS (Sponsor's SSN) CHAMPVA (VA File #) GROUP HEALTH PLAN (SSN or ID) FECA BLK LUNG (SSN) OTHER (ID)

1a. INSURED'S I.D. NUMBER (FOR PROGRAM IN ITEM 1)

2. PATIENT'S NAME (Last Name, First Name, Middle Initial)

3. PATIENT'S BIRTH DATE MM DD YY SEX M F

4. INSURED'S NAME (Last Name, First Name, Middle Initial)

5. PATIENT'S ADDRESS (No. Street)

6. PATIENT RELATIONSHIP TO INSURED Self Spouse Child Other

7. INSURED'S ADDRESS (No. Street)

CITY STATE

8. PATIENT STATUS Single Married Other

CITY STATE

ZIP CODE TELEPHONE (Include Area Code) ( )

Employed Full-Time Student Part-Time Student

ZIP CODE TELEPHONE (INCLUDE AREA CODE) ( )

9. OTHER INSURED'S NAME (Last Name, First Name, Middle Initial)

10. IS PATIENT'S CONDITION RELATED TO:

11. INSURED'S POLICY GROUP OR FECA NUMBER

a. OTHER INSURED'S POLICY OR GROUP NUMBER

a. EMPLOYMENT? (CURRENT OR PREVIOUS) YES NO

a. INSURED'S DATE OF BIRTH MM DD YY SEX M F

b. OTHER INSURED'S DATE OF BIRTH MM DD YY SEX M F

b. AUTO ACCIDENT? YES NO PLACE (State)

b. EMPLOYER'S NAME OR SCHOOL NAME

c. EMPLOYER'S NAME OR SCHOOL NAME

c. OTHER ACCIDENT? YES NO

c. INSURANCE PLAN NAME OR PROGRAM NAME

d. INSURANCE PLAN NAME OR PROGRAM NAME

10d. RESERVED FOR LOCAL USE

d. IS THERE ANOTHER HEALTH BENEFIT PLAN? YES NO If yes, return to and complete item 9 a – d.

READ BACK OF FORM BEFORE COMPLETING & SIGNING THIS FORM.

12. PATIENT'S OR AUTHORIZED PERSON'S SIGNATURE I authorize the release of any medical or other information necessary to process this claim. I also request payment of government benefits either to myself or to the party who accepts assignment below.

SIGNED ______ DATE ______

13. INSURED'S OR AUTHORIZED PERSON'S SIGNATURE I authorize payment of medical benefits to the undersigned physician or supplier for services described below.

SIGNED ______

PATIENT AND INSURED INFORMATION

14. DATE OF CURRENT: MM DD YY ILLNESS (First symptom) OR INJURY (Accident) OR PREGNANCY (LMP)

15. IF PATIENT HAS HAD SAME OR SIMILAR ILLNESS, GIVE FIRST DATE MM DD YY

16. DATES PATIENT UNABLE TO WORK IN CURRENT OCCUPATION FROM MM DD YY TO MM DD YY

17. NAME OF REFERRING PHYSICIAN OR OTHER SOURCE

17a. I.D. NUMBER OF REFERRING PHYSICIAN

18. HOSPITALIZATION DATES RELATED TO CURRENT SERVICES FROM MM DD YY TO MM DD YY

19. RESERVED FOR LOCAL USE

20. OUTSIDE LAB? YES NO $ CHARGES

21. DIAGNOSIS OR NATURE OF ILLNESS OR INJURY. (RELATE ITEMS 1, 2, 3, OR 4 TO ITEM 24E BY LINE)

1. ___ . __
2. ___ . __
3. ___ . __
4. ___ . __

22. MEDICAID RESUBMISSION CODE ORIGINAL REF. NO.

23. PRIOR AUTHORIZATION NUMBER

24. A DATE(S) OF SERVICE From MM DD YY To MM DD YY	B Place of Service	C Type of Service	D PROCEDURES, SERVICES, OR SUPPLIES (Explain Unusual Circumstances) CPT/HCPCS MODIFIER	E DIAGNOSIS CODE	F $ CHARGES	G DAYS OR UNITS	H EPSDT Family Plan	I EMG	J COB	K RESERVED FOR LOCAL USE
1										
2										
3										
4										
5										
6										

25. FEDERAL TAX I.D. NUMBER SSN EIN

26. PATIENT'S ACCOUNT NO.

27. ACCEPT ASSIGNMENT? (For govt. claims, see back) YES NO

28. TOTAL CHARGE $

29. AMOUNT PAID $

30. BALANCE DUE $

31. SIGNATURE OF PHYSICIAN OR SUPPLIER INCLUDING DEGREES OR CREDENTIALS (I certify that the statements on the reverse apply to this bill and are made a part thereof.)

SIGNED DATE

32. NAME AND ADDRESS OF FACILITY WHERE SERVICES WERE RENDERED (If other than home or office)

33. PHYSICIAN'S, SUPPLIER'S BILLING NAME, ADDRESS, ZIP CODE & PHONE #

PIN# GRP#

PHYSICIAN OR SUPPLIER INFORMATION

(SAMPLE ONLY - NOT APPROVED FOR USE)

PLEASE PRINT OR TYPE

SAMPLE FORM 1500
SAMPLE FORM 1500 SAMPLE FORM 1500

Case Study 15-b

DATE	REMARKS				
11/20/YYYY					
PATIENT			CHART #	SEX	BIRTHDATE
Sharon W. Casey 333-55-7979			15-b	F	10/06/1970
MAILING ADDRESS	CITY	STATE	ZIP	HOME PHONE	WORK PHONE
483 Oakdale Avenue	Anywhere	US	12345	(101) 333-5555	
EMPLOYER	ADDRESS		PATIENT STATUS		
			MARRIED DIVORCED SINGLE (X) STUDENT OTHER		
INSURANCE: PRIMARY	ID#	GROUP	SECONDARY POLICY		
Medicaid	22334455				
POLICYHOLDER NAME	BIRTHDATE	RELATIONSHIP	POLICYHOLDER NAME	BIRTHDATE	RELATIONSHIP
SUPPLEMENTAL PLAN			EMPLOYER		
POLICYHOLDER NAME	BIRTHDATE	RELATIONSHIP	DIAGNOSIS		CODE
			1. Excessive menstruation		626.2
EMPLOYER			2. Irregular menstrual cycle		626.4
			3.		
REFERRING PHYSICIAN UPIN/SSN			4.		
Donald L. Givings, M.D.	DLG1234				
PLACE OF SERVICE	Office				

PROCEDURES	CODE	CHARGE
1. Office Consult Level III	99243	$85.00
2.		
3.		
4.		
5.		
6.		

SPECIAL NOTES			
TOTAL CHARGES	PAYMENTS	ADJUSTMENTS	BALANCE
$85.00	-0-	-0-	$85.00
RETURN VISIT		PHYSICIAN SIGNATURE	
One month		Maria C Section, M.D.	

MEDICARE # M1234
MEDICAID # MCS1234
BCBS # 11223

MARIA C. SECTION, M.D. OB/GYN
11 MADEN LANE, ANYWHERE, US 12345
PHONE NUMBER (101)111-5555

EIN # 11669977
SSN # 444-22-1234
UPIN # MS1234

PLEASE
DO NOT
STAPLE
IN THIS
AREA

(SAMPLE ONLY - NOT APPROVED FOR USE)

CARRIER

PICA

HEALTH INSURANCE CLAIM FORM

PICA

1. MEDICARE (Medicare #) MEDICAID (Medicaid #) CHAMPUS (Sponsor's SSN) CHAMPVA (VA File #) GROUP HEALTH PLAN (SSN or ID) FECA BLK LUNG (SSN) OTHER (ID)

1a. INSURED'S I.D. NUMBER (FOR PROGRAM IN ITEM 1)

2. PATIENT'S NAME (Last Name, First Name, Middle Initial)

3. PATIENT'S BIRTH DATE MM DD YY SEX M F

4. INSURED'S NAME (Last Name, First Name, Middle Initial)

5. PATIENT'S ADDRESS (No. Street)

6. PATIENT RELATIONSHIP TO INSURED Self Spouse Child Other

7. INSURED'S ADDRESS (No. Street)

CITY STATE

8. PATIENT STATUS Single Married Other

CITY STATE

ZIP CODE TELEPHONE (Include Area Code) ( )

Employed Full-Time Student Part-Time Student

ZIP CODE TELEPHONE (INCLUDE AREA CODE) ( )

9. OTHER INSURED'S NAME (Last Name, First Name, Middle Initial)

10. IS PATIENT'S CONDITION RELATED TO:

11. INSURED'S POLICY GROUP OR FECA NUMBER

a. OTHER INSURED'S POLICY OR GROUP NUMBER

a. EMPLOYMENT? (CURRENT OR PREVIOUS) YES NO

a. INSURED'S DATE OF BIRTH MM DD YY SEX M F

b. OTHER INSURED'S DATE OF BIRTH MM DD YY SEX M F

b. AUTO ACCIDENT? PLACE (State) YES NO

b. EMPLOYER'S NAME OR SCHOOL NAME

c. EMPLOYER'S NAME OR SCHOOL NAME

c. OTHER ACCIDENT? YES NO

c. INSURANCE PLAN NAME OR PROGRAM NAME

d. INSURANCE PLAN NAME OR PROGRAM NAME

10d. RESERVED FOR LOCAL USE

d. IS THERE ANOTHER HEALTH BENEFIT PLAN? YES NO If yes, return to and complete item 9 a – d.

READ BACK OF FORM BEFORE COMPLETING & SIGNING THIS FORM.

12. PATIENT'S OR AUTHORIZED PERSON'S SIGNATURE I authorize the release of any medical or other information necessary to process this claim. I also request payment of government benefits either to myself or to the party who accepts assignment below.

SIGNED ______ DATE ______

13. INSURED'S OR AUTHORIZED PERSON'S SIGNATURE I authorize payment of medical benefits to the undersigned physician or supplier for services described below.

SIGNED ______

PATIENT AND INSURED INFORMATION

14. DATE OF CURRENT: MM DD YY ILLNESS (First symptom) OR INJURY (Accident) OR PREGNANCY (LMP)

15. IF PATIENT HAS HAD SAME OR SIMILAR ILLNESS, GIVE FIRST DATE MM DD YY

16. DATES PATIENT UNABLE TO WORK IN CURRENT OCCUPATION FROM MM DD YY TO MM DD YY

17. NAME OF REFERRING PHYSICIAN OR OTHER SOURCE

17a. I.D. NUMBER OF REFERRING PHYSICIAN

18. HOSPITALIZATION DATES RELATED TO CURRENT SERVICES FROM MM DD YY TO MM DD YY

19. RESERVED FOR LOCAL USE

20. OUTSIDE LAB? YES NO $ CHARGES

21. DIAGNOSIS OR NATURE OF ILLNESS OR INJURY. (RELATE ITEMS 1, 2, 3, OR 4 TO ITEM 24E BY LINE)

1. ___ . __
2. ___ . __
3. ___ . __
4. ___ . __

22. MEDICAID RESUBMISSION CODE ORIGINAL REF. NO.

23. PRIOR AUTHORIZATION NUMBER

24.	A DATE(S) OF SERVICE From MM DD YY To MM DD YY	B Place of Service	C Type of Service	D PROCEDURES, SERVICES, OR SUPPLIES (Explain Unusual Circumstances) CPT/HCPCS MODIFIER	E DIAGNOSIS CODE	F $ CHARGES	G DAYS OR UNITS	H EPSDT Family Plan	I EMG	J COB	K RESERVED FOR LOCAL USE
1											
2											
3											
4											
5											
6											

25. FEDERAL TAX I.D. NUMBER SSN EIN

26. PATIENT'S ACCOUNT NO.

27. ACCEPT ASSIGNMENT? (For govt. claims, see back) YES NO

28. TOTAL CHARGE $

29. AMOUNT PAID $

30. BALANCE DUE $

31. SIGNATURE OF PHYSICIAN OR SUPPLIER INCLUDING DEGREES OR CREDENTIALS (I certify that the statements on the reverse apply to this bill and are made a part thereof.)

SIGNED DATE

32. NAME AND ADDRESS OF FACILITY WHERE SERVICES WERE RENDERED (If other than home or office)

33. PHYSICIAN'S, SUPPLIER'S BILLING NAME, ADDRESS, ZIP CODE & PHONE #

PIN# GRP#

PHYSICIAN OR SUPPLIER INFORMATION

(SAMPLE ONLY - NOT APPROVED FOR USE)

PLEASE PRINT OR TYPE

SAMPLE FORM 1500
SAMPLE FORM 1500 SAMPLE FORM 1500

Case Study 15-c

DATE	REMARKS
06/19/YYYY	

PATIENT	CHART #	SEX	BIRTHDATE
Fred R. Jones 384-66-4535	15-c	M	01/05/1949

MAILING ADDRESS	CITY	STATE	ZIP	HOME PHONE	WORK PHONE
444 Taylor Avenue	Anywhere	US	12345	(101) 333-5555	

EMPLOYER	ADDRESS	PATIENT STATUS
		X (DIVORCED) — MARRIED DIVORCED SINGLE STUDENT OTHER

INSURANCE: PRIMARY	ID#	GROUP	SECONDARY POLICY
Medicaid	55771122		

POLICYHOLDER NAME	BIRTHDATE	RELATIONSHIP	POLICYHOLDER NAME	BIRTHDATE	RELATIONSHIP

SUPPLEMENTAL PLAN	EMPLOYER

POLICYHOLDER NAME	BIRTHDATE	RELATIONSHIP

EMPLOYER

REFERRING PHYSICIAN UPIN/SSN

DIAGNOSIS	CODE
1. Difficulty in walking	719.70
2.	
3.	
4.	

PLACE OF SERVICE Office

PROCEDURES	CODE	CHARGE
1. Est. patient OV Level III	99213	$75.00
2.		
3.		
4.		
5.		
6.		

SPECIAL NOTES

Refer patient to a Podiatrist

TOTAL CHARGES	PAYMENTS	ADJUSTMENTS	BALANCE
$75.00	-0-	-0-	$75.00

RETURN VISIT	PHYSICIAN SIGNATURE
3 months	Donald L. Givings, M.D.

MEDICARE # D1234
MEDICAID # DLG1234
BCBS # 12345

DONALD L. GIVINGS, M.D.
11350 MEDICAL DRIVE, ANYWHERE, US 12345
PHONE NUMBER (101)111-5555

EIN # 11123456
SSN # 123-12-1234
UPIN # DG1234

PLEASE
DO NOT
STAPLE
IN THIS
AREA

(SAMPLE ONLY - NOT APPROVED FOR USE)

CARRIER

PICA

HEALTH INSURANCE CLAIM FORM

PICA

1. MEDICARE (Medicare #) MEDICAID (Medicaid #) CHAMPUS (Sponsor's SSN) CHAMPVA (VA File #) GROUP HEALTH PLAN (SSN or ID) FECA BLK LUNG (SSN) OTHER (ID)

1a. INSURED'S I.D. NUMBER (FOR PROGRAM IN ITEM 1)

2. PATIENT'S NAME (Last Name, First Name, Middle Initial)

3. PATIENT'S BIRTH DATE MM DD YY SEX M F

4. INSURED'S NAME (Last Name, First Name, Middle Initial)

5. PATIENT'S ADDRESS (No. Street)

6. PATIENT RELATIONSHIP TO INSURED Self Spouse Child Other

7. INSURED'S ADDRESS (No. Street)

CITY STATE

8. PATIENT STATUS Single Married Other

CITY STATE

ZIP CODE TELEPHONE (Include Area Code) ( )

Employed Full-Time Student Part-Time Student

ZIP CODE TELEPHONE (INCLUDE AREA CODE) ( )

9. OTHER INSURED'S NAME (Last Name, First Name, Middle Initial)

10. IS PATIENT'S CONDITION RELATED TO:

11. INSURED'S POLICY GROUP OR FECA NUMBER

a. OTHER INSURED'S POLICY OR GROUP NUMBER

a. EMPLOYMENT? (CURRENT OR PREVIOUS) YES NO

a. INSURED'S DATE OF BIRTH MM DD YY SEX M F

b. OTHER INSURED'S DATE OF BIRTH MM DD YY SEX M F

b. AUTO ACCIDENT? YES NO PLACE (State)

b. EMPLOYER'S NAME OR SCHOOL NAME

c. EMPLOYER'S NAME OR SCHOOL NAME

c. OTHER ACCIDENT? YES NO

c. INSURANCE PLAN NAME OR PROGRAM NAME

d. INSURANCE PLAN NAME OR PROGRAM NAME

10d. RESERVED FOR LOCAL USE

d. IS THERE ANOTHER HEALTH BENEFIT PLAN? YES NO If yes, return to and complete item 9 a – d.

READ BACK OF FORM BEFORE COMPLETING & SIGNING THIS FORM.

12. PATIENT'S OR AUTHORIZED PERSON'S SIGNATURE I authorize the release of any medical or other information necessary to process this claim. I also request payment of government benefits either to myself or to the party who accepts assignment below.

SIGNED DATE

13. INSURED'S OR AUTHORIZED PERSON'S SIGNATURE I authorize payment of medical benefits to the undersigned physician or supplier for services described below.

SIGNED

PATIENT AND INSURED INFORMATION

14. DATE OF CURRENT: MM DD YY ILLNESS (First symptom) OR INJURY (Accident) OR PREGNANCY (LMP)

15. IF PATIENT HAS HAD SAME OR SIMILAR ILLNESS, GIVE FIRST DATE MM DD YY

16. DATES PATIENT UNABLE TO WORK IN CURRENT OCCUPATION FROM MM DD YY TO MM DD YY

17. NAME OF REFERRING PHYSICIAN OR OTHER SOURCE

17a. I.D. NUMBER OF REFERRING PHYSICIAN

18. HOSPITALIZATION DATES RELATED TO CURRENT SERVICES FROM MM DD YY TO MM DD YY

19. RESERVED FOR LOCAL USE

20. OUTSIDE LAB? YES NO $ CHARGES

21. DIAGNOSIS OR NATURE OF ILLNESS OR INJURY. (RELATE ITEMS 1, 2, 3, OR 4 TO ITEM 24E BY LINE)

1. ___ . __

3. ___ . __

2. ___ . __

4. ___ . __

22. MEDICAID RESUBMISSION CODE ORIGINAL REF. NO.

23. PRIOR AUTHORIZATION NUMBER

24.	A DATE(S) OF SERVICE From MM DD YY	To MM DD YY	B Place of Service	C Type of Service	D PROCEDURES, SERVICES, OR SUPPLIES (Explain Unusual Circumstances) CPT/HCPCS | MODIFIER	E DIAGNOSIS CODE	F $ CHARGES	G DAYS OR UNITS	H EPSDT Family Plan	I EMG	J COB	K RESERVED FOR LOCAL USE
1												
2												
3												
4												
5												
6												

25. FEDERAL TAX I.D. NUMBER SSN EIN

26. PATIENT'S ACCOUNT NO.

27. ACCEPT ASSIGNMENT? (For govt. claims, see back) YES NO

28. TOTAL CHARGE $

29. AMOUNT PAID $

30. BALANCE DUE $

31. SIGNATURE OF PHYSICIAN OR SUPPLIER INCLUDING DEGREES OR CREDENTIALS (I certify that the statements on the reverse apply to this bill and are made a part thereof.)

SIGNED DATE

32. NAME AND ADDRESS OF FACILITY WHERE SERVICES WERE RENDERED (If other than home or office)

33. PHYSICIAN'S, SUPPLIER'S BILLING NAME, ADDRESS, ZIP CODE & PHONE #

PIN# GRP#

PHYSICIAN OR SUPPLIER INFORMATION

(SAMPLE ONLY - NOT APPROVED FOR USE)

PLEASE PRINT OR TYPE

SAMPLE FORM 1500
SAMPLE FORM 1500 SAMPLE FORM 1500

Case Study 15-d

DATE	REMARKS
06/23/YYYY	

PATIENT	CHART #	SEX	BIRTHDATE
Fred R. Jones 384-66-4535	15-d	M	01/05/1949

MAILING ADDRESS	CITY	STATE	ZIP	HOME PHONE	WORK PHONE
444 Taylor Avenue	Anywhere	US	12345	(101) 333-5555	

EMPLOYER	ADDRESS	PATIENT STATUS
		X MARRIED DIVORCED SINGLE STUDENT OTHER

INSURANCE: PRIMARY	ID#	GROUP	SECONDARY POLICY
Medicaid	55771122		

POLICYHOLDER NAME	BIRTHDATE	RELATIONSHIP	POLICYHOLDER NAME	BIRTHDATE	RELATIONSHIP

SUPPLEMENTAL PLAN	EMPLOYER

POLICYHOLDER NAME	BIRTHDATE	RELATIONSHIP

EMPLOYER

REFERRING PHYSICIAN UPIN/SSN: Donald L. Givings, M.D. DLG1234

DIAGNOSIS	CODE
1. Fracture, great toe	826.0
2.	
3.	
4.	

PLACE OF SERVICE: Office

PROCEDURES	CODE	CHARGE
1. Office Consult Level II	99242	$75.00
2. Toe Xray 2 views	73660	$50.00
3. Closed treatment of fracture, great toe	28490	$65.00
4.		
5.		
6.		

SPECIAL NOTES

TOTAL CHARGES	PAYMENTS	ADJUSTMENTS	BALANCE
$190.00	-0-	-0-	$190.00

RETURN VISIT	PHYSICIAN SIGNATURE
	John F. Walker, D.P.M.

MEDICARE # J2234
MEDICAID # JFW1234
BCBS # 12345

JOHN F. WALKER, D.P.M. PODIATRY
546 FOOTHILL PLACE, ANYWHERE, US 12345
PHONE NUMBER (101)111-5555

EIN # 11993377
SSN # 657-12-4454
UPIN # JW1234

PLEASE DO NOT STAPLE IN THIS AREA

PICA

(SAMPLE ONLY - NOT APPROVED FOR USE)

CARRIER

HEALTH INSURANCE CLAIM FORM

PICA

1. MEDICARE (Medicare #) | MEDICAID (Medicaid #) | CHAMPUS (Sponsor's SSN) | CHAMPVA (VA File #) | GROUP HEALTH PLAN (SSN or ID) | FECA BLK LUNG (SSN) | OTHER (ID)

1a. INSURED'S I.D. NUMBER (FOR PROGRAM IN ITEM 1)

2. PATIENT'S NAME (Last Name, First Name, Middle Initial)

3. PATIENT'S BIRTH DATE MM DD YY SEX M F

4. INSURED'S NAME (Last Name, First Name, Middle Initial)

5. PATIENT'S ADDRESS (No. Street)

6. PATIENT RELATIONSHIP TO INSURED Self Spouse Child Other

7. INSURED'S ADDRESS (No. Street)

CITY STATE

8. PATIENT STATUS Single Married Other

CITY STATE

ZIP CODE TELEPHONE (Include Area Code) ( )

Employed Full-Time Student Part-Time Student

ZIP CODE TELEPHONE (INCLUDE AREA CODE) ( )

9. OTHER INSURED'S NAME (Last Name, First Name, Middle Initial)

10. IS PATIENT'S CONDITION RELATED TO:

11. INSURED'S POLICY GROUP OR FECA NUMBER

a. OTHER INSURED'S POLICY OR GROUP NUMBER

a. EMPLOYMENT? (CURRENT OR PREVIOUS) YES NO

a. INSURED'S DATE OF BIRTH MM DD YY SEX M F

b. OTHER INSURED'S DATE OF BIRTH MM DD YY SEX M F

b. AUTO ACCIDENT? PLACE (State) YES NO

b. EMPLOYER'S NAME OR SCHOOL NAME

c. EMPLOYER'S NAME OR SCHOOL NAME

c. OTHER ACCIDENT? YES NO

c. INSURANCE PLAN NAME OR PROGRAM NAME

d. INSURANCE PLAN NAME OR PROGRAM NAME

10d. RESERVED FOR LOCAL USE

d. IS THERE ANOTHER HEALTH BENEFIT PLAN? YES NO If yes, return to and complete item 9 a – d.

READ BACK OF FORM BEFORE COMPLETING & SIGNING THIS FORM.

12. PATIENT'S OR AUTHORIZED PERSON'S SIGNATURE I authorize the release of any medical or other information necessary to process this claim. I also request payment of government benefits either to myself or to the party who accepts assignment below.

SIGNED DATE

13. INSURED'S OR AUTHORIZED PERSON'S SIGNATURE I authorize payment of medical benefits to the undersigned physician or supplier for services described below.

SIGNED

PATIENT AND INSURED INFORMATION

14. DATE OF CURRENT: MM DD YY ILLNESS (First symptom) OR INJURY (Accident) OR PREGNANCY (LMP)

15. IF PATIENT HAS HAD SAME OR SIMILAR ILLNESS, GIVE FIRST DATE MM DD YY

16. DATES PATIENT UNABLE TO WORK IN CURRENT OCCUPATION FROM MM DD YY TO MM DD YY

17. NAME OF REFERRING PHYSICIAN OR OTHER SOURCE

17a. I.D. NUMBER OF REFERRING PHYSICIAN

18. HOSPITALIZATION DATES RELATED TO CURRENT SERVICES FROM MM DD YY TO MM DD YY

19. RESERVED FOR LOCAL USE

20. OUTSIDE LAB? YES NO $ CHARGES

21. DIAGNOSIS OR NATURE OF ILLNESS OR INJURY. (RELATE ITEMS 1, 2, 3, OR 4 TO ITEM 24E BY LINE)

1. ___ . __ 3. ___ . __

2. ___ . __ 4. ___ . __

22. MEDICAID RESUBMISSION CODE ORIGINAL REF. NO.

23. PRIOR AUTHORIZATION NUMBER

24. A DATE(S) OF SERVICE From MM DD YY To MM DD YY	B Place of Service	C Type of Service	D PROCEDURES, SERVICES, OR SUPPLIES (Explain Unusual Circumstances) CPT/HCPCS MODIFIER	E DIAGNOSIS CODE	F $ CHARGES	G DAYS OR UNITS	H EPSDT Family Plan	I EMG	J COB	K RESERVED FOR LOCAL USE
1										
2										
3										
4										
5										
6										

25. FEDERAL TAX I.D. NUMBER SSN EIN

26. PATIENT'S ACCOUNT NO.

27. ACCEPT ASSIGNMENT? (For govt. claims, see back) YES NO

28. TOTAL CHARGE $

29. AMOUNT PAID $

30. BALANCE DUE $

31. SIGNATURE OF PHYSICIAN OR SUPPLIER INCLUDING DEGREES OR CREDENTIALS (I certify that the statements on the reverse apply to this bill and are made a part thereof.)

SIGNED DATE

32. NAME AND ADDRESS OF FACILITY WHERE SERVICES WERE RENDERED (If other than home or office)

33. PHYSICIAN'S, SUPPLIER'S BILLING NAME, ADDRESS, ZIP CODE & PHONE #

PIN# GRP#

PHYSICIAN OR SUPPLIER INFORMATION

(SAMPLE ONLY - NOT APPROVED FOR USE)

PLEASE PRINT OR TYPE

SAMPLE FORM 1500
SAMPLE FORM 1500 SAMPLE FORM 1500

Case Study 15-e

DATE	REMARKS
07/18/YYYY	

PATIENT	CHART #	SEX	BIRTHDATE
Richard J. Davis 123-55-7979	15-e	M	03/10/1994

MAILING ADDRESS	CITY	STATE	ZIP	HOME PHONE	WORK PHONE
3764 Ravenwood Ave	Anywhere	US	12345	(101) 333-5555	

EMPLOYER	ADDRESS	PATIENT STATUS
		MARRIED DIVORCED SINGLE STUDENT OTHER

INSURANCE: PRIMARY	ID#	GROUP	SECONDARY POLICY
Medicaid	77557755		

POLICYHOLDER NAME	BIRTHDATE	RELATIONSHIP	POLICYHOLDER NAME	BIRTHDATE	RELATIONSHIP

SUPPLEMENTAL PLAN	EMPLOYER

POLICYHOLDER NAME	BIRTHDATE	RELATIONSHIP

EMPLOYER

REFERRING PHYSICIAN UPIN/SSN

DIAGNOSIS	CODE
1. Routine child health check	V20.2
2.	
3.	
4.	

PLACE OF SERVICE Office

PROCEDURES	CODE	CHARGE
1. Preventive medicine Est. Patient 5-11 years	99393	$60.00
2. DTaP	90700	$40.00
3. MMR	90707	$55.00
4. OPV	90712	$25.00
5. Immunization administration (x3)	90471	$25.00
6.	90472	$25.00
	90472	$25.00

SPECIAL NOTES

TOTAL CHARGES	PAYMENTS	ADJUSTMENTS	BALANCE
$255.00	-0-	-0-	$255.00

RETURN VISIT	PHYSICIAN SIGNATURE
	Donald L. Givings, M.D.

MEDICARE # D1234
MEDICAID # DLG1234
BCBS # 12345

DONALD L. GIVINGS, M.D.
11350 MEDICAL DRIVE, ANYWHERE, US 12345
PHONE NUMBER (101)111-5555

EIN # 11123456
SSN # 123-12-1234
UPIN # DG1234

PLEASE
DO NOT
STAPLE
IN THIS
AREA

(SAMPLE ONLY - NOT APPROVED FOR USE)

CARRIER

PICA

HEALTH INSURANCE CLAIM FORM

PICA

1. MEDICARE (Medicare #) MEDICAID (Medicaid #) CHAMPUS (Sponsor's SSN) CHAMPVA (VA File #) GROUP HEALTH PLAN (SSN or ID) FECA BLK LUNG (SSN) OTHER (ID)

1a. INSURED'S I.D. NUMBER (FOR PROGRAM IN ITEM 1)

2. PATIENT'S NAME (Last Name, First Name, Middle Initial)

3. PATIENT'S BIRTH DATE MM DD YY SEX M F

4. INSURED'S NAME (Last Name, First Name, Middle Initial)

5. PATIENT'S ADDRESS (No. Street)

6. PATIENT RELATIONSHIP TO INSURED Self Spouse Child Other

7. INSURED'S ADDRESS (No. Street)

CITY STATE

8. PATIENT STATUS Single Married Other

CITY STATE

ZIP CODE TELEPHONE (Include Area Code) ( )

Employed Full-Time Student Part-Time Student

ZIP CODE TELEPHONE (INCLUDE AREA CODE) ( )

9. OTHER INSURED'S NAME (Last Name, First Name, Middle Initial)

10. IS PATIENT'S CONDITION RELATED TO:

11. INSURED'S POLICY GROUP OR FECA NUMBER

a. OTHER INSURED'S POLICY OR GROUP NUMBER

a. EMPLOYMENT? (CURRENT OR PREVIOUS) YES NO

a. INSURED'S DATE OF BIRTH MM DD YY SEX M F

b. OTHER INSURED'S DATE OF BIRTH MM DD YY SEX M F

b. AUTO ACCIDENT? YES NO PLACE (State)

b. EMPLOYER'S NAME OR SCHOOL NAME

c. EMPLOYER'S NAME OR SCHOOL NAME

c. OTHER ACCIDENT? YES NO

c. INSURANCE PLAN NAME OR PROGRAM NAME

d. INSURANCE PLAN NAME OR PROGRAM NAME

10d. RESERVED FOR LOCAL USE

d. IS THERE ANOTHER HEALTH BENEFIT PLAN? YES NO If yes, return to and complete item 9 a – d.

READ BACK OF FORM BEFORE COMPLETING & SIGNING THIS FORM.

12. PATIENT'S OR AUTHORIZED PERSON'S SIGNATURE I authorize the release of any medical or other information necessary to process this claim. I also request payment of government benefits either to myself or to the party who accepts assignment below.

SIGNED DATE

13. INSURED'S OR AUTHORIZED PERSON'S SIGNATURE I authorize payment of medical benefits to the undersigned physician or supplier for services described below.

SIGNED

PATIENT AND INSURED INFORMATION

14. DATE OF CURRENT: MM DD YY ILLNESS (First symptom) OR INJURY (Accident) OR PREGNANCY (LMP)

15. IF PATIENT HAS HAD SAME OR SIMILAR ILLNESS, GIVE FIRST DATE MM DD YY

16. DATES PATIENT UNABLE TO WORK IN CURRENT OCCUPATION FROM MM DD YY TO MM DD YY

17. NAME OF REFERRING PHYSICIAN OR OTHER SOURCE

17a. I.D. NUMBER OF REFERRING PHYSICIAN

18. HOSPITALIZATION DATES RELATED TO CURRENT SERVICES FROM MM DD YY TO MM DD YY

19. RESERVED FOR LOCAL USE

20. OUTSIDE LAB? YES NO $ CHARGES

21. DIAGNOSIS OR NATURE OF ILLNESS OR INJURY. (RELATE ITEMS 1, 2, 3, OR 4 TO ITEM 24E BY LINE)

1. ___ . __

2. ___ . __

3. ___ . __

4. ___ . __

22. MEDICAID RESUBMISSION CODE ORIGINAL REF. NO.

23. PRIOR AUTHORIZATION NUMBER

24. A DATE(S) OF SERVICE From MM DD YY To MM DD YY	B Place of Service	C Type of Service	D PROCEDURES, SERVICES, OR SUPPLIES (Explain Unusual Circumstances) CPT/HCPCS MODIFIER	E DIAGNOSIS CODE	F $ CHARGES	G DAYS OR UNITS	H EPSDT Family Plan	I EMG	J COB	K RESERVED FOR LOCAL USE
1										
2										
3										
4										
5										
6										

25. FEDERAL TAX I.D. NUMBER SSN EIN

26. PATIENT'S ACCOUNT NO.

27. ACCEPT ASSIGNMENT? (For govt. claims, see back) YES NO

28. TOTAL CHARGE $

29. AMOUNT PAID $

30. BALANCE DUE $

31. SIGNATURE OF PHYSICIAN OR SUPPLIER INCLUDING DEGREES OR CREDENTIALS (I certify that the statements on the reverse apply to this bill and are made a part thereof.)

SIGNED DATE

32. NAME AND ADDRESS OF FACILITY WHERE SERVICES WERE RENDERED (If other than home or office)

33. PHYSICIAN'S, SUPPLIER'S BILLING NAME, ADDRESS, ZIP CODE & PHONE #

PIN# GRP#

PHYSICIAN OR SUPPLIER INFORMATION

(SAMPLE ONLY - NOT APPROVED FOR USE)

PLEASE PRINT OR TYPE

SAMPLE FORM 1500
SAMPLE FORM 1500 SAMPLE FORM 1500

Case Study 15-f

DATE	REMARKS
09/17/YYYY	

PATIENT		CHART #	SEX	BIRTHDATE
Dolores Giovanni	234-56-7891	15-f	F	10/22/1966

MAILING ADDRESS	CITY	STATE	ZIP	HOME PHONE	WORK PHONE
384 Beverly Avenue	Anywhere	US	12345	(101) 333-5555	

EMPLOYER	ADDRESS	PATIENT STATUS
		MARRIED DIVORCED (X) SINGLE STUDENT OTHER

INSURANCE: PRIMARY	ID#	GROUP	SECONDARY POLICY
Medicare	88776655		

POLICYHOLDER NAME	BIRTHDATE	RELATIONSHIP	POLICYHOLDER NAME	BIRTHDATE	RELATIONSHIP

SUPPLEMENTAL PLAN	EMPLOYER

POLICYHOLDER NAME	BIRTHDATE	RELATIONSHIP

EMPLOYER

REFERRING PHYSICIAN UPIN/SSN

DIAGNOSIS	CODE
1. E. coli, unspecified	008.00
2.	
3.	
4.	

PLACE OF SERVICE Mercy Hospital, Anywhere St., Anywhere, US 12345, Medicaid PIN# MHS2244

PROCEDURES	CODE	CHARGE
1. Initial Hosp. Level III 09/13/YYYY	99223	$175.00
2. Subsq. Hosp. Level III 09/14/YYYY, 09/15/YYYY, 09/16/YYYY	99233	Each @ $85.00
3. Hosp. Discharge more than 30 min. 09/17/YYYY	99239	$100.00
4.		
5.		
6.		

SPECIAL NOTES

TOTAL CHARGES	PAYMENTS	ADJUSTMENTS	BALANCE
$530.00	-0-	-0-	$530.00

RETURN VISIT	PHYSICIAN SIGNATURE
	Donald L. Givings, M.D.

MEDICARE # D1234
MEDICAID # DLG1234
BCBS # 12345

DONALD L. GIVINGS, M.D.
11350 MEDICAL DRIVE, ANYWHERE, US 12345
PHONE NUMBER (101)111-5555

EIN # 11-123456
SSN # 123-12-1234
UPIN # DG1234

PLEASE
DO NOT
STAPLE
IN THIS
AREA

(SAMPLE ONLY - NOT APPROVED FOR USE)

CARRIER

PICA

HEALTH INSURANCE CLAIM FORM

PICA

1. MEDICARE (Medicare #) MEDICAID (Medicaid #) CHAMPUS (Sponsor's SSN) CHAMPVA (VA File #) GROUP HEALTH PLAN (SSN or ID) FECA BLK LUNG (SSN) OTHER (ID)

1a. INSURED'S I.D. NUMBER (FOR PROGRAM IN ITEM 1)

2. PATIENT'S NAME (Last Name, First Name, Middle Initial)

3. PATIENT'S BIRTH DATE MM DD YY SEX M F

4. INSURED'S NAME (Last Name, First Name, Middle Initial)

5. PATIENT'S ADDRESS (No. Street)

6. PATIENT RELATIONSHIP TO INSURED Self Spouse Child Other

7. INSURED'S ADDRESS (No. Street)

CITY STATE

8. PATIENT STATUS Single Married Other

CITY STATE

ZIP CODE TELEPHONE (Include Area Code) ( )

Employed Full-Time Student Part-Time Student

ZIP CODE TELEPHONE (INCLUDE AREA CODE) ( )

9. OTHER INSURED'S NAME (Last Name, First Name, Middle Initial)

10. IS PATIENT'S CONDITION RELATED TO:

11. INSURED'S POLICY GROUP OR FECA NUMBER

a. OTHER INSURED'S POLICY OR GROUP NUMBER

a. EMPLOYMENT? (CURRENT OR PREVIOUS) YES NO

a. INSURED'S DATE OF BIRTH MM DD YY SEX M F

b. OTHER INSURED'S DATE OF BIRTH MM DD YY SEX M F

b. AUTO ACCIDENT? PLACE (State) YES NO

b. EMPLOYER'S NAME OR SCHOOL NAME

c. EMPLOYER'S NAME OR SCHOOL NAME

c. OTHER ACCIDENT? YES NO

c. INSURANCE PLAN NAME OR PROGRAM NAME

d. INSURANCE PLAN NAME OR PROGRAM NAME

10d. RESERVED FOR LOCAL USE

d. IS THERE ANOTHER HEALTH BENEFIT PLAN? YES NO If yes, return to and complete item 9 a – d.

READ BACK OF FORM BEFORE COMPLETING & SIGNING THIS FORM.

12. PATIENT'S OR AUTHORIZED PERSON'S SIGNATURE I authorize the release of any medical or other information necessary to process this claim. I also request payment of government benefits either to myself or to the party who accepts assignment below.

SIGNED DATE

13. INSURED'S OR AUTHORIZED PERSON'S SIGNATURE I authorize payment of medical benefits to the undersigned physician or supplier for services described below.

SIGNED

PATIENT AND INSURED INFORMATION

14. DATE OF CURRENT: MM DD YY ILLNESS (First symptom) OR INJURY (Accident) OR PREGNANCY (LMP)

15. IF PATIENT HAS HAD SAME OR SIMILAR ILLNESS, GIVE FIRST DATE MM DD YY

16. DATES PATIENT UNABLE TO WORK IN CURRENT OCCUPATION FROM MM DD YY TO MM DD YY

17. NAME OF REFERRING PHYSICIAN OR OTHER SOURCE

17a. I.D. NUMBER OF REFERRING PHYSICIAN

18. HOSPITALIZATION DATES RELATED TO CURRENT SERVICES FROM MM DD YY TO MM DD YY

19. RESERVED FOR LOCAL USE

20. OUTSIDE LAB? YES NO $ CHARGES

21. DIAGNOSIS OR NATURE OF ILLNESS OR INJURY. (RELATE ITEMS 1, 2, 3, OR 4 TO ITEM 24E BY LINE)

1. ___ . __ 3. ___ . __

2. ___ . __ 4. ___ . __

22. MEDICAID RESUBMISSION CODE ORIGINAL REF. NO.

23. PRIOR AUTHORIZATION NUMBER

24. A DATE(S) OF SERVICE From MM DD YY To MM DD YY	B Place of Service	C Type of Service	D PROCEDURES, SERVICES, OR SUPPLIES (Explain Unusual Circumstances) CPT/HCPCS MODIFIER	E DIAGNOSIS CODE	F $ CHARGES	G DAYS OR UNITS	H EPSDT Family Plan	I EMG	J COB	K RESERVED FOR LOCAL USE
1										
2										
3										
4										
5										
6										

25. FEDERAL TAX I.D. NUMBER SSN EIN

26. PATIENT'S ACCOUNT NO.

27. ACCEPT ASSIGNMENT? (For govt. claims, see back) YES NO

28. TOTAL CHARGE $

29. AMOUNT PAID $

30. BALANCE DUE $

31. SIGNATURE OF PHYSICIAN OR SUPPLIER INCLUDING DEGREES OR CREDENTIALS (I certify that the statements on the reverse apply to this bill and are made a part thereof.)

SIGNED DATE

32. NAME AND ADDRESS OF FACILITY WHERE SERVICES WERE RENDERED (If other than home or office)

33. PHYSICIAN'S, SUPPLIER'S BILLING NAME, ADDRESS, ZIP CODE & PHONE #

PIN# GRP#

PHYSICIAN OR SUPPLIER INFORMATION

(SAMPLE ONLY - NOT APPROVED FOR USE)

PLEASE PRINT OR TYPE

SAMPLE FORM 1500
SAMPLE FORM 1500 SAMPLE FORM 1500

TRICARE

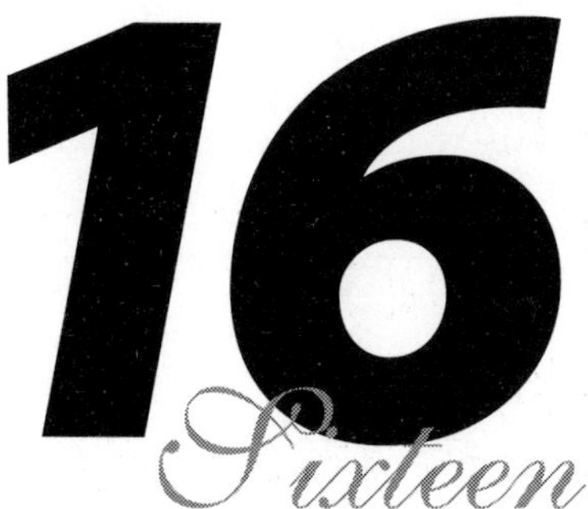

HISTORY OF CHAMPUS AND DEVELOPMENT OF TRICARE

1. Complete the following sentences.
   a. TRICARE is a health care program for ______________________________.
   b. The Military Health Services System is the entire health care system ______________________________.

TRICARE ADMINISTRATION

2. What is the name of the office that coordinates and administers the TRICARE program?

   ____

3. Where do you send TRICARE claims? ______________________________

TRICARE OPTIONS

4. List three TRICARE health care options.
   a. ______________________________
   b. ______________________________
   c. ______________________________

5. Match the insurance terms in the first column with the definitions in the second column. Write the correct letter in each blank.

   _______ TRICARE Prime — a. PPO

   _______ TRICARE Extra — b. fee-for-service

   _______ TRICARE Standard — c. HMO

6. Which of the three TRICARE options provides comprehensive health care benefits at the lowest cost?

   ____

7. Who guides TRICARE Prime members through the health care system and coordinates all specialty medical needs? ______________________________

8. Briefly describe the *catastrophic cap benefit.* ____

____

9. No enrollment is required to be covered by ____.

10. When is the Point-of-Service option activated for a TRICARE Prime Beneficiary?

____

11. For each question, enter **Y** for yes or **N** for no on the line provided.

    ________ a. Are TRICARE Extra network providers allowed to balance bill?

    ________ b. Are TRICARE Extra enrollees allowed to seek health care services from an MTF?

    ________ c. Are TRICARE Standard enrollees responsible for deductibles and cost-shares?

    ________ d. Are there any enrollment requirements for TRICARE Standard?

    ________ e. Do TRICARE Standard participating providers have to accept the TRICARE Standard allowable charge as payment in full?

TRICARE AS A SECONDARY PAYER

12. Briefly describe when TRICARE is used as a secondary payer. ______________________________

____

TRICARE LIMITING CHARGES

13. All TRICARE NonPAR providers are subject to a ____________________ ____________________ of 15% above the TRICARE Fee Schedule for PAR providers.

14. State the exceptions to the 15% limiting charge.

____

____

TRICARE BILLING INFORMATION

15. When sending claims to the TRICARE carrier, be sure to use both the ____________________ ____________________ ____________________ number and its associated zip code.

16. TRICARE is based in ___. (Circle the correct answer.)

    a. California

    b. Colorado

    c. New York

    d. None of the above

17. Changes in general benefits are enacted by ___. (Circle the correct answer.)

  a. HCFA
  b. the military
  c. the United States Congress
  d. none of the above

18. The form used to file a TRICARE claim is ___. (Circle the correct answer.)

  a. HCFA-1450
  b. HCFA-1500
  c. different for each catchment area
  d. any of the above

19. For mental health cases, a TRICARE Treatment Report must be filed with a claim for more than ___ outpatient visits in any calendar year. (Circle the correct answer.)

  a. 25
  b. 30
  c. 45
  d. none of the above

20. Claims will be denied if they are filed more than ___ months after the date of service for outpatient care. (Circle the correct answer.)

  a. 6
  b. 9
  c. 12
  d. 18

21. Which of the following TRICARE plans require(s) payment of enrollment fees? (Circle the correct answer.)

  a. TRICARE Prime
  b. TRICARE Standard
  c. TRICARE Extra
  d. all of the above

22. All deductibles are applied in the government's fiscal year which runs from ___. (Circle the correct answer.)

  a. July 1 of one year to June 30 of the next
  b. October 1 of one year to September 30 of the next
  c. January 1 to December 31 of the same year

Critical Thinking

23. Write a paragraph describing the *Good Faith Policy*.

____

____

____

24. If a TRICARE patient is being transferred within six months, should the yes or no box contain an "X" in Block 27 of the HCFA-1500 claim form? __________ Why? ______________________________

____

25. What words should be written across the top of the claim form when filing services that fall under the special handicap benefits? ______________________________

26. What words should be written on the envelope when filing services for hospice care?

____

27. If a TRICARE claim has been filed with no response for 45 days, who should be contacted?

____

Know Your Acronyms

28. Define the following acronyms:

    a. PCM ______________________________
    b. CRI ______________________________
    c. TSC ______________________________
    d. HCF ______________________________
    e. TMA ______________________________
    f. DEERS ______________________________
    g. MTF ______________________________
    h. NAS ______________________________
    i. LA ______________________________
    j. MHSS ______________________________
    k. HA ______________________________
    l. PMO ______________________________
    m. NMOP ______________________________
    n. TPR ______________________________
    o. FEHBP ______________________________
    p. BSR ______________________________
    q. BCAC ______________________________
    r. FI ______________________________
    s. PFPWD ______________________________
    t. CHAMPVA ______________________________
    u. OHI ______________________________

EXERCISES

1. Complete Case Studies 16-a through 16-e using the blank claim form provided. Follow the step-by-step instructions in the textbook to properly complete the claim form. If a patient has secondary coverage, complete an additional claim form using secondary directions from the textbook. You may choose to use a pencil so corrections can be made.

Case Study 16-a

DATE	REMARKS
11/05/YYYY	Duty Station Address 111 Army Base, Aberdeen MD 21040

PATIENT		CHART #	SEX	BIRTHDATE
Jeffrey D. Heem	234-55-6789	16-a	M	05/05/1964

MAILING ADDRESS	CITY	STATE	ZIP	HOME PHONE	WORK PHONE
333 Heavenly Place	Anywhere	US	12345	(101) 333-5555	

EMPLOYER	ADDRESS	PATIENT STATUS
US Army	See Remarks	X MARRIED DIVORCED SINGLE STUDENT OTHER

INSURANCE: PRIMARY	ID#	GROUP	SECONDARY POLICY
TRICARE Standard	234-55-6789		

POLICYHOLDER NAME	BIRTHDATE	RELATIONSHIP	POLICYHOLDER NAME	BIRTHDATE	RELATIONSHIP
		Self			

SUPPLEMENTAL PLAN	EMPLOYER

POLICYHOLDER NAME	BIRTHDATE	RELATIONSHIP	DIAGNOSIS	CODE
			1. Acute sinusitis, frontal	461.1
EMPLOYER			2. Sore throat	784.1
			3.	
REFERRING PHYSICIAN UPIN/SSN			4.	

PLACE OF SERVICE Office

PROCEDURES	CODE	CHARGE
1. New patient OV Level II	99202	$70.00
2.		
3.		
4.		
5.		
6.		

SPECIAL NOTES

TOTAL CHARGES	PAYMENTS	ADJUSTMENTS	BALANCE
$70.00	-0-	-0-	$70.00

RETURN VISIT	PHYSICIAN SIGNATURE
	Donald L. Givings, M.D.

MEDICARE # D1234
MEDICAID # DLG1234
BCBS # 12345

DONALD L. GIVINGS, M.D.
11350 MEDICAL DRIVE, ANYWHERE, US 12345
PHONE NUMBER (101)111-5555

EIN # 11123456
SSN # 123-12-1234
UPIN # DG1234
GRP # DG12345

PLEASE
DO NOT
STAPLE
IN THIS
AREA

(SAMPLE ONLY - NOT APPROVED FOR USE)

CARRIER

PICA

HEALTH INSURANCE CLAIM FORM

PICA

1. MEDICARE (Medicare #) MEDICAID (Medicaid #) CHAMPUS (Sponsor's SSN) CHAMPVA (VA File #) GROUP HEALTH PLAN (SSN or ID) FECA BLK LUNG (SSN) OTHER (ID)

1a. INSURED'S I.D. NUMBER (FOR PROGRAM IN ITEM 1)

2. PATIENT'S NAME (Last Name, First Name, Middle Initial)

3. PATIENT'S BIRTH DATE MM DD YY SEX M F

4. INSURED'S NAME (Last Name, First Name, Middle Initial)

5. PATIENT'S ADDRESS (No. Street)

6. PATIENT RELATIONSHIP TO INSURED Self Spouse Child Other

7. INSURED'S ADDRESS (No. Street)

CITY STATE

8. PATIENT STATUS Single Married Other

CITY STATE

ZIP CODE TELEPHONE (Include Area Code) ( )

Employed Full-Time Student Part-Time Student

ZIP CODE TELEPHONE (INCLUDE AREA CODE) ( )

9. OTHER INSURED'S NAME (Last Name, First Name, Middle Initial)

10. IS PATIENT'S CONDITION RELATED TO:

11. INSURED'S POLICY GROUP OR FECA NUMBER

a. OTHER INSURED'S POLICY OR GROUP NUMBER

a. EMPLOYMENT? (CURRENT OR PREVIOUS) YES NO

a. INSURED'S DATE OF BIRTH MM DD YY SEX M F

b. OTHER INSURED'S DATE OF BIRTH MM DD YY SEX M F

b. AUTO ACCIDENT? PLACE (State) YES NO

b. EMPLOYER'S NAME OR SCHOOL NAME

c. EMPLOYER'S NAME OR SCHOOL NAME

c. OTHER ACCIDENT? YES NO

c. INSURANCE PLAN NAME OR PROGRAM NAME

d. INSURANCE PLAN NAME OR PROGRAM NAME

10d. RESERVED FOR LOCAL USE

d. IS THERE ANOTHER HEALTH BENEFIT PLAN? YES NO If yes, return to and complete item 9 a – d.

READ BACK OF FORM BEFORE COMPLETING & SIGNING THIS FORM.

12. PATIENT'S OR AUTHORIZED PERSON'S SIGNATURE I authorize the release of any medical or other information necessary to process this claim. I also request payment of government benefits either to myself or to the party who accepts assignment below.

SIGNED ______ DATE ______

13. INSURED'S OR AUTHORIZED PERSON'S SIGNATURE I authorize payment of medical benefits to the undersigned physician or supplier for services described below.

SIGNED ______

PATIENT AND INSURED INFORMATION

14. DATE OF CURRENT: MM DD YY ILLNESS (First symptom) OR INJURY (Accident) OR PREGNANCY (LMP)

15. IF PATIENT HAS HAD SAME OR SIMILAR ILLNESS, GIVE FIRST DATE MM DD YY

16. DATES PATIENT UNABLE TO WORK IN CURRENT OCCUPATION FROM MM DD YY TO MM DD YY

17. NAME OF REFERRING PHYSICIAN OR OTHER SOURCE

17a. I.D. NUMBER OF REFERRING PHYSICIAN

18. HOSPITALIZATION DATES RELATED TO CURRENT SERVICES FROM MM DD YY TO MM DD YY

19. RESERVED FOR LOCAL USE

20. OUTSIDE LAB? YES NO $ CHARGES

21. DIAGNOSIS OR NATURE OF ILLNESS OR INJURY. (RELATE ITEMS 1, 2, 3, OR 4 TO ITEM 24E BY LINE)

1. ___ . __
2. ___ . __
3. ___ . __
4. ___ . __

22. MEDICAID RESUBMISSION CODE ORIGINAL REF. NO.

23. PRIOR AUTHORIZATION NUMBER

24. A DATE(S) OF SERVICE From MM DD YY To MM DD YY	B Place of Service	C Type of Service	D PROCEDURES, SERVICES, OR SUPPLIES (Explain Unusual Circumstances) CPT/HCPCS MODIFIER	E DIAGNOSIS CODE	F $ CHARGES	G DAYS OR UNITS	H EPSDT Family Plan	I EMG	J COB	K RESERVED FOR LOCAL USE
1										
2										
3										
4										
5										
6										

25. FEDERAL TAX I.D. NUMBER SSN EIN

26. PATIENT'S ACCOUNT NO.

27. ACCEPT ASSIGNMENT? (For govt. claims, see back) YES NO

28. TOTAL CHARGE $

29. AMOUNT PAID $

30. BALANCE DUE $

31. SIGNATURE OF PHYSICIAN OR SUPPLIER INCLUDING DEGREES OR CREDENTIALS (I certify that the statements on the reverse apply to this bill and are made a part thereof.)

SIGNED DATE

32. NAME AND ADDRESS OF FACILITY WHERE SERVICES WERE RENDERED (If other than home or office)

33. PHYSICIAN'S, SUPPLIER'S BILLING NAME, ADDRESS, ZIP CODE & PHONE #

PIN# GRP#

PHYSICIAN OR SUPPLIER INFORMATION

(SAMPLE ONLY - NOT APPROVED FOR USE)

PLEASE PRINT OR TYPE

SAMPLE FORM 1500
SAMPLE FORM 1500 SAMPLE FORM 1500

Case Study 16-b

DATE	REMARKS				
06/22/YYYY	Duty Station Address Dept. 21 Naval Station, Anywhere US 23456				

PATIENT		CHART #	SEX	BIRTHDATE
Dana S. Bright	456-77-2345	16-b	F	07/05/1971

MAILING ADDRESS	CITY	STATE	ZIP	HOME PHONE	WORK PHONE
28 Upton Circle	Anywhere	US	12345	(101) 333-5555	

EMPLOYER	ADDRESS	PATIENT STATUS
		X MARRIED DIVORCED SINGLE STUDENT OTHER

INSURANCE: PRIMARY	ID#	GROUP	SECONDARY POLICY
TRICARE Extra	567-56-5757		

POLICYHOLDER NAME	BIRTHDATE	RELATIONSHIP	POLICYHOLDER NAME	BIRTHDATE	RELATIONSHIP
Ron L. Bright	8/12/70	Spouse			

SUPPLEMENTAL PLAN	EMPLOYER

POLICYHOLDER NAME	BIRTHDATE	RELATIONSHIP	DIAGNOSIS	CODE
			1. Chronic cholecystitis	575.11
EMPLOYER			2.	
US Navy (See duty address in remarks)			3.	
REFERRING PHYSICIAN UPIN/SSN			4.	

PLACE OF SERVICE Office

PROCEDURES	CODE	CHARGE
1. Est. patient Level IV	99214	$85.00
2.		
3.		
4.		
5.		
6.		

SPECIAL NOTES

Refer patient to Dr. Kutter

TOTAL CHARGES	PAYMENTS	ADJUSTMENTS	BALANCE
$85.00	-0-	-0-	$85.00

RETURN VISIT	PHYSICIAN SIGNATURE
	Donald L. Givings, M.D.

MEDICARE # D1234 MEDICAID # DLG1234 BCBS # 12345	**DONALD L. GIVINGS, M.D.** **11350 MEDICAL DRIVE, ANYWHERE, US 12345** **PHONE NUMBER (101)111-5555**	EIN # 11123456 SSN # 123-12-1234 UPIN # DG1234 GRP # DG12345

PLEASE
DO NOT
STAPLE
IN THIS
AREA

(SAMPLE ONLY - NOT APPROVED FOR USE)

CARRIER

PICA

HEALTH INSURANCE CLAIM FORM

PICA

1. MEDICARE (Medicare #) MEDICAID (Medicaid #) CHAMPUS (Sponsor's SSN) CHAMPVA (VA File #) GROUP HEALTH PLAN (SSN or ID) FECA BLK LUNG (SSN) OTHER (ID)

1a. INSURED'S I.D. NUMBER (FOR PROGRAM IN ITEM 1)

2. PATIENT'S NAME (Last Name, First Name, Middle Initial)

3. PATIENT'S BIRTH DATE MM DD YY SEX M F

4. INSURED'S NAME (Last Name, First Name, Middle Initial)

5. PATIENT'S ADDRESS (No. Street)

6. PATIENT RELATIONSHIP TO INSURED Self Spouse Child Other

7. INSURED'S ADDRESS (No. Street)

CITY STATE

8. PATIENT STATUS Single Married Other

CITY STATE

ZIP CODE TELEPHONE (Include Area Code) ( )

Employed Full-Time Student Part-Time Student

ZIP CODE TELEPHONE (INCLUDE AREA CODE) ( )

9. OTHER INSURED'S NAME (Last Name, First Name, Middle Initial)

10. IS PATIENT'S CONDITION RELATED TO:

11. INSURED'S POLICY GROUP OR FECA NUMBER

a. OTHER INSURED'S POLICY OR GROUP NUMBER

a. EMPLOYMENT? (CURRENT OR PREVIOUS) YES NO

a. INSURED'S DATE OF BIRTH MM DD YY SEX M F

b. OTHER INSURED'S DATE OF BIRTH MM DD YY SEX M F

b. AUTO ACCIDENT? PLACE (State) YES NO

b. EMPLOYER'S NAME OR SCHOOL NAME

c. EMPLOYER'S NAME OR SCHOOL NAME

c. OTHER ACCIDENT? YES NO

c. INSURANCE PLAN NAME OR PROGRAM NAME

d. INSURANCE PLAN NAME OR PROGRAM NAME

10d. RESERVED FOR LOCAL USE

d. IS THERE ANOTHER HEALTH BENEFIT PLAN? YES NO If yes, return to and complete item 9 a – d.

READ BACK OF FORM BEFORE COMPLETING & SIGNING THIS FORM.

12. PATIENT'S OR AUTHORIZED PERSON'S SIGNATURE I authorize the release of any medical or other information necessary to process this claim. I also request payment of government benefits either to myself or to the party who accepts assignment below.

SIGNED ______________ DATE ______________

13. INSURED'S OR AUTHORIZED PERSON'S SIGNATURE I authorize payment of medical benefits to the undersigned physician or supplier for services described below.

SIGNED ______________

PATIENT AND INSURED INFORMATION

14. DATE OF CURRENT: MM DD YY ILLNESS (First symptom) OR INJURY (Accident) OR PREGNANCY (LMP)

15. IF PATIENT HAS HAD SAME OR SIMILAR ILLNESS, GIVE FIRST DATE MM DD YY

16. DATES PATIENT UNABLE TO WORK IN CURRENT OCCUPATION FROM MM DD YY TO MM DD YY

17. NAME OF REFERRING PHYSICIAN OR OTHER SOURCE

17a. I.D. NUMBER OF REFERRING PHYSICIAN

18. HOSPITALIZATION DATES RELATED TO CURRENT SERVICES FROM MM DD YY TO MM DD YY

19. RESERVED FOR LOCAL USE

20. OUTSIDE LAB? YES NO $ CHARGES

21. DIAGNOSIS OR NATURE OF ILLNESS OR INJURY. (RELATE ITEMS 1, 2, 3, OR 4 TO ITEM 24E BY LINE)

1. ___ . __ 3. ___ . __

2. ___ . __ 4. ___ . __

22. MEDICAID RESUBMISSION CODE ORIGINAL REF. NO.

23. PRIOR AUTHORIZATION NUMBER

24. A DATE(S) OF SERVICE From MM DD YY	To MM DD YY	B Place of Service	C Type of Service	D PROCEDURES, SERVICES, OR SUPPLIES (Explain Unusual Circumstances) CPT/HCPCS MODIFIER	E DIAGNOSIS CODE	F $ CHARGES	G DAYS OR UNITS	H EPSDT Family Plan	I EMG	J COB	K RESERVED FOR LOCAL USE
1											
2											
3											
4											
5											
6											

25. FEDERAL TAX I.D. NUMBER SSN EIN

26. PATIENT'S ACCOUNT NO.

27. ACCEPT ASSIGNMENT? (For govt. claims, see back) YES NO

28. TOTAL CHARGE $

29. AMOUNT PAID $

30. BALANCE DUE $

31. SIGNATURE OF PHYSICIAN OR SUPPLIER INCLUDING DEGREES OR CREDENTIALS (I certify that the statements on the reverse apply to this bill and are made a part thereof.)

SIGNED DATE

32. NAME AND ADDRESS OF FACILITY WHERE SERVICES WERE RENDERED (If other than home or office)

33. PHYSICIAN'S, SUPPLIER'S BILLING NAME, ADDRESS, ZIP CODE & PHONE #

PIN# GRP#

PHYSICIAN OR SUPPLIER INFORMATION

(SAMPLE ONLY - NOT APPROVED FOR USE)

PLEASE PRINT OR TYPE

SAMPLE FORM 1500
SAMPLE FORM 1500 SAMPLE FORM 1500

Case Study 16-c

DATE	REMARKS
06/29/YYYY	Duty Station Address Dept. 21 Naval Station, Anywhere US 23456

PATIENT		CHART #	SEX	BIRTHDATE
Dana S. Bright	456-77-2345	16-c	F	07/05/1971

MAILING ADDRESS	CITY	STATE	ZIP	HOME PHONE	WORK PHONE
28 Upton Circle	Anywhere	US	12345	(101) 333-5555	

EMPLOYER	ADDRESS	PATIENT STATUS
		X MARRIED DIVORCED SINGLE STUDENT OTHER

INSURANCE: PRIMARY	ID#	GROUP	SECONDARY POLICY
TRICARE Extra	567-56-5757		

POLICYHOLDER NAME	BIRTHDATE	RELATIONSHIP	POLICYHOLDER NAME	BIRTHDATE	RELATIONSHIP
Ron L. Bright	8/12/70	Spouse			

SUPPLEMENTAL PLAN	EMPLOYER

POLICYHOLDER NAME	BIRTHDATE	RELATIONSHIP

EMPLOYER
US Navy (See duty address in remarks)

REFERRING PHYSICIAN UPIN/SSN
Donald L. Givings, M.D. 11-123456

DIAGNOSIS	CODE
1. Chronic cholecystitis	575.11
2.	
3.	
4.	

PLACE OF SERVICE Mercy Hospital, Anywhere St., Anywhere, US 12345 (Outpatient)

PROCEDURES	CODE	CHARGE
1. Laparoscopic cholecystectomy 6/29/YYYY	56340	$2,300.00
2.		
3.		
4.		
5.		
6.		

SPECIAL NOTES
Send a letter to Dr. Givings thanking him for this referral

TOTAL CHARGES	PAYMENTS	ADJUSTMENTS	BALANCE
$2,300.00	-0-	-0-	$2,300.00

RETURN VISIT	PHYSICIAN SIGNATURE
	Jonathan B. Kutter, M.D.

MEDICARE # J1234 MEDICAID # JBK1234 BCBS # 12885	**JONATHAN B. KUTTER, M.D. SURGEON** **339 WOODLAND PLACE, ANYWHERE, US 12345** **PHONE NUMBER (101)111-5555**	EIN # 11556677 SSN # 245-12-1234 UPIN # JK1234 GRP # JK12345

PLEASE DO NOT STAPLE IN THIS AREA

(SAMPLE ONLY - NOT APPROVED FOR USE)

CARRIER

PICA

HEALTH INSURANCE CLAIM FORM

PICA

1. MEDICARE (Medicare #) MEDICAID (Medicaid #) CHAMPUS (Sponsor's SSN) CHAMPVA (VA File #) GROUP HEALTH PLAN (SSN or ID) FECA BLK LUNG (SSN) OTHER (ID)

1a. INSURED'S I.D. NUMBER (FOR PROGRAM IN ITEM 1)

2. PATIENT'S NAME (Last Name, First Name, Middle Initial)

3. PATIENT'S BIRTH DATE MM DD YY SEX M F

4. INSURED'S NAME (Last Name, First Name, Middle Initial)

5. PATIENT'S ADDRESS (No. Street)

6. PATIENT RELATIONSHIP TO INSURED Self Spouse Child Other

7. INSURED'S ADDRESS (No. Street)

CITY STATE

8. PATIENT STATUS Single Married Other

CITY STATE

ZIP CODE TELEPHONE (Include Area Code) ( )

Employed Full-Time Student Part-Time Student

ZIP CODE TELEPHONE (INCLUDE AREA CODE) ( )

9. OTHER INSURED'S NAME (Last Name, First Name, Middle Initial)

10. IS PATIENT'S CONDITION RELATED TO:

11. INSURED'S POLICY GROUP OR FECA NUMBER

a. OTHER INSURED'S POLICY OR GROUP NUMBER

a. EMPLOYMENT? (CURRENT OR PREVIOUS) YES NO

a. INSURED'S DATE OF BIRTH MM DD YY SEX M F

b. OTHER INSURED'S DATE OF BIRTH MM DD YY SEX M F

b. AUTO ACCIDENT? YES NO PLACE (State)

b. EMPLOYER'S NAME OR SCHOOL NAME

c. EMPLOYER'S NAME OR SCHOOL NAME

c. OTHER ACCIDENT? YES NO

c. INSURANCE PLAN NAME OR PROGRAM NAME

d. INSURANCE PLAN NAME OR PROGRAM NAME

10d. RESERVED FOR LOCAL USE

d. IS THERE ANOTHER HEALTH BENEFIT PLAN? YES NO If yes, return to and complete item 9 a – d.

READ BACK OF FORM BEFORE COMPLETING & SIGNING THIS FORM.

12. PATIENT'S OR AUTHORIZED PERSON'S SIGNATURE I authorize the release of any medical or other information necessary to process this claim. I also request payment of government benefits either to myself or to the party who accepts assignment below.

SIGNED DATE

13. INSURED'S OR AUTHORIZED PERSON'S SIGNATURE I authorize payment of medical benefits to the undersigned physician or supplier for services described below.

SIGNED

PATIENT AND INSURED INFORMATION

14. DATE OF CURRENT: MM DD YY ILLNESS (First symptom) OR INJURY (Accident) OR PREGNANCY (LMP)

15. IF PATIENT HAS HAD SAME OR SIMILAR ILLNESS, GIVE FIRST DATE MM DD YY

16. DATES PATIENT UNABLE TO WORK IN CURRENT OCCUPATION FROM MM DD YY TO MM DD YY

17. NAME OF REFERRING PHYSICIAN OR OTHER SOURCE

17a. I.D. NUMBER OF REFERRING PHYSICIAN

18. HOSPITALIZATION DATES RELATED TO CURRENT SERVICES FROM MM DD YY TO MM DD YY

19. RESERVED FOR LOCAL USE

20. OUTSIDE LAB? YES NO $ CHARGES

21. DIAGNOSIS OR NATURE OF ILLNESS OR INJURY. (RELATE ITEMS 1, 2, 3, OR 4 TO ITEM 24E BY LINE)

1. ___ . __ 3. ___ . __

2. ___ . __ 4. ___ . __

22. MEDICAID RESUBMISSION CODE ORIGINAL REF. NO.

23. PRIOR AUTHORIZATION NUMBER

24. A DATE(S) OF SERVICE From MM DD YY To MM DD YY	B Place of Service	C Type of Service	D PROCEDURES, SERVICES, OR SUPPLIES (Explain Unusual Circumstances) CPT/HCPCS MODIFIER	E DIAGNOSIS CODE	F $ CHARGES	G DAYS OR UNITS	H EPSDT Family Plan	I EMG	J COB	K RESERVED FOR LOCAL USE
1										
2										
3										
4										
5										
6										

25. FEDERAL TAX I.D. NUMBER SSN EIN

26. PATIENT'S ACCOUNT NO.

27. ACCEPT ASSIGNMENT? (For govt. claims, see back) YES NO

28. TOTAL CHARGE $

29. AMOUNT PAID $

30. BALANCE DUE $

31. SIGNATURE OF PHYSICIAN OR SUPPLIER INCLUDING DEGREES OR CREDENTIALS (I certify that the statements on the reverse apply to this bill and are made a part thereof.)

SIGNED DATE

32. NAME AND ADDRESS OF FACILITY WHERE SERVICES WERE RENDERED (If other than home or office)

33. PHYSICIAN'S, SUPPLIER'S BILLING NAME, ADDRESS, ZIP CODE & PHONE #

PIN# GRP#

PHYSICIAN OR SUPPLIER INFORMATION

(SAMPLE ONLY - NOT APPROVED FOR USE)

PLEASE PRINT OR TYPE

SAMPLE FORM 1500
SAMPLE FORM 1500 SAMPLE FORM 1500

Case Study 16-d

DATE			REMARKS			
04/12/YYYY						

PATIENT		CHART #	SEX	BIRTHDATE
Odel M. Ryer Jr.	464-44-4646	16-d	M	04/28/1949

MAILING ADDRESS	CITY	STATE	ZIP	HOME PHONE	WORK PHONE
484 Pinewood Ave.	Anywhere	US	12345	(101) 333-5555	

EMPLOYER	ADDRESS	PATIENT STATUS
US Air Force Retired	Anywhere US	X MARRIED DIVORCED SINGLE STUDENT OTHER

INSURANCE: PRIMARY	ID#	GROUP	SECONDARY POLICY
TRICARE Standard	464-44-4646		

POLICYHOLDER NAME	BIRTHDATE	RELATIONSHIP	POLICYHOLDER NAME	BIRTHDATE	RELATIONSHIP
		Self			

SUPPLEMENTAL PLAN	EMPLOYER

POLICYHOLDER NAME	BIRTHDATE	RELATIONSHIP	DIAGNOSIS	CODE
			1. Heartburn	787.1
EMPLOYER			2.	
			3.	
REFERRING PHYSICIAN UPIN/SSN			4.	

PLACE OF SERVICE Office

PROCEDURES	CODE	CHARGE
1. Est. patient OV Level I	99211	$55.00
2.		
3.		
4.		
5.		
6.		

SPECIAL NOTES

TOTAL CHARGES	PAYMENTS	ADJUSTMENTS	BALANCE
$55.00	-0-	-0-	$55.00

RETURN VISIT	PHYSICIAN SIGNATURE
PRN	Donald L. Givings, M.D.

MEDICARE # D1234
MEDICAID # DLG1234
BCBS # 12345

DONALD L. GIVINGS, M.D.
11350 MEDICAL DRIVE, ANYWHERE, US 12345
PHONE NUMBER (101)111-5555

EIN # 11123456
SSN # 123-12-1234
UPIN # DG1234
GRP # DG12345

PLEASE
DO NOT
STAPLE
IN THIS
AREA

(SAMPLE ONLY - NOT APPROVED FOR USE)

CARRIER

PICA

HEALTH INSURANCE CLAIM FORM

PICA

1. MEDICARE (Medicare #) MEDICAID (Medicaid #) CHAMPUS (Sponsor's SSN) CHAMPVA (VA File #) GROUP HEALTH PLAN (SSN or ID) FECA BLK LUNG (SSN) OTHER (ID)

1a. INSURED'S I.D. NUMBER (FOR PROGRAM IN ITEM 1)

2. PATIENT'S NAME (Last Name, First Name, Middle Initial)

3. PATIENT'S BIRTH DATE MM DD YY SEX M F

4. INSURED'S NAME (Last Name, First Name, Middle Initial)

5. PATIENT'S ADDRESS (No. Street)

6. PATIENT RELATIONSHIP TO INSURED Self Spouse Child Other

7. INSURED'S ADDRESS (No. Street)

CITY STATE

8. PATIENT STATUS Single Married Other

CITY STATE

ZIP CODE TELEPHONE (Include Area Code) ( )

Employed Full-Time Student Part-Time Student

ZIP CODE TELEPHONE (INCLUDE AREA CODE) ( )

9. OTHER INSURED'S NAME (Last Name, First Name, Middle Initial)

10. IS PATIENT'S CONDITION RELATED TO:

11. INSURED'S POLICY GROUP OR FECA NUMBER

a. OTHER INSURED'S POLICY OR GROUP NUMBER

a. EMPLOYMENT? (CURRENT OR PREVIOUS) YES NO

a. INSURED'S DATE OF BIRTH MM DD YY SEX M F

b. OTHER INSURED'S DATE OF BIRTH MM DD YY SEX M F

b. AUTO ACCIDENT? PLACE (State) YES NO

b. EMPLOYER'S NAME OR SCHOOL NAME

c. EMPLOYER'S NAME OR SCHOOL NAME

c. OTHER ACCIDENT? YES NO

c. INSURANCE PLAN NAME OR PROGRAM NAME

d. INSURANCE PLAN NAME OR PROGRAM NAME

10d. RESERVED FOR LOCAL USE

d. IS THERE ANOTHER HEALTH BENEFIT PLAN? YES NO If yes, return to and complete item 9 a – d.

READ BACK OF FORM BEFORE COMPLETING & SIGNING THIS FORM.

12. PATIENT'S OR AUTHORIZED PERSON'S SIGNATURE I authorize the release of any medical or other information necessary to process this claim. I also request payment of government benefits either to myself or to the party who accepts assignment below.

SIGNED DATE

13. INSURED'S OR AUTHORIZED PERSON'S SIGNATURE I authorize payment of medical benefits to the undersigned physician or supplier for services described below.

SIGNED

PATIENT AND INSURED INFORMATION

14. DATE OF CURRENT: MM DD YY ILLNESS (First symptom) OR INJURY (Accident) OR PREGNANCY (LMP)

15. IF PATIENT HAS HAD SAME OR SIMILAR ILLNESS, GIVE FIRST DATE MM DD YY

16. DATES PATIENT UNABLE TO WORK IN CURRENT OCCUPATION FROM MM DD YY TO MM DD YY

17. NAME OF REFERRING PHYSICIAN OR OTHER SOURCE

17a. I.D. NUMBER OF REFERRING PHYSICIAN

18. HOSPITALIZATION DATES RELATED TO CURRENT SERVICES FROM MM DD YY TO MM DD YY

19. RESERVED FOR LOCAL USE

20. OUTSIDE LAB? YES NO $ CHARGES

21. DIAGNOSIS OR NATURE OF ILLNESS OR INJURY. (RELATE ITEMS 1, 2, 3, OR 4 TO ITEM 24E BY LINE)

1. ___ . ___

2. ___ . ___

3. ___ . ___

4. ___ . ___

22. MEDICAID RESUBMISSION CODE ORIGINAL REF. NO.

23. PRIOR AUTHORIZATION NUMBER

24. A DATE(S) OF SERVICE From MM DD YY To MM DD YY	B Place of Service	C Type of Service	D PROCEDURES, SERVICES, OR SUPPLIES (Explain Unusual Circumstances) CPT/HCPCS MODIFIER	E DIAGNOSIS CODE	F $ CHARGES	G DAYS OR UNITS	H EPSDT Family Plan	I EMG	J COB	K RESERVED FOR LOCAL USE
1										
2										
3										
4										
5										
6										

25. FEDERAL TAX I.D. NUMBER SSN EIN

26. PATIENT'S ACCOUNT NO.

27. ACCEPT ASSIGNMENT? (For govt. claims, see back) YES NO

28. TOTAL CHARGE $

29. AMOUNT PAID $

30. BALANCE DUE $

31. SIGNATURE OF PHYSICIAN OR SUPPLIER INCLUDING DEGREES OR CREDENTIALS (I certify that the statements on the reverse apply to this bill and are made a part thereof.)

SIGNED DATE

32. NAME AND ADDRESS OF FACILITY WHERE SERVICES WERE RENDERED (If other than home or office)

33. PHYSICIAN'S, SUPPLIER'S BILLING NAME, ADDRESS, ZIP CODE & PHONE #

PIN# GRP#

PHYSICIAN OR SUPPLIER INFORMATION

(SAMPLE ONLY - NOT APPROVED FOR USE)

PLEASE PRINT OR TYPE

SAMPLE FORM 1500
SAMPLE FORM 1500 SAMPLE FORM 1500

Case Study 16-e

DATE	REMARKS
06/11/YYYY	Father is stationed at 555 Regiment Way, Anywhere US 12345

PATIENT		CHART #	SEX	BIRTHDATE
Annalisa M. Faris	456-77-5555	16-e	F	04/04/1999

MAILING ADDRESS	CITY	STATE	ZIP	HOME PHONE	WORK PHONE
394 Myriam Court	Anywhere	US	12345	(101) 333-5555	

EMPLOYER	ADDRESS	PATIENT STATUS
		MARRIED DIVORCED SINGLE (X) STUDENT OTHER

INSURANCE: PRIMARY	ID#	GROUP	SECONDARY POLICY
TRICARE Prime	323-23-3333		

POLICYHOLDER NAME	BIRTHDATE	RELATIONSHIP	POLICYHOLDER NAME	BIRTHDATE	RELATIONSHIP
Nacir R. Faris	6/21/75	Father			

SUPPLEMENTAL PLAN	EMPLOYER

POLICYHOLDER NAME | BIRTHDATE | RELATIONSHIP

EMPLOYER: US Army (See duty address in remarks)

REFERRING PHYSICIAN UPIN/SSN:

DIAGNOSIS	CODE
1. Chills with fever	780.6
2. Lethargy	780.7
3. Loss of appetite	783.0
4. Loss of weight	783.2

PLACE OF SERVICE: Mercy Hospital, Anywhere Street, Anywhere, US 12345

PROCEDURES		CODE	CHARGE
1. Initial Hosp. Level V	06/02/YYYY	99225	$200.00
2. Subsq. Hosp. Level III	06/03/YYYY	99233	85.00
3. Subsq. Hosp. Level III	06/04/YYYY	99233	85.00
4. Subsq. Hosp. Level III	06/05/YYYY	99233	85.00
5. Subsq. Hosp. Level II	06/06/YYYY	99232	75.00
6. Subsq. Hosp. Level II	06/07/YYYY	99232	75.00
7. Subsq. Hosp. Level II	06/08/YYYY	99232	75.00

SPECIAL NOTES
Admission authorization # D50123
Patient was discharged 06/11/YYYY but not seen

TOTAL CHARGES	PAYMENTS	ADJUSTMENTS	BALANCE
$680.00	-0-	-0-	$680.00

RETURN VISIT	PHYSICIAN SIGNATURE
	Donald L. Givings, M.D.

DONALD L. GIVINGS, M.D.
11350 MEDICAL DRIVE, ANYWHERE, US 12345
PHONE NUMBER (101)111-5555

MEDICARE # D1234
MEDICAID # DLG1234
BCBS # 12345

EIN # 11123456
SSN # 123-12-1234
UPIN # DG1234
GRP # DG1234

PLEASE
DO NOT
STAPLE
IN THIS
AREA

(SAMPLE ONLY - NOT APPROVED FOR USE)

CARRIER

PICA

HEALTH INSURANCE CLAIM FORM

PICA

1. MEDICARE (Medicare #) MEDICAID (Medicaid #) CHAMPUS (Sponsor's SSN) CHAMPVA (VA File #) GROUP HEALTH PLAN (SSN or ID) FECA BLK LUNG (SSN) OTHER (ID)

1a. INSURED'S I.D. NUMBER (FOR PROGRAM IN ITEM 1)

2. PATIENT'S NAME (Last Name, First Name, Middle Initial)

3. PATIENT'S BIRTH DATE MM DD YY SEX M F

4. INSURED'S NAME (Last Name, First Name, Middle Initial)

5. PATIENT'S ADDRESS (No. Street)

6. PATIENT RELATIONSHIP TO INSURED Self Spouse Child Other

7. INSURED'S ADDRESS (No. Street)

CITY STATE

8. PATIENT STATUS Single Married Other

CITY STATE

ZIP CODE TELEPHONE (Include Area Code) ( )

Employed Full-Time Student Part-Time Student

ZIP CODE TELEPHONE (INCLUDE AREA CODE) ( )

9. OTHER INSURED'S NAME (Last Name, First Name, Middle Initial)

10. IS PATIENT'S CONDITION RELATED TO:

11. INSURED'S POLICY GROUP OR FECA NUMBER

a. OTHER INSURED'S POLICY OR GROUP NUMBER

a. EMPLOYMENT? (CURRENT OR PREVIOUS) YES NO

a. INSURED'S DATE OF BIRTH MM DD YY SEX M F

b. OTHER INSURED'S DATE OF BIRTH MM DD YY SEX M F

b. AUTO ACCIDENT? PLACE (State) YES NO

b. EMPLOYER'S NAME OR SCHOOL NAME

c. EMPLOYER'S NAME OR SCHOOL NAME

c. OTHER ACCIDENT? YES NO

c. INSURANCE PLAN NAME OR PROGRAM NAME

d. INSURANCE PLAN NAME OR PROGRAM NAME

10d. RESERVED FOR LOCAL USE

d. IS THERE ANOTHER HEALTH BENEFIT PLAN? YES NO If yes, return to and complete item 9 a – d.

READ BACK OF FORM BEFORE COMPLETING & SIGNING THIS FORM.

12. PATIENT'S OR AUTHORIZED PERSON'S SIGNATURE I authorize the release of any medical or other information necessary to process this claim. I also request payment of government benefits either to myself or to the party who accepts assignment below.

SIGNED ______ DATE ______

13. INSURED'S OR AUTHORIZED PERSON'S SIGNATURE I authorize payment of medical benefits to the undersigned physician or supplier for services described below.

SIGNED ______

PATIENT AND INSURED INFORMATION

14. DATE OF CURRENT: MM DD YY ILLNESS (First symptom) OR INJURY (Accident) OR PREGNANCY (LMP)

15. IF PATIENT HAS HAD SAME OR SIMILAR ILLNESS, GIVE FIRST DATE MM DD YY

16. DATES PATIENT UNABLE TO WORK IN CURRENT OCCUPATION FROM MM DD YY TO MM DD YY

17. NAME OF REFERRING PHYSICIAN OR OTHER SOURCE

17a. I.D. NUMBER OF REFERRING PHYSICIAN

18. HOSPITALIZATION DATES RELATED TO CURRENT SERVICES FROM MM DD YY TO MM DD YY

19. RESERVED FOR LOCAL USE

20. OUTSIDE LAB? YES NO $ CHARGES

21. DIAGNOSIS OR NATURE OF ILLNESS OR INJURY. (RELATE ITEMS 1, 2, 3, OR 4 TO ITEM 24E BY LINE)

1. ___ . __
2. ___ . __
3. ___ . __
4. ___ . __

22. MEDICAID RESUBMISSION CODE ORIGINAL REF. NO.

23. PRIOR AUTHORIZATION NUMBER

24. A DATE(S) OF SERVICE From MM DD YY To MM DD YY	B Place of Service	C Type of Service	D PROCEDURES, SERVICES, OR SUPPLIES (Explain Unusual Circumstances) CPT/HCPCS MODIFIER	E DIAGNOSIS CODE	F $ CHARGES	G DAYS OR UNITS	H EPSDT Family Plan	I EMG	J COB	K RESERVED FOR LOCAL USE
1										
2										
3										
4										
5										
6										

25. FEDERAL TAX I.D. NUMBER SSN EIN

26. PATIENT'S ACCOUNT NO.

27. ACCEPT ASSIGNMENT? (For govt. claims, see back) YES NO

28. TOTAL CHARGE $

29. AMOUNT PAID $

30. BALANCE DUE $

31. SIGNATURE OF PHYSICIAN OR SUPPLIER INCLUDING DEGREES OR CREDENTIALS (I certify that the statements on the reverse apply to this bill and are made a part thereof.)

SIGNED DATE

32. NAME AND ADDRESS OF FACILITY WHERE SERVICES WERE RENDERED (If other than home or office)

33. PHYSICIAN'S, SUPPLIER'S BILLING NAME, ADDRESS, ZIP CODE & PHONE #

PIN# GRP#

PHYSICIAN OR SUPPLIER INFORMATION

(SAMPLE ONLY - NOT APPROVED FOR USE)

PLEASE PRINT OR TYPE

SAMPLE FORM 1500
SAMPLE FORM 1500 SAMPLE FORM 1500

Workers' Compensation

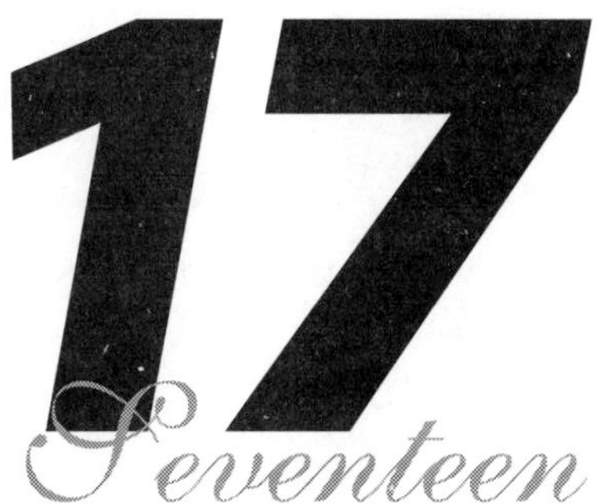

INTRODUCTION

1. Describe reimbursement procedures for employee care (e.g., for on-the-job injuries) before the enactment of workers' compensation laws.

____

____

____

____

____

2. State the threefold philosophy behind the establishment of workers' compensation laws.

   a. _______________
   b. _______________
   c. _______________

FEDERAL COMPENSATION PROGRAMS

3. The Black Lung Benefits Act provides workers' compensation for _____ suffering from "black lung."

4. If a patient has been injured at work, how can the provider find the mailing address of the district office for submission of injury reports and claims? _______________

STATE-SPONSORED COVERAGE

5. List four types of coverage that have emerged from state legislatures.

   a. _______________
   b. _______________
   c. _______________
   d. _______________

6. The cost of workers' compensation has skyrocketed, causing many employers to turn long-term cases over to ___. (Circle the correct answer.)

   a. Medicare

   b. Medicaid

   c. managed care programs

   d. none of the above

7. What is the name of the government agency responsible for administering the workers' compensation law and handling appeals for claims that have been denied? (Circle the correct answer.)

   a. State Compensation Fund

   b. State Compensation Department

   c. State Compensation Division

   d. none of the above

ELIGIBILITY

8. List three occupations in which coverage for stress-related disorders has been awarded.

   a. ____________________

   b. ____________________

   c. ____________________

9. Give two situations of when an employee would qualify for workers' compensation even though he/she was not physically on company property. (Do not use examples given in the textbook.)

   ____

   ____

   ____

   ____

   ____

   ____

   ____

CLASSIFICATION OF ON-THE-JOB INJURIES

10. List five classifications of workers' compensation cases mandated by federal law.

   a. ____________________

   b. ____________________

   c. ____________________

   d. ____________________

   e. ____________________

11. For each item, enter **T** for a true statement or **F** for a false statement on the line provided.

_______ a. Medical claims with no disability are filed for minor injuries when the worker is treated and able to return to work within a few days.

_______ b. Temporary disability claims cover medical treatment for injuries and disorders but not payment for lost income.

_______ c. Permanent disability refers to the employee's degree of injury.

_______ d. Vocational rehabilitation claims cover the expense of vocational retraining.

12. Describe the difference between **disability precluding heavy lifting** and **disability precluding very heavy lifting**. ____

____

13. Match the terminology describing pain in the first column with the definitions in the second column. Write the correct letter in each blank.

_______ minimal pain	a. tolerable, but there may be some limitations in performance of assigned duties
_______ slight pain	b. precludes any activity that precipitates pain
_______ moderate pain	c. tolerable, but there may be marked handicapping of performance
_______ severe pain	d. annoyance, but will not handicap the performance of the patient's work

14. How are death benefits computed? ____

OSHA ACT OF 1970

15. Why was OSHA enacted by Congress? ____

16. What is the name of the vaccination that must be administered to each worker who might be exposed to infectious materials? ____

17. Comprehensive records of all vaccinations received and any accidental exposure incidents must be kept for ___ years. (Circle the correct answer.)

    a. 5
    b. 10
    c. 15
    d. 20

SPECIAL HANDLING OF WORKERS' COMPENSATION CASES

18. If a patient has workers' compensation and the amount charged for the treatment is greater than the approved reimbursement for the treatment, can the provider balance bill the patient? ____________

Critical Thinking

19. Why is it important to maintain separate files on patients who receive treatment from the same provider for both work-related disorders and regular medical care?

____

____

____

____

____

FIRST REPORT OF INJURY

20. When should the First Report of Injury form be completed? ____

____

21. List four parties who should receive a copy of a First Report of Injury form.

    a. ____
    b. ____
    c. ____
    d. ____

22. Explain why there is no patient signature line on the First Report of Injury form.

____

____

____

23. What is the time limit for filing the First Report of Injury form? ____

____

24. If an employer disputes the legitimacy of a claim, should the provider still file the First Report of Injury form? ____________

25. When a patient receives written notice of denial of the claim from the employer, the patient is required to file an appeal with the ___. (Circle the correct answer.)

    a. employer
    b. state Workers' Compensation Commission/Board
    c. insurance carrier
    d. all of the above

PROGRESS REPORTS

26. What is the purpose of the Progress Report? ____

____

27. What should be done with a file or case number once it is assigned by the carrier or the Workers' Compensation Commission/Board? ____________________________________

____

BILLING INFORMATION NOTES

28. Which of the following injured workers may be eligible for federal compensation plans? (Circle the correct answer/answers.)
   a. coal miners
   b. military employees
   c. federal employees
   d. all of the above

29. Which of the following can be designated a fiscal agent by state law and the corporation involved? (Circle the correct answer.)
   a. the State Compensation Fund
   b. a private, commercial insurance carrier
   c. the employer's special company capital funds set aside for compensation cases
   d. any of the above

30. What is the deductible for workers' compensation claims? ________________________

31. What is the copayment for workers' compensation claims? ________________________

Know Your Acronyms

32. Define the following acronyms:
   a. OSHA ____
   b. MSDS ____
   c. FECA ____
   d. FELA ____
   e. LHWCA ____

EXERCISES

1. Complete Case Studies 17-a through 17-f using the blank claim forms provided. Follow the step-by-step instructions in the textbook to properly complete each claim form. If a patient has secondary coverage, complete an additional claim form using secondary directions from the textbook. You may choose to use a pencil so corrections can be made.

Case Study 17-a

DATE	REMARKS
02/03/YYYY	Injured today at work, no assigned claim number

PATIENT		CHART #	SEX	BIRTHDATE
Sandy S. Grand	444-55-6666	17-a	F	12/03/1972

MAILING ADDRESS	CITY	STATE	ZIP	HOME PHONE	WORK PHONE
109 Darling Road	Anywhere	US	12345	(101) 333-5555	(101) 444-5555

EMPLOYER	ADDRESS		PATIENT STATUS
Starport Fitness Center	Anywhere	US	MARRIED DIVORCED SINGLE (X) STUDENT OTHER

INSURANCE: PRIMARY	ID#	GROUP	SECONDARY POLICY
Workers Trust			

POLICYHOLDER NAME	BIRTHDATE	RELATIONSHIP	POLICYHOLDER NAME	BIRTHDATE	RELATIONSHIP
		Self			

SUPPLEMENTAL PLAN	EMPLOYER

POLICYHOLDER NAME	BIRTHDATE	RELATIONSHIP

EMPLOYER

REFERRING PHYSICIAN UPIN/SSN

DIAGNOSIS	CODE
1. Wrist fracture, closed	814.00
2. Fall from chair	E884.2
3.	
4.	

PLACE OF SERVICE Office

PROCEDURES	CODE	CHARGE
1. New patient OV Level IV	99204	$100.00
2.		
3.		
4.		
5.		
6.		
7.		

SPECIAL NOTES
Patient cannot return to work until seen by the Orthopedist, Dr. Breaker

TOTAL CHARGES	PAYMENTS	ADJUSTMENTS	BALANCE
$100.00	-0-	-0-	$100.00

RETURN VISIT	PHYSICIAN SIGNATURE
	Donald L. Givings, M.D.

MEDICARE # D1234
MEDICAID # DLG1234
BCBS # 12345

DONALD L. GIVINGS, M.D.
11350 MEDICAL DRIVE, ANYWHERE, US 12345
PHONE NUMBER (101)111-5555

EIN # 11123456
SSN # 123-12-1234
UPIN # DG1234
GRP # DG12345

PLEASE
DO NOT
STAPLE
IN THIS
AREA

(SAMPLE ONLY - NOT APPROVED FOR USE)

CARRIER

PICA

HEALTH INSURANCE CLAIM FORM

PICA

1. MEDICARE (Medicare #) MEDICAID (Medicaid #) CHAMPUS (Sponsor's SSN) CHAMPVA (VA File #) GROUP HEALTH PLAN (SSN or ID) FECA BLK LUNG (SSN) OTHER (ID)

1a. INSURED'S I.D. NUMBER (FOR PROGRAM IN ITEM 1)

2. PATIENT'S NAME (Last Name, First Name, Middle Initial)

3. PATIENT'S BIRTH DATE MM DD YY SEX M F

4. INSURED'S NAME (Last Name, First Name, Middle Initial)

5. PATIENT'S ADDRESS (No. Street)

6. PATIENT RELATIONSHIP TO INSURED Self Spouse Child Other

7. INSURED'S ADDRESS (No. Street)

CITY STATE

8. PATIENT STATUS Single Married Other

CITY STATE

ZIP CODE TELEPHONE (Include Area Code) ( )

Employed Full-Time Student Part-Time Student

ZIP CODE TELEPHONE (INCLUDE AREA CODE) ( )

9. OTHER INSURED'S NAME (Last Name, First Name, Middle Initial)

10. IS PATIENT'S CONDITION RELATED TO:

11. INSURED'S POLICY GROUP OR FECA NUMBER

a. OTHER INSURED'S POLICY OR GROUP NUMBER

a. EMPLOYMENT? (CURRENT OR PREVIOUS) YES NO

a. INSURED'S DATE OF BIRTH MM DD YY SEX M F

b. OTHER INSURED'S DATE OF BIRTH MM DD YY SEX M F

b. AUTO ACCIDENT? PLACE (State) YES NO

b. EMPLOYER'S NAME OR SCHOOL NAME

c. EMPLOYER'S NAME OR SCHOOL NAME

c. OTHER ACCIDENT? YES NO

c. INSURANCE PLAN NAME OR PROGRAM NAME

d. INSURANCE PLAN NAME OR PROGRAM NAME

10d. RESERVED FOR LOCAL USE

d. IS THERE ANOTHER HEALTH BENEFIT PLAN? YES NO If yes, return to and complete item 9 a – d.

READ BACK OF FORM BEFORE COMPLETING & SIGNING THIS FORM.

12. PATIENT'S OR AUTHORIZED PERSON'S SIGNATURE I authorize the release of any medical or other information necessary to process this claim. I also request payment of government benefits either to myself or to the party who accepts assignment below.

SIGNED ____________ DATE ____________

13. INSURED'S OR AUTHORIZED PERSON'S SIGNATURE I authorize payment of medical benefits to the undersigned physician or supplier for services described below.

SIGNED ____________

PATIENT AND INSURED INFORMATION

14. DATE OF CURRENT: MM DD YY ◀ ILLNESS (First symptom) OR INJURY (Accident) OR PREGNANCY (LMP)

15. IF PATIENT HAS HAD SAME OR SIMILAR ILLNESS, GIVE FIRST DATE MM DD YY

16. DATES PATIENT UNABLE TO WORK IN CURRENT OCCUPATION FROM MM DD YY TO MM DD YY

17. NAME OF REFERRING PHYSICIAN OR OTHER SOURCE

17a. I.D. NUMBER OF REFERRING PHYSICIAN

18. HOSPITALIZATION DATES RELATED TO CURRENT SERVICES FROM MM DD YY TO MM DD YY

19. RESERVED FOR LOCAL USE

20. OUTSIDE LAB? YES NO $ CHARGES

21. DIAGNOSIS OR NATURE OF ILLNESS OR INJURY. (RELATE ITEMS 1, 2, 3, OR 4 TO ITEM 24E BY LINE)

1. ____ . __

2. ____ . __

3. ____ . __

4. ____ . __

22. MEDICAID RESUBMISSION CODE ORIGINAL REF. NO.

23. PRIOR AUTHORIZATION NUMBER

24. A DATE(S) OF SERVICE From MM DD YY To MM DD YY	B Place of Service	C Type of Service	D PROCEDURES, SERVICES, OR SUPPLIES (Explain Unusual Circumstances) CPT/HCPCS MODIFIER	E DIAGNOSIS CODE	F $ CHARGES	G DAYS OR UNITS	H EPSDT Family Plan	I EMG	J COB	K RESERVED FOR LOCAL USE
1										
2										
3										
4										
5										
6										

25. FEDERAL TAX I.D. NUMBER SSN EIN

26. PATIENT'S ACCOUNT NO.

27. ACCEPT ASSIGNMENT? (For govt. claims, see back) YES NO

28. TOTAL CHARGE $

29. AMOUNT PAID $

30. BALANCE DUE $

31. SIGNATURE OF PHYSICIAN OR SUPPLIER INCLUDING DEGREES OR CREDENTIALS (I certify that the statements on the reverse apply to this bill and are made a part thereof.)

SIGNED DATE

32. NAME AND ADDRESS OF FACILITY WHERE SERVICES WERE RENDERED (If other than home or office)

33. PHYSICIAN'S, SUPPLIER'S BILLING NAME, ADDRESS, ZIP CODE & PHONE #

PIN# GRP#

PHYSICIAN OR SUPPLIER INFORMATION

(SAMPLE ONLY - NOT APPROVED FOR USE)

PLEASE PRINT OR TYPE

SAMPLE FORM 1500
SAMPLE FORM 1500 SAMPLE FORM 1500

Case Study 17-b

DATE	REMARKS
02/05/YYYY	Patient may return to work 2/12/YYYY

PATIENT		CHART #	SEX	BIRTHDATE
Sandy S. Grand	444-55-6666	17-b	F	12/03/1972

MAILING ADDRESS	CITY	STATE	ZIP	HOME PHONE	WORK PHONE
109 Darling Road	Anywhere	US	12345	(101) 333-5555	(101) 444-5555

EMPLOYER	ADDRESS		PATIENT STATUS
Starport Fitness Center	Anywhere	US	MARRIED DIVORCED SINGLE (X) STUDENT OTHER

INSURANCE: PRIMARY	ID#	GROUP	SECONDARY POLICY
Workers Trust	CLR5457		

POLICYHOLDER NAME	BIRTHDATE	RELATIONSHIP	POLICYHOLDER NAME	BIRTHDATE	RELATIONSHIP
		Self			

SUPPLEMENTAL PLAN	EMPLOYER

POLICYHOLDER NAME	BIRTHDATE	RELATIONSHIP

EMPLOYER

DIAGNOSIS	CODE
1. Wrist fracture, closed	814.00
2. Fall from chair	E884.2
3.	
4.	

REFERRING PHYSICIAN UPIN/SSN	
Donald L. Givings, M.D.	123-12-1234

PLACE OF SERVICE Office

PROCEDURES	CODE	CHARGE
1. Office consult Level IV	99244	$95.00
2. Xray wrist, complete	73110	$75.00
3. Application of cast, hand and lower forearm	29085	$50.00
4.		
5.		
6.		
7.		

SPECIAL NOTES

Date of injury: 02/03/YYYY

TOTAL CHARGES	PAYMENTS	ADJUSTMENTS	BALANCE
$220.00	-0-	-0-	$220.00

RETURN VISIT	PHYSICIAN SIGNATURE
2 weeks	*Elliot A. Breaker, M.D.*

MEDICARE # E1234
MEDICAID # EAB1234
BCBS # 48489

Elliot A. Breaker, M.D. Orthopedist
5124 PHARMACY DRIVE, ANYWHERE, US 12345
PHONE NUMBER (101)111-5555

EIN # 11997755
SSN # 223-22-1222
UPIN # EB1234
GRP # EB12345

PLEASE
DO NOT
STAPLE
IN THIS
AREA

(SAMPLE ONLY - NOT APPROVED FOR USE)

CARRIER

PICA

HEALTH INSURANCE CLAIM FORM

PICA

1. MEDICARE (Medicare #) MEDICAID (Medicaid #) CHAMPUS (Sponsor's SSN) CHAMPVA (VA File #) GROUP HEALTH PLAN (SSN or ID) FECA BLK LUNG (SSN) OTHER (ID)

1a. INSURED'S I.D. NUMBER (FOR PROGRAM IN ITEM 1)

2. PATIENT'S NAME (Last Name, First Name, Middle Initial)

3. PATIENT'S BIRTH DATE MM DD YY SEX M F

4. INSURED'S NAME (Last Name, First Name, Middle Initial)

5. PATIENT'S ADDRESS (No. Street)

6. PATIENT RELATIONSHIP TO INSURED Self Spouse Child Other

7. INSURED'S ADDRESS (No. Street)

CITY STATE

8. PATIENT STATUS Single Married Other

CITY STATE

ZIP CODE TELEPHONE (Include Area Code) ( )

Employed Full-Time Student Part-Time Student

ZIP CODE TELEPHONE (INCLUDE AREA CODE) ( )

9. OTHER INSURED'S NAME (Last Name, First Name, Middle Initial)

10. IS PATIENT'S CONDITION RELATED TO:

11. INSURED'S POLICY GROUP OR FECA NUMBER

a. OTHER INSURED'S POLICY OR GROUP NUMBER

a. EMPLOYMENT? (CURRENT OR PREVIOUS) YES NO

a. INSURED'S DATE OF BIRTH MM DD YY SEX M F

b. OTHER INSURED'S DATE OF BIRTH MM DD YY SEX M F

b. AUTO ACCIDENT? PLACE (State) YES NO

b. EMPLOYER'S NAME OR SCHOOL NAME

c. EMPLOYER'S NAME OR SCHOOL NAME

c. OTHER ACCIDENT? YES NO

c. INSURANCE PLAN NAME OR PROGRAM NAME

d. INSURANCE PLAN NAME OR PROGRAM NAME

10d. RESERVED FOR LOCAL USE

d. IS THERE ANOTHER HEALTH BENEFIT PLAN? YES NO If yes, return to and complete item 9 a – d.

READ BACK OF FORM BEFORE COMPLETING & SIGNING THIS FORM.

12. PATIENT'S OR AUTHORIZED PERSON'S SIGNATURE I authorize the release of any medical or other information necessary to process this claim. I also request payment of government benefits either to myself or to the party who accepts assignment below.

SIGNED DATE

13. INSURED'S OR AUTHORIZED PERSON'S SIGNATURE I authorize payment of medical benefits to the undersigned physician or supplier for services described below.

SIGNED

PATIENT AND INSURED INFORMATION

14. DATE OF CURRENT: MM DD YY ILLNESS (First symptom) OR INJURY (Accident) OR PREGNANCY (LMP)

15. IF PATIENT HAS HAD SAME OR SIMILAR ILLNESS, GIVE FIRST DATE MM DD YY

16. DATES PATIENT UNABLE TO WORK IN CURRENT OCCUPATION FROM MM DD YY TO MM DD YY

17. NAME OF REFERRING PHYSICIAN OR OTHER SOURCE

17a. I.D. NUMBER OF REFERRING PHYSICIAN

18. HOSPITALIZATION DATES RELATED TO CURRENT SERVICES FROM MM DD YY TO MM DD YY

19. RESERVED FOR LOCAL USE

20. OUTSIDE LAB? YES NO $ CHARGES

21. DIAGNOSIS OR NATURE OF ILLNESS OR INJURY. (RELATE ITEMS 1, 2, 3, OR 4 TO ITEM 24E BY LINE)

1. ___ . ___
2. ___ . ___
3. ___ . ___
4. ___ . ___

22. MEDICAID RESUBMISSION CODE ORIGINAL REF. NO.

23. PRIOR AUTHORIZATION NUMBER

24.	A DATE(S) OF SERVICE From MM DD YY	To MM DD YY	B Place of Service	C Type of Service	D PROCEDURES, SERVICES, OR SUPPLIES (Explain Unusual Circumstances) CPT/HCPCS MODIFIER	E DIAGNOSIS CODE	F $ CHARGES	G DAYS OR UNITS	H EPSDT Family Plan	I EMG	J COB	K RESERVED FOR LOCAL USE
1												
2												
3												
4												
5												
6												

PHYSICIAN OR SUPPLIER INFORMATION

25. FEDERAL TAX I.D. NUMBER SSN EIN

26. PATIENT'S ACCOUNT NO.

27. ACCEPT ASSIGNMENT? (For govt. claims, see back) YES NO

28. TOTAL CHARGE $

29. AMOUNT PAID $

30. BALANCE DUE $

31. SIGNATURE OF PHYSICIAN OR SUPPLIER INCLUDING DEGREES OR CREDENTIALS (I certify that the statements on the reverse apply to this bill and are made a part thereof.)

SIGNED DATE

32. NAME AND ADDRESS OF FACILITY WHERE SERVICES WERE RENDERED (If other than home or office)

33. PHYSICIAN'S, SUPPLIER'S BILLING NAME, ADDRESS, ZIP CODE & PHONE #

PIN# GRP#

(SAMPLE ONLY - NOT APPROVED FOR USE)

PLEASE PRINT OR TYPE

SAMPLE FORM 1500
SAMPLE FORM 1500 SAMPLE FORM 1500

Case Study 17-c

DATE	REMARKS
05/12/YYYY	Patient injured at end of shift today

PATIENT		CHART #	SEX	BIRTHDATE
Marianna D. Holland	494-55-6969	17-c	F	11/05/1977

MAILING ADDRESS	CITY	STATE	ZIP	HOME PHONE	WORK PHONE
509 Dutch Street	Anywhere	US	12345	(101) 333-5555	(101) 444-5555

EMPLOYER	ADDRESS	PATIENT STATUS
Hair Etc.	Anywhere US	X MARRIED DIVORCED SINGLE STUDENT OTHER

INSURANCE: PRIMARY	ID#	GROUP	SECONDARY POLICY
Workers Shield	BA6788		

POLICYHOLDER NAME	BIRTHDATE	RELATIONSHIP	POLICYHOLDER NAME	BIRTHDATE	RELATIONSHIP
		Self			

SUPPLEMENTAL PLAN	EMPLOYER

POLICYHOLDER NAME	BIRTHDATE	RELATIONSHIP	DIAGNOSIS	CODE
			1. Fracture, nasal bones, closed	802.0
EMPLOYER			2.	
			3.	
REFERRING PHYSICIAN UPIN/SSN			4.	

PLACE OF SERVICE Office

PROCEDURES	CODE	CHARGE
1. New patient OV Level III	99203	$80.00
2.		
3.		
4.		
5.		
6.		

SPECIAL NOTES

Patient may return to work 5/16/YYYY

TOTAL CHARGES	PAYMENTS	ADJUSTMENTS	BALANCE
$80.00	-0-	-0-	$80.00

RETURN VISIT	PHYSICIAN SIGNATURE
PRN	Donald L. Givings, M.D.

DONALD L. GIVINGS, M.D.
11350 MEDICAL DRIVE, ANYWHERE, US 12345
PHONE NUMBER (101)111-5555

MEDICARE # D1234
MEDICAID # DLG1234
BCBS # 12345

EIN # 11123456
SSN # 123-12-1234
UPIN # DG1234
GRP # DG12345

PLEASE
DO NOT
STAPLE
IN THIS
AREA

(SAMPLE ONLY - NOT APPROVED FOR USE)

CARRIER

PICA

HEALTH INSURANCE CLAIM FORM

PICA

1. MEDICARE (Medicare #) | MEDICAID (Medicaid #) | CHAMPUS (Sponsor's SSN) | CHAMPVA (VA File #) | GROUP HEALTH PLAN (SSN or ID) | FECA BLK LUNG (SSN) | OTHER (ID)

1a. INSURED'S I.D. NUMBER (FOR PROGRAM IN ITEM 1)

2. PATIENT'S NAME (Last Name, First Name, Middle Initial)

3. PATIENT'S BIRTH DATE MM DD YY — SEX M F

4. INSURED'S NAME (Last Name, First Name, Middle Initial)

5. PATIENT'S ADDRESS (No. Street)

6. PATIENT RELATIONSHIP TO INSURED — Self, Spouse, Child, Other

7. INSURED'S ADDRESS (No. Street)

CITY — STATE

8. PATIENT STATUS — Single, Married, Other; Employed, Full-Time Student, Part-Time Student

CITY — STATE

ZIP CODE — TELEPHONE (Include Area Code) ( )

ZIP CODE — TELEPHONE (INCLUDE AREA CODE) ( )

9. OTHER INSURED'S NAME (Last Name, First Name, Middle Initial)

10. IS PATIENT'S CONDITION RELATED TO:

11. INSURED'S POLICY GROUP OR FECA NUMBER

a. OTHER INSURED'S POLICY OR GROUP NUMBER

a. EMPLOYMENT? (CURRENT OR PREVIOUS) — YES, NO

a. INSURED'S DATE OF BIRTH MM DD YY — SEX M F

b. OTHER INSURED'S DATE OF BIRTH MM DD YY — SEX M F

b. AUTO ACCIDENT? — YES, NO — PLACE (State)

b. EMPLOYER'S NAME OR SCHOOL NAME

c. EMPLOYER'S NAME OR SCHOOL NAME

c. OTHER ACCIDENT? — YES, NO

c. INSURANCE PLAN NAME OR PROGRAM NAME

d. INSURANCE PLAN NAME OR PROGRAM NAME

10d. RESERVED FOR LOCAL USE

d. IS THERE ANOTHER HEALTH BENEFIT PLAN? — YES, NO — If yes, return to and complete item 9 a – d.

READ BACK OF FORM BEFORE COMPLETING & SIGNING THIS FORM.

12. PATIENT'S OR AUTHORIZED PERSON'S SIGNATURE I authorize the release of any medical or other information necessary to process this claim. I also request payment of government benefits either to myself or to the party who accepts assignment below.

SIGNED ______ DATE ______

13. INSURED'S OR AUTHORIZED PERSON'S SIGNATURE I authorize payment of medical benefits to the undersigned physician or supplier for services described below.

SIGNED ______

PATIENT AND INSURED INFORMATION

14. DATE OF CURRENT: MM DD YY — ILLNESS (First symptom) OR INJURY (Accident) OR PREGNANCY (LMP)

15. IF PATIENT HAS HAD SAME OR SIMILAR ILLNESS, GIVE FIRST DATE MM DD YY

16. DATES PATIENT UNABLE TO WORK IN CURRENT OCCUPATION — FROM MM DD YY — TO MM DD YY

17. NAME OF REFERRING PHYSICIAN OR OTHER SOURCE

17a. I.D. NUMBER OF REFERRING PHYSICIAN

18. HOSPITALIZATION DATES RELATED TO CURRENT SERVICES — FROM MM DD YY — TO MM DD YY

19. RESERVED FOR LOCAL USE

20. OUTSIDE LAB? — YES, NO — $ CHARGES

21. DIAGNOSIS OR NATURE OF ILLNESS OR INJURY. (RELATE ITEMS 1, 2, 3, OR 4 TO ITEM 24E BY LINE)

1. ___ . __
2. ___ . __
3. ___ . __
4. ___ . __

22. MEDICAID RESUBMISSION CODE — ORIGINAL REF. NO.

23. PRIOR AUTHORIZATION NUMBER

24.	A DATE(S) OF SERVICE From MM DD YY	To MM DD YY	B Place of Service	C Type of Service	D PROCEDURES, SERVICES, OR SUPPLIES (Explain Unusual Circumstances) CPT/HCPCS MODIFIER	E DIAGNOSIS CODE	F $ CHARGES	G DAYS OR UNITS	H EPSDT Family Plan	I EMG	J COB	K RESERVED FOR LOCAL USE
1												
2												
3												
4												
5												
6												

25. FEDERAL TAX I.D. NUMBER — SSN EIN

26. PATIENT'S ACCOUNT NO.

27. ACCEPT ASSIGNMENT? (For govt. claims, see back) — YES, NO

28. TOTAL CHARGE $

29. AMOUNT PAID $

30. BALANCE DUE $

31. SIGNATURE OF PHYSICIAN OR SUPPLIER INCLUDING DEGREES OR CREDENTIALS (I certify that the statements on the reverse apply to this bill and are made a part thereof.)

SIGNED DATE

32. NAME AND ADDRESS OF FACILITY WHERE SERVICES WERE RENDERED (If other than home or office)

33. PHYSICIAN'S, SUPPLIER'S BILLING NAME, ADDRESS, ZIP CODE & PHONE #

PIN# — GRP#

PHYSICIAN OR SUPPLIER INFORMATION

(SAMPLE ONLY - NOT APPROVED FOR USE)

PLEASE PRINT OR TYPE

SAMPLE FORM 1500
SAMPLE FORM 1500 SAMPLE FORM 1500

Case Study 17-d

DATE	REMARKS
10/10/YYYY	Injured yesterday at work

PATIENT		CHART #	SEX	BIRTHDATE
Thomas J. Buffett	363-44-5858	17-d	M	12/03/1965

MAILING ADDRESS	CITY	STATE	ZIP	HOME PHONE	WORK PHONE
12 Hauser Drive	Anywhere	US	12345	(101) 333-5555	(101) 444-5555

EMPLOYER	ADDRESS	PATIENT STATUS
Start Packing Real Estate	Anywhere US	X MARRIED DIVORCED SINGLE STUDENT OTHER

INSURANCE: PRIMARY	ID#	GROUP	SECONDARY POLICY
Workers Guard	WC4958		

POLICYHOLDER NAME	BIRTHDATE	RELATIONSHIP	POLICYHOLDER NAME	BIRTHDATE	RELATIONSHIP
		Self			

SUPPLEMENTAL PLAN	EMPLOYER

POLICYHOLDER NAME BIRTHDATE RELATIONSHIP

EMPLOYER

REFERRING PHYSICIAN UPIN/SSN

DIAGNOSIS	CODE
1. Ankle sprain, deltoid	845.01
2.	
3.	
4.	

PLACE OF SERVICE Office

PROCEDURES	CODE	CHARGE
1. New patient OV Level II	99202	$70.00
2.		
3.		
4.		
5.		
6.		

SPECIAL NOTES

Patient may return to work tomorrow

TOTAL CHARGES	PAYMENTS	ADJUSTMENTS	BALANCE
$70.00	$0.00	$0.00	$70.00

RETURN VISIT	PHYSICIAN SIGNATURE
PRN	Donald L. Givings, M.D.

MEDICARE # D1234
MEDICAID # DLG1234
BCBS # 12345

DONALD L. GIVINGS, M.D.
11350 MEDICAL DRIVE, ANYWHERE, US 12345
PHONE NUMBER (101)111-5555

EIN # 11123456
SSN # 123-12-1234
UPIN # DG1234
GRP # DG12345

PLEASE
DO NOT
STAPLE
IN THIS
AREA

(SAMPLE ONLY - NOT APPROVED FOR USE)

CARRIER

PICA

HEALTH INSURANCE CLAIM FORM

PICA

PATIENT AND INSURED INFORMATION

1. MEDICARE (Medicare #) MEDICAID (Medicaid #) CHAMPUS (Sponsor's SSN) CHAMPVA (VA File #) GROUP HEALTH PLAN (SSN or ID) FECA BLK LUNG (SSN) OTHER (ID)

1a. INSURED'S I.D. NUMBER (FOR PROGRAM IN ITEM 1)

2. PATIENT'S NAME (Last Name, First Name, Middle Initial)

3. PATIENT'S BIRTH DATE MM DD YY SEX M F

4. INSURED'S NAME (Last Name, First Name, Middle Initial)

5. PATIENT'S ADDRESS (No. Street)

6. PATIENT RELATIONSHIP TO INSURED Self Spouse Child Other

7. INSURED'S ADDRESS (No. Street)

CITY STATE

8. PATIENT STATUS Single Married Other

CITY STATE

ZIP CODE TELEPHONE (Include Area Code) ( )

Employed Full-Time Student Part-Time Student

ZIP CODE TELEPHONE (INCLUDE AREA CODE) ( )

9. OTHER INSURED'S NAME (Last Name, First Name, Middle Initial)

10. IS PATIENT'S CONDITION RELATED TO:

11. INSURED'S POLICY GROUP OR FECA NUMBER

a. OTHER INSURED'S POLICY OR GROUP NUMBER

a. EMPLOYMENT? (CURRENT OR PREVIOUS) YES NO

a. INSURED'S DATE OF BIRTH MM DD YY SEX M F

b. OTHER INSURED'S DATE OF BIRTH MM DD YY SEX M F

b. AUTO ACCIDENT? PLACE (State) YES NO

b. EMPLOYER'S NAME OR SCHOOL NAME

c. EMPLOYER'S NAME OR SCHOOL NAME

c. OTHER ACCIDENT? YES NO

c. INSURANCE PLAN NAME OR PROGRAM NAME

d. INSURANCE PLAN NAME OR PROGRAM NAME

10d. RESERVED FOR LOCAL USE

d. IS THERE ANOTHER HEALTH BENEFIT PLAN? YES NO If yes, return to and complete item 9 a – d.

READ BACK OF FORM BEFORE COMPLETING & SIGNING THIS FORM.

12. PATIENT'S OR AUTHORIZED PERSON'S SIGNATURE I authorize the release of any medical or other information necessary to process this claim. I also request payment of government benefits either to myself or to the party who accepts assignment below.

SIGNED ____________ DATE ____________

13. INSURED'S OR AUTHORIZED PERSON'S SIGNATURE I authorize payment of medical benefits to the undersigned physician or supplier for services described below.

SIGNED ____________

PHYSICIAN OR SUPPLIER INFORMATION

14. DATE OF CURRENT: MM DD YY ILLNESS (First symptom) OR INJURY (Accident) OR PREGNANCY (LMP)

15. IF PATIENT HAS HAD SAME OR SIMILAR ILLNESS, GIVE FIRST DATE MM DD YY

16. DATES PATIENT UNABLE TO WORK IN CURRENT OCCUPATION FROM MM DD YY TO MM DD YY

17. NAME OF REFERRING PHYSICIAN OR OTHER SOURCE

17a. I.D. NUMBER OF REFERRING PHYSICIAN

18. HOSPITALIZATION DATES RELATED TO CURRENT SERVICES FROM MM DD YY TO MM DD YY

19. RESERVED FOR LOCAL USE

20. OUTSIDE LAB? YES NO $ CHARGES

21. DIAGNOSIS OR NATURE OF ILLNESS OR INJURY. (RELATE ITEMS 1, 2, 3, OR 4 TO ITEM 24E BY LINE)

1. ___ . __ 3. ___ . __

2. ___ . __ 4. ___ . __

22. MEDICAID RESUBMISSION CODE ORIGINAL REF. NO.

23. PRIOR AUTHORIZATION NUMBER

24. A DATE(S) OF SERVICE From MM DD YY	To MM DD YY	B Place of Service	C Type of Service	D PROCEDURES, SERVICES, OR SUPPLIES (Explain Unusual Circumstances) CPT/HCPCS MODIFIER	E DIAGNOSIS CODE	F $ CHARGES	G DAYS OR UNITS	H EPSDT Family Plan	I EMG	J COB	K RESERVED FOR LOCAL USE
1											
2											
3											
4											
5											
6											

25. FEDERAL TAX I.D. NUMBER SSN EIN

26. PATIENT'S ACCOUNT NO.

27. ACCEPT ASSIGNMENT? (For govt. claims, see back) YES NO

28. TOTAL CHARGE $

29. AMOUNT PAID $

30. BALANCE DUE $

31. SIGNATURE OF PHYSICIAN OR SUPPLIER INCLUDING DEGREES OR CREDENTIALS (I certify that the statements on the reverse apply to this bill and are made a part thereof.)

SIGNED DATE

32. NAME AND ADDRESS OF FACILITY WHERE SERVICES WERE RENDERED (If other than home or office)

33. PHYSICIAN'S, SUPPLIER'S BILLING NAME, ADDRESS, ZIP CODE & PHONE #

PIN# GRP#

(SAMPLE ONLY - NOT APPROVED FOR USE)

PLEASE PRINT OR TYPE

SAMPLE FORM 1500
SAMPLE FORM 1500 SAMPLE FORM 1500

Case Study 17-e

DATE	REMARKS
07/16/YYYY	Patient was seen in the ER today. Injury occurred at work this morning

PATIENT		CHART #	SEX	BIRTHDATE
Priscilla R. Shepard	456-78-9999	17-e	F	07/15/1956

MAILING ADDRESS	CITY	STATE	ZIP	HOME PHONE	WORK PHONE
23 Easy Street	Anywhere	US	12345	(101) 333-5555	(101) 444-5555

EMPLOYER	ADDRESS		PATIENT STATUS
Ultimate Cleaners	Anywhere	US	MARRIED DIVORCED SINGLE (X) STUDENT OTHER

INSURANCE: PRIMARY	ID#	GROUP	SECONDARY POLICY
Workers Prompt	MA4958		

POLICYHOLDER NAME	BIRTHDATE	RELATIONSHIP	POLICYHOLDER NAME	BIRTHDATE	RELATIONSHIP
		Self			

SUPPLEMENTAL PLAN	EMPLOYER

POLICYHOLDER NAME	BIRTHDATE	RELATIONSHIP

EMPLOYER

REFERRING PHYSICIAN UPIN/SSN

DIAGNOSIS	CODE
1. Open wound shoulder complicated	880.10
2.	
3.	
4.	

PLACE OF SERVICE Mercy Hospital, Anywhere Street, Anywhere, US 12345

PROCEDURES	CODE	CHARGE
1. ER Visit Level III	99283	$150.00
2.		
3.		
4.		
5.		
6.		

SPECIAL NOTES

Patient is to be admitted in the morning

TOTAL CHARGES	PAYMENTS	ADJUSTMENTS	BALANCE
$150.00	$0.00	$0.00	$150.00

RETURN VISIT	PHYSICIAN SIGNATURE
	Donald L. Givings, M.D.

MEDICARE # D1234
MEDICAID # DLG1234
BCBS # 12345

DONALD L. GIVINGS, M.D.
11350 MEDICAL DRIVE, ANYWHERE, US 12345
PHONE NUMBER (101)111-5555

EIN # 11123456
SSN # 123-12-1234
UPIN # DG1234
GRP # DG12345

PLEASE
DO NOT
STAPLE
IN THIS
AREA

(SAMPLE ONLY - NOT APPROVED FOR USE)

CARRIER

PICA

HEALTH INSURANCE CLAIM FORM

PICA

1. MEDICARE (Medicare #) MEDICAID (Medicaid #) CHAMPUS (Sponsor's SSN) CHAMPVA (VA File #) GROUP HEALTH PLAN (SSN or ID) FECA BLK LUNG (SSN) OTHER (ID)

1a. INSURED'S I.D. NUMBER (FOR PROGRAM IN ITEM 1)

2. PATIENT'S NAME (Last Name, First Name, Middle Initial)

3. PATIENT'S BIRTH DATE MM DD YY SEX M F

4. INSURED'S NAME (Last Name, First Name, Middle Initial)

5. PATIENT'S ADDRESS (No. Street)

6. PATIENT RELATIONSHIP TO INSURED Self Spouse Child Other

7. INSURED'S ADDRESS (No. Street)

CITY STATE

8. PATIENT STATUS Single Married Other

CITY STATE

ZIP CODE TELEPHONE (Include Area Code) ( )

Employed Full-Time Student Part-Time Student

ZIP CODE TELEPHONE (INCLUDE AREA CODE) ( )

9. OTHER INSURED'S NAME (Last Name, First Name, Middle Initial)

10. IS PATIENT'S CONDITION RELATED TO:

11. INSURED'S POLICY GROUP OR FECA NUMBER

a. OTHER INSURED'S POLICY OR GROUP NUMBER

a. EMPLOYMENT? (CURRENT OR PREVIOUS) YES NO

a. INSURED'S DATE OF BIRTH MM DD YY SEX M F

b. OTHER INSURED'S DATE OF BIRTH MM DD YY SEX M F

b. AUTO ACCIDENT? YES NO PLACE (State)

b. EMPLOYER'S NAME OR SCHOOL NAME

c. EMPLOYER'S NAME OR SCHOOL NAME

c. OTHER ACCIDENT? YES NO

c. INSURANCE PLAN NAME OR PROGRAM NAME

d. INSURANCE PLAN NAME OR PROGRAM NAME

10d. RESERVED FOR LOCAL USE

d. IS THERE ANOTHER HEALTH BENEFIT PLAN? YES NO If yes, return to and complete item 9 a – d.

READ BACK OF FORM BEFORE COMPLETING & SIGNING THIS FORM.

12. PATIENT'S OR AUTHORIZED PERSON'S SIGNATURE I authorize the release of any medical or other information necessary to process this claim. I also request payment of government benefits either to myself or to the party who accepts assignment below.

SIGNED DATE

13. INSURED'S OR AUTHORIZED PERSON'S SIGNATURE I authorize payment of medical benefits to the undersigned physician or supplier for services described below.

SIGNED

PATIENT AND INSURED INFORMATION

14. DATE OF CURRENT: MM DD YY ILLNESS (First symptom) OR INJURY (Accident) OR PREGNANCY (LMP)

15. IF PATIENT HAS HAD SAME OR SIMILAR ILLNESS, GIVE FIRST DATE MM DD YY

16. DATES PATIENT UNABLE TO WORK IN CURRENT OCCUPATION FROM MM DD YY TO MM DD YY

17. NAME OF REFERRING PHYSICIAN OR OTHER SOURCE

17a. I.D. NUMBER OF REFERRING PHYSICIAN

18. HOSPITALIZATION DATES RELATED TO CURRENT SERVICES FROM MM DD YY TO MM DD YY

19. RESERVED FOR LOCAL USE

20. OUTSIDE LAB? YES NO $ CHARGES

21. DIAGNOSIS OR NATURE OF ILLNESS OR INJURY. (RELATE ITEMS 1, 2, 3, OR 4 TO ITEM 24E BY LINE)

1. ___ . __ 3. ___ . __

2. ___ . __ 4. ___ . __

22. MEDICAID RESUBMISSION CODE ORIGINAL REF. NO.

23. PRIOR AUTHORIZATION NUMBER

24. A DATE(S) OF SERVICE From MM DD YY To MM DD YY	B Place of Service	C Type of Service	D PROCEDURES, SERVICES, OR SUPPLIES (Explain Unusual Circumstances) CPT/HCPCS MODIFIER	E DIAGNOSIS CODE	F $ CHARGES	G DAYS OR UNITS	H EPSDT Family Plan	I EMG	J COB	K RESERVED FOR LOCAL USE
1										
2										
3										
4										
5										
6										

25. FEDERAL TAX I.D. NUMBER SSN EIN

26. PATIENT'S ACCOUNT NO.

27. ACCEPT ASSIGNMENT? (For govt. claims, see back) YES NO

28. TOTAL CHARGE $

29. AMOUNT PAID $

30. BALANCE DUE $

31. SIGNATURE OF PHYSICIAN OR SUPPLIER INCLUDING DEGREES OR CREDENTIALS (I certify that the statements on the reverse apply to this bill and are made a part thereof.)

SIGNED DATE

32. NAME AND ADDRESS OF FACILITY WHERE SERVICES WERE RENDERED (If other than home or office)

33. PHYSICIAN'S, SUPPLIER'S BILLING NAME, ADDRESS, ZIP CODE & PHONE #

PIN# GRP#

PHYSICIAN OR SUPPLIER INFORMATION

(SAMPLE ONLY - NOT APPROVED FOR USE)

PLEASE PRINT OR TYPE

SAMPLE FORM 1500
SAMPLE FORM 1500 SAMPLE FORM 1500

Case Study 17-f

DATE: 07/21/YYYY
REMARKS:

PATIENT: Priscilla R. Shepard 456-78-9999
CHART #: 17-f
SEX: F
BIRTHDATE: 07/15/1956

MAILING ADDRESS: 23 Easy Street
CITY: Anywhere
STATE: US
ZIP: 12345
HOME PHONE: (101) 333-5555
WORK PHONE: (101) 444-5555

EMPLOYER: Ultimate Cleaners
ADDRESS: Anywhere US
PATIENT STATUS: MARRIED DIVORCED SINGLE (X) STUDENT OTHER

INSURANCE: PRIMARY: Workers Prompt
ID#: MA4958
GROUP:
SECONDARY POLICY:

POLICYHOLDER NAME:
BIRTHDATE:
RELATIONSHIP: Self
POLICYHOLDER NAME:
BIRTHDATE:
RELATIONSHIP:

SUPPLEMENTAL PLAN:
EMPLOYER:

POLICYHOLDER NAME:
BIRTHDATE:
RELATIONSHIP:

EMPLOYER:

REFERRING PHYSICIAN UPIN/SSN:

DIAGNOSIS	CODE
1. Open wound, shoulder, complicated	880.10
2.	
3.	
4.	

PLACE OF SERVICE: Mercy Hospital, Anywhere Street, Anywhere, US 12345

PROCEDURES		CODE	CHARGE
1. Initial Visit Level III	07/17/YYYY	99223	$150.00
2. Subsq. Hosp. Level II	07/18/YYYY	99232	$75.00
3. Subsq. Hosp. Level II	07/19/YYYY	99232	$75.00
4. Hosp. Discharge 45 min.	07/20/YYYY	99239	$75.00
5.			
6.			

SPECIAL NOTES: Date of injury 07/16/YYYY

TOTAL CHARGES	PAYMENTS	ADJUSTMENTS	BALANCE
$375.00	$0.00	$0.00	$375.00

RETURN VISIT:
PHYSICIAN SIGNATURE: Donald L. Givings, M.D.

MEDICARE # D1234
MEDICAID # DLG1234
BCBS # 12345

DONALD L. GIVINGS, M.D.
11350 MEDICAL DRIVE, ANYWHERE, US 12345
PHONE NUMBER (101)111-5555

EIN # 11123456
SSN # 123-12-1234
UPIN # DG1234
GRP # DG12345

PLEASE
DO NOT
STAPLE
IN THIS
AREA

(SAMPLE ONLY - NOT APPROVED FOR USE)

CARRIER

PICA

HEALTH INSURANCE CLAIM FORM

PICA

1. MEDICARE (Medicare #) MEDICAID (Medicaid #) CHAMPUS (Sponsor's SSN) CHAMPVA (VA File #) GROUP HEALTH PLAN (SSN or ID) FECA BLK LUNG (SSN) OTHER (ID)

1a. INSURED'S I.D. NUMBER (FOR PROGRAM IN ITEM 1)

2. PATIENT'S NAME (Last Name, First Name, Middle Initial)

3. PATIENT'S BIRTH DATE MM DD YY SEX M F

4. INSURED'S NAME (Last Name, First Name, Middle Initial)

5. PATIENT'S ADDRESS (No. Street)

6. PATIENT RELATIONSHIP TO INSURED Self Spouse Child Other

7. INSURED'S ADDRESS (No. Street)

CITY STATE

8. PATIENT STATUS Single Married Other

CITY STATE

ZIP CODE TELEPHONE (Include Area Code) ( )

Employed Full-Time Student Part-Time Student

ZIP CODE TELEPHONE (INCLUDE AREA CODE) ( )

9. OTHER INSURED'S NAME (Last Name, First Name, Middle Initial)

10. IS PATIENT'S CONDITION RELATED TO:

11. INSURED'S POLICY GROUP OR FECA NUMBER

a. OTHER INSURED'S POLICY OR GROUP NUMBER

a. EMPLOYMENT? (CURRENT OR PREVIOUS) YES NO

a. INSURED'S DATE OF BIRTH MM DD YY SEX M F

b. OTHER INSURED'S DATE OF BIRTH MM DD YY SEX M F

b. AUTO ACCIDENT? PLACE (State) YES NO

b. EMPLOYER'S NAME OR SCHOOL NAME

c. EMPLOYER'S NAME OR SCHOOL NAME

c. OTHER ACCIDENT? YES NO

c. INSURANCE PLAN NAME OR PROGRAM NAME

d. INSURANCE PLAN NAME OR PROGRAM NAME

10d. RESERVED FOR LOCAL USE

d. IS THERE ANOTHER HEALTH BENEFIT PLAN? YES NO If yes, return to and complete item 9 a – d.

READ BACK OF FORM BEFORE COMPLETING & SIGNING THIS FORM.

12. PATIENT'S OR AUTHORIZED PERSON'S SIGNATURE I authorize the release of any medical or other information necessary to process this claim. I also request payment of government benefits either to myself or to the party who accepts assignment below.

SIGNED DATE

13. INSURED'S OR AUTHORIZED PERSON'S SIGNATURE I authorize payment of medical benefits to the undersigned physician or supplier for services described below.

SIGNED

PATIENT AND INSURED INFORMATION

14. DATE OF CURRENT: MM DD YY ILLNESS (First symptom) OR INJURY (Accident) OR PREGNANCY (LMP)

15. IF PATIENT HAS HAD SAME OR SIMILAR ILLNESS, GIVE FIRST DATE MM DD YY

16. DATES PATIENT UNABLE TO WORK IN CURRENT OCCUPATION MM DD YY FROM MM DD YY TO

17. NAME OF REFERRING PHYSICIAN OR OTHER SOURCE

17a. I.D. NUMBER OF REFERRING PHYSICIAN

18. HOSPITALIZATION DATES RELATED TO CURRENT SERVICES MM DD YY FROM MM DD YY TO

19. RESERVED FOR LOCAL USE

20. OUTSIDE LAB? YES NO $ CHARGES

21. DIAGNOSIS OR NATURE OF ILLNESS OR INJURY. (RELATE ITEMS 1, 2, 3, OR 4 TO ITEM 24E BY LINE)

1. ___ . __ 3. ___ . __

2. ___ . __ 4. ___ . __

22. MEDICAID RESUBMISSION CODE ORIGINAL REF. NO.

23. PRIOR AUTHORIZATION NUMBER

24.	A DATE(S) OF SERVICE From MM DD YY	To MM DD YY	B Place of Service	C Type of Service	D PROCEDURES, SERVICES, OR SUPPLIES (Explain Unusual Circumstances) CPT/HCPCS MODIFIER	E DIAGNOSIS CODE	F $ CHARGES	G DAYS OR UNITS	H EPSDT Family Plan	I EMG	J COB	K RESERVED FOR LOCAL USE
1												
2												
3												
4												
5												
6												

25. FEDERAL TAX I.D. NUMBER SSN EIN

26. PATIENT'S ACCOUNT NO.

27. ACCEPT ASSIGNMENT? (For govt. claims, see back) YES NO

28. TOTAL CHARGE $

29. AMOUNT PAID $

30. BALANCE DUE $

31. SIGNATURE OF PHYSICIAN OR SUPPLIER INCLUDING DEGREES OR CREDENTIALS (I certify that the statements on the reverse apply to this bill and are made a part thereof.)

SIGNED DATE

32. NAME AND ADDRESS OF FACILITY WHERE SERVICES WERE RENDERED (If other than home or office)

33. PHYSICIAN'S, SUPPLIER'S BILLING NAME, ADDRESS, ZIP CODE & PHONE #

PIN# GRP#

PHYSICIAN OR SUPPLIER INFORMATION

(SAMPLE ONLY - NOT APPROVED FOR USE)

PLEASE PRINT OR TYPE

SAMPLE FORM 1500
SAMPLE FORM 1500 SAMPLE FORM 1500